Depression in Special Populations

Editors

WARREN Y.K. NG
KAREN DINEEN WAGNER

CHILD AND ADOLESCENT PSYCHIATRIC CLINICS OF NORTH AMERICA

www.childpsych.theclinics.com

Consulting Editor
TODD E. PETERS

July 2019 • Volume 28 • Number 3

ELSEVIER

1600 John F. Kennedy Boulevard • Suite 1800 • Philadelphia, Pennsylvania, 19103-2899

http://www.theclinics.com

CHILD AND ADOLESCENT PSYCHIATRIC CLINICS OF NORTH AMERICA Volume 28, Number 3
July 2019 ISSN 1056–4993, ISBN-13: 978-0-323-68205-3

Editor: Lauren Boyle
Developmental Editor: Kristen Helm

Child and Adolescent Psychiatric Clinics of North America (ISSN 1056-4993) is published quarterly by Elsevier Inc., 360 Park Avenue South, New York, NY 10010-1710. Months of issue are January, April, July, and October. Business and Editorial Offices: 1600 John F. Kennedy Boulevard, Suite 1800, Philadelphia, PA 19103-2899. Periodicals postage paid at New York, NY and additional mailing offices. Subscription prices are $335.00 per year (US individuals), $627.00 per year (US institutions), $100.00 per year (US students), $388.00 per year (Canadian individuals), $762.00 per year (Canadian institutions), $200.00 per year (Canadian students), $446.00 per year (international individuals), $762.00 per year (international institutions), and $200.00 per year (international students). International air speed delivery is included in all *Clinics* subscription prices. All prices are subject to change without notice. **POSTMASTER:** Send address changes to *Child and Adolescent Psychiatric Clinics of North America*, Elsevier Health Sciences Division, Subscription Customer Service, 3251 Riverport Lane, Maryland Heights, MO 63043. **Customer Service: 1-800-654-2452 (U.S. and Canada); 314-447-8871 (outside U.S. and Canada). Fax: 314-447-8029. E-mail:** JournalsCustomer Service-usa@elsevier.com **(for print support) or** journalsonlinesupport-usa@elsevier.com **(for online support).**

Reprints. For copies of 100 or more of articles in this publication, please contact the Commercial Reprints Department, Elsevier Inc., 360 Park Avenue South, New York, New York 10010-1710 Tel.: 212-633-3874; Fax: 212-633-3820, E-mail: reprints@elsevier.com.

Child and Adolescent Psychiatric Clinics of North America is covered in *MEDLINE/PubMed (Index Medicus), ISI, SSCI, Research Alert, Social Search, Current Contents,* and *EMBASE/Excerpta Medica.*

Contributors

CONSULTING EDITOR

TODD E. PETERS, MD, FAPA
Medical Director, Child and Adolescent Services, Chief Medical Information Officer
(CMIO), Sheppard Pratt Health System, Sheppard Pratt Physicians PA Clinical Operations
Liaison, Baltimore, Maryland

EDITORS

WARREN Y. K. NG, MD, MPH
Associate Professor of Psychiatry, Division of Child and Adolescent Psychiatry,
Columbia University Irving Medical Center, NewYork-Presbyterian Hospital, New York,
New York

KAREN DINEEN WAGNER, MD, PhD
Professor and Chair, Department of Psychiatry and Behavioral Sciences, Titus Harris
Chair, Harry K. Davis Professor, University of Texas Medical Branch, President, American
Academy of Child and Adolescent Psychiatry (2017-2019), University of Texas Medical
Branch, Galveston, Texas

AUTHORS

ALKA ANEJA, MD
Medical Director, Department of Psychiatry, Fremont Hospital, Fremont, California

REGINA BARONIA, MD
Research Associate, Department of Psychiatry, Texas Tech University Health Sciences
Center, Lubbock, Texas

TAMI D. BENTON, MD
Chair of Psychiatry, The Children's Hospital of Philadelphia, Associate Professor,
Department of Psychiatry, Perelman School of Medicine, University of Pennsylvania,
Philadelphia, Pennsylvania

STEPHANIE BRENNAN, MD
Senior Resident, Department of Pediatrics, Texas Tech University Health Sciences Center,
Lubbock, Texas

ALEXANDRA CANETTI, MD
Program Medical Director, Special Needs Clinic and School Based Mental Health
Program, Assistant Professor of Psychiatry, Division of Child and Adolescent Psychiatry,
Columbia University Irving Medical Center, New York, New York

VIVIEN CHAN, MD, DFAPA, DFAACAP
Chief of Mental Health Clinics, Student Health Center, University of California Irvine, Irvine, California; Clinical Professor, Department of Psychiatry and Human Behavior, UCI Health, Orange, California; Community Mental Health Psychiatrist, Center for Resiliency, Wellness and Education, Children, Youth, Prevention and Intervention Behavioral Services, Orange County Healthcare Agency, Orange, California

ALEXIS CHAVEZ, MD
Child and Adolescent Psychiatry Fellow, Department of Psychiatry, University of Colorado, Anschutz, Aurora, Colorado

JUDITH A. COHEN, MD
Professor of Psychiatry, Drexel University College of Medicine, Allegheny Health Network, Pittsburgh, Pennsylvania

MILANGEL T. CONCEPCION ZAYAS, MD, MPH
Clinical Assistant Professor of Psychiatry, Dartmouth Geisel School of Medicine, Dartmouth-Hitchcock Medical Center, Staff Psychiatrist, West Central Behavioral Health

STEPHEN J. COZZA, MD
Professor of Psychiatry, Associate Director, Center for the Study of Traumatic Stress, Uniformed Services University of the Health Sciences, Potomac, Maryland

LISA M. CULLINS, MD
Child and Adolescent Psychiatrist, Adjunct Assistant Professor of Behavioral Sciences and Pediatrics, George Washington University School of Medicine, Washington, DC

REBECCA SUSAN DAILY, MD, DFAPA, DFAACAP, FAPA
St Elizabeth's Hospitals, The Rainbolt Family Chair in Child Psychiatry, Vice Chairman of Child and Adolescent Psychiatry, Assistant Professor, Oklahoma City, Oklahoma

MICHAEL D. DE BELLIS, MD, MPH
Director, Healthy Childhood Brain Development and Developmental Traumatology Research Program, Professor, Department of Psychiatry and Behavioral Sciences, Duke University Medical Center, Durham, North Carolina

JENNIFER DERENNE, MD, DFAACAP
Psychiatric Director of Inpatient Eating Disorders, Comprehensive Care Program, Clinical Associate Professor of Psychiatry and Behavioral Sciences, Division of Child and Adolescent Psychiatry, Lucile Packard Children's Hospital at Stanford, Stanford University, Palo Alto, California

JOSEPH G. DOUGHERTY, MD
Program Director, Child and Adolescent Psychiatry Fellowship, Walter Reed National Military Medical Center, Washington, DC

JANA DREYZEHNER, MD
Founder and CEO, Life Connect Health, Consulting Psychiatrist, Tennessee School for the Deaf, Knoxville, Tennessee

LISA R. FORTUNA, MD, MPH
Director, Child and Adolescent Psychiatry, Boston Medical Center, Assistant Professor of Psychiatry, Boston University School of Medicine, Boston, Massachusetts

D. CATHERINE FUCHS, MD, DFAACAP
Professor of Psychiatry and Behavioral Sciences and Pediatrics, Division of Child and Adolescent Psychiatry, Vanderbilt University Medical Center, Vanderbilt Child and Adolescent Psychiatry, Nashville, Tennessee

KAREN A. GOLDBERG, MD
Medical Director, Behavioral Health Services, eQHealth Solutions, Tampa, Florida

KATHERINE GOTHAM, PhD
Assistant Professor, Department of Psychiatry and Behavioral Sciences, Vanderbilt University Medical Center, Nashville, Tennessee

ANTHONY P.S. GUERRERO, MD
Professor of Psychiatry, Clinical Professor of Pediatrics, Chair, Department of Psychiatry, Director, Child and Adolescent Psychiatry Division, University of Hawai'i, John A. Burns School of Medicine, Honolulu, Hawaii

GLORIA T. HAN, MA
Doctoral Candidate, Department of Psychology, Vanderbilt University, Nashville, Tennessee

SARAH E. HERBERT, MD, MSW
Clinical Associate Professor, Department of Psychiatry and Behavioral Sciences, Morehouse School of Medicine, Atlanta, Georgia

JESSE D. HINCKLEY, MD, PhD
Fellow, Division of Substance Dependence, Department of Psychiatry, University of Colorado School of Medicine, Aurora, Colorado

NADIA JASSIM, BS, MFA
School Mental Health Team, Division of Child and Adolescent Psychiatry, Lucile Packard Children's Hospital at Stanford, Stanford University School of Medicine, Stanford, California

BRANDON JOHNSON, MD
Attending Psychiatrist, CARES, Director of Faculty Practice in Psychiatry, Mount Sinai St. Luke's Hospital, Assistant Professor of Psychiatry, Icahn School of Medicine at Mount Sinai, New York, New York

SHASHANK V. JOSHI, MD
School Mental Health Team, Associate Professor and Director of Training, Division of Child and Adolescent Psychiatry, Lucile Packard Children's Hospital at Stanford, Stanford University School of Medicine, Stanford, California

NIRANJAN KARNIK, MD, PhD
The Cynthia Oudejans Harris Professor of Psychiatry and Associate Dean for Community Behavioral Health, Rush Medical College, Rush University Medical Center, Chicago, Illinois

WARREN Y. K. NG, MD, MPH
Associate Professor of Psychiatry, Division of Child and Adolescent Psychiatry, Columbia University Irving Medical Center, NewYork-Presbyterian Hospital, New York, New York

IAN KODISH, MD, PhD
Department of Psychiatry and Behavioral Sciences, University of Washington School of Medicine, Seattle, Washington

SCOTT LEIBOWITZ, MD
Medical Director of Behavioral Health, THRIVE Gender Development Program, Nationwide Children's Hospital, Clinical Associate Professor, The Ohio State University College of Medicine, Columbus, Ohio

DENISE LEUNG, MD
Program Medical Director, Child and Adolescent Psychiatry Community Services, Assistant Professor of Psychiatry, Division of Child and Adolescent Psychiatry, Columbia University Irving Medical Center, New York, New York

RICHARD LIVINGSTON, MD
Professor of Psychiatry, University of Arkansas College of Medicine, Little Rock, Arkansas

NASUH MALAS, MD, MPH
Director of Pediatric Consultation-Liaison Psychiatry, Assistant Professor, Departments of Psychiatry, and Pediatrics and Communicable Diseases, University of Michigan Medical School, Ann Arbor, Michigan

NITHYA MANI, MD
Fellow in Child and Adolescent Psychiatry, Lucile Packard Children's Hospital at Stanford, Stanford University School of Medicine, Stanford, California

SHALICE McKNIGHT, DO
Child and Adolescent Psychiatrist, Fort Belvoir Community Hospital, Fort Belvoir, Virginia

JESSICA MOORE, MD
The University of Texas Southwestern Medical Center, Dallas, Texas

WYNNE MORGAN, MD
Assistant Professor, Department of Psychiatry, Division of Child and Adolescent Psychiatry, University of Massachusetts Medical School, Worcester, Massachusetts

MICHAEL W. NAYLOR, MD
Professor of Clinical Psychiatry, Department of Psychiatry, The University of Illinois at Chicago, Institute for Juvenile Research, Chicago, Illinois

KATE B. NOONER, PhD
Director of the Trauma and Resilience Laboratory, Associate Professor, Department of Psychology, University of North Carolina Wilmington, Wilmington, North Carolina

DOUGLAS K. NOVINS, MD
Professor, Vice Chair, and Director, Division of Child and Adolescent Psychiatry, Department of Psychiatry, Cannon Y. and Lyndia Harvey Chair in Child and Adolescent Psychiatry, Chair, Pediatric Mental Health Institute, Children's Hospital Colorado, University of Colorado School of Medicine, Professor of Community and Behavioral Health, Centers for American Indian and Alaska Native Health, Colorado School of Public Health, Aurora, Colorado

MARYLAND PAO, MD
Chief of Psychiatry Consultation-Liaison Service, Clinical Director of the National Institute of Mental Health (NIMH), Intramural Research Program, National Institutes of Health, National Institute of Mental Health, Clinical Research Center, Bethesda, Maryland

FLORENCIA PEZZIMENTI, MEd
Research Assistant, Department of Psychiatry and Behavioral Sciences, Vanderbilt University Medical Center, Nashville, Tennessee

SIGITA PLIOPLYS, MD
Head of Pediatric Neuropsychiatry Program, Professor, Department of Child and
Adolescent Psychiatry, Ann and Robert H. Lurie Children's Hospital of Chicago,
Northwestern University Feinberg School of Medicine, Chicago, Illinois

UJJWAL RAMTEKKAR, MD, MPE, MBA
Associate Medical Director, Partners for Kids, Nationwide Children's Hospital, Columbus,
Ohio

LAURA RICHARDSON, MD, MPH
Department of Pediatrics, University of Washington School of Medicine, Seattle
Children's Research Institute, Seattle, Washington

PAULA RIGGS, MD
Professor and Vice Chair, Division of Substance Dependence, Department of Psychiatry,
University of Colorado School of Medicine, Aurora, Colorado

DAVID E. ROTH, MD, FAAP, FAPA
Medical Director, Mind & Body Works, Inc., Honolulu, Hawaii

JEANETTE M. SCHEID, MD, PhD
Associate Professor, Department of Psychiatry, Michigan State University, East Lansing,
Michigan

ABIGAIL SCHLESINGER, MD
UPMC Western Psychiatric Hospital, UPMC Children's Hospital of Pittsburgh, University
of Pittsburgh School of Medicine, Wexford, Pennsylvania

MARTINE M. SOLAGES, MD
Child and Adolescent Psychiatrist, Pediatrician, Silver Spring, Maryland

RACHEL M. SULLIVAN, MD
Associate Program Director, Psychiatry Residency, Tripler Army Medical Center,
Assistant Professor, Uniformed Services University of the Health Sciences, Mililani,
Hawaii

ROMA A. VASA, MD
Associate Professor, Department of Psychiatry and Behavioral Sciences, Johns Hopkins
University School of Medicine, Kennedy Krieger Institute, Baltimore, Maryland

SARAH MALLARD WAKEFIELD, MD
Assistant Professor, Department of Psychiatry, School of Medicine, Texas Tech
University Health Sciences Center, Texas Tech University, Lubbock, Texas

JOHN T. WALKUP, MD
Head, Child and Adolescent Psychiatry, Margaret C. Osterman Professor in Child and
Adolescent Psychiatry, Professor of Psychiatry and Behavioral Sciences, Northwestern
University Feinberg School of Medicine, Ann & Robert H. Lurie Children's Hospital of
Chicago, Chicago, Illinois

SOFIJA ZEKOVIĆ-ROTH, LAc, DOM
Clinical Director, Mind & Body Works, Inc., Honolulu, Hawaii

Contents

> Maltreatment affects 9.1 to 17.1 of every 1000 US children and adolescents. Maltreated youth are at high risk for depression. Clinicians should screen young patients for maltreatment history. Depressed maltreated youth are at high risk for treatment resistance. Combination treatment with selective serotonin reuptake inhibitors and cognitive behavior therapy (CBT) with a trauma-informed approach should be considered for depressed maltreated youth. Behavioral management can be integrated with trauma-focused CBT to treat the externalizing disorders that commonly occur in maltreated depressed youth. If one approach is unsuccessful, a change to another medication or type of evidence-based psychotherapy or intervention is indicated.

> Child maltreatment presents a significant public health challenge and is strongly associated with development of depression during childhood and adolescence. Not all abused or neglected children are in the child welfare system, but most children in the foster care system have a history of maltreatment. Involvement with the child welfare system presents an additional risk for psychopathology. The role of child maltreatment and child welfare involvement in development of depression in children and adolescents is reviewed and effective treatments are discussed. Clinicians working with foster children must collaborate with care providers and other stakeholders to enhance the child's placement permanence.

> Creative collaborative approaches are required to meet the demands of managing depression in youth. Primary care providers are well positioned to engage depressed youth and their families, yet often lack the training, access to psychiatric providers, and the reimbursement structure to support their efforts. Child and adolescent psychiatrists are encouraged to support pediatricians in establishing more robust systems to provide screening and effective treatment interventions, particularly for youth at higher risk. Several models of collaborative care are described, in addition to their emerging evidence-base, in an effort to disseminate evolving treatment strategies that can drive implementation of effective collaborative approaches.

> Justice-involved youth are at exceedingly high risk of trauma exposure, multisystem involvement, and mental health distress, including depression. Justice-involved youth carry with them both a high symptom burden and a high cost to society. Both could be reduced through evidence-based prevention and treatment strategies. Effective treatment of mental disorders may reduce future justice involvement, whereas lack of treatment increases likelihood of justice involvement into adulthood. Multiple effective programs exist to improve the lives of justice-involved youth and subsequently decrease the cost to society of detaining and adjudicating these youth within the juvenile justice system.

> There are special considerations when treating depression in the children of military families, due to both unique stressors and unique access to treatment and support resources. This article provides a brief overview of the history of military family care, an understanding of ongoing efforts to provide excellent and timely care for these children, and an understanding of the unique stressors and challenges that the depressed military child faces. The Department of Defense is dedicated to providing for the unique needs of military children and providing robust services to care for these children and their families.

> In this article, the authors make a compelling case that all clinicians who treat youth with depressive disorders should embrace strategies to engage with school staff to best serve their patients in the classroom. Because these disorders have a high incidence in the school population (13% of US teens experienced at least 1 major depressive episode in 2016), this can affect learning, social interactions, and classroom engagement. Several approaches are highlighted for assessment of depressive symptoms, intervention and treatment in school settings, and prevention strategies, including depression education curricula and programs promoting subjective well-being, such as positive psychology and mindfulness.

> Transitional age youth with a history of mood disorders, such as major depressive disorder, are uniquely vulnerable to clinical destabilization and relapse in the context of life transition. Moving from a structured adolescence to a more independent and potentially more demanding young adult life can result in worsening symptoms and barriers to effective help-seeking. Transitional age youth newly diagnosed are exposed to their first course of treatment of a potentially chronic condition. This article describes the challenges inherent in navigating this life transition, and also offers strategies to promote a successful "launch" into adulthood.

The benefits and acceptability of using telepsychiatry to provide psychiatric treatment to youth in their homes, schools, primary care provider offices, juvenile correction centers, and residential facilities are well established. Telepsychiatry removes geographic barriers between patients and providers and improves the access to and ease of receiving quality care. Effective telepsychiatrists use strategic room staging, enhanced nonverbal communication, and technical experience to ensure sessions provide an authentic treatment experience and strong provider-patient alliances are forged. When the telepsychiatry venue is used properly, sessions feel authentic and pediatric treatment outcomes meet and sometimes exceed those of sessions conducted in traditional venues.

Depression is both common and impactful in youth with autism spectrum disorder (ASD) and is swiftly growing in recognition as a major public health concern within the autism community. This article is intended to provide a brief overview of the prevalence, impact, presentation, and risk factors associated with cooccurring depression in children and adolescents with ASD. Clinical guidelines for the assessment and treatment of depression in the ASD population are offered in line with the small existing evidence base.

Depression has been shown to be more prevalent in deaf and hard of hearing (DHH) youth than in their hearing peers. This increase in vulnerability likely stems from communicative barriers in a hearing world and adverse experiences related to stigma and discrimination. There are a variety of factors to consider in the assessment and treatment of depression in DHH youth. Additional attention, research, and resources are needed to support children and their families early on in life to reduce the impact associated with deafness, and to improve prevention and treatment of depression in this vulnerable population.

Depression risk is 2 to 3 times higher in medically ill youth compared with the general pediatric population. The relationship between medical illness and depression is bidirectional with significant contributions from psychological, developmental, illness-related, familial, and treatment factors. This article discusses the presentation, early identification, evaluation, and management of depression in medically ill youth and identifies specific risk factors and reviewing selected medical illness-specific considerations.

Depression and human immunodeficiency virus disease are common co-
occurring conditions among youth living with human immunodeficiency vi-
rus/AIDS. Depression serves as a risk factor for contracting the disease
and for nonadherence to medications and adherence to safe sex practices. Although new infections are decreasing nationally, subpopulations
of youths continue to have the highest rates of new infections, specifically
ethnic and sexual minority youths. Depression contributes to poor health
outcomes for youths with human immunodeficiency virus disease.
Evidence-based psychotherapy and pharmacotherapy for depression
are effective treatments. Integrated care with medical and mental health
provides the best care for this population of youth.

Substance use disorders (SUDs) are commonly co-occurring among adolescents with depression. Integrated treatment is important given treatment
implications and increased rates of suicidality. All adolescents should be
screened for SUD using Screening, Brief Intervention, and Referral to Treatment. Review of randomized controlled trials in adolescents reveals
motivational enhancement therapy/cognitive behavioral therapy is an
evidence-based intervention and should be considered first-line treatment.
If depression does not improve, fluoxetine should be considered, as it is
well-tolerated in substance-involved adolescents with depression. Adolescents who do not show improvement in SUD or who have severe SUD
should be referred to evidence-based SUD treatment.

This article reviews the risk and protective factors, symptom presentation,
and the significant interface of spirituality and religion of depression in African American and black Caribbean children and adolescents and their
families. The article provides practical implications for diagnosis and treatment of depression in this special population of youth.

This article reviews the risk and protective factors and symptom presentation of depression in Latino and immigrant refugee children and adolescents. The significance of culture, linguistics, and community in the
emergence of depression in Latino and immigrant refugee children and adolescents and their families is explored. The article provides practical implications for diagnosis and treatment of depression in this special
population of youth.

CHILD AND ADOLESCENT PSYCHIATRIC CLINICS

ISSUE OF RELATED INTEREST

Psychiatric Clinics of North America June 2018 (Vol. 41, No. 2)
Psychodynamic Psychiatry
Thomas N. Franklin, *Editor*
Available at http://www.psych.theclinics.com/

AACAP Members: Please go to www.jaacap.org for information on access to the Child and Adolescent Psychiatric Clinics. *Resident* Members of AACAP: Special access information is available at www.childpsych.theclinics.com.

THE CLINICS ARE AVAILABLE ONLINE!
Access your subscription at:
www.theclinics.com

Preface

Depression in Special Populations

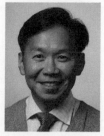   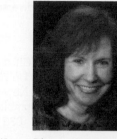

Warren Y.K. Ng, MD, MPH   Karen Dineen Wagner, MD, PhD
Editors

Depression affects the promise of the future for children and adolescents, by interfering with how they learn, develop, socialize, and fulfill their potential. Screening, early intervention, and treatment are key components to address depression in youth. Depression can have its onset in preschool children with reported prevalence rates rising to 11% in adolescents. The Youth Risk Behavior Surveillance survey found that 28.5% of high school students, aged 14 to 18 years, reported that they felt sad or hopeless every day for over 2 weeks. There were differences in gender and ethnicity, with female students and Hispanic students reporting higher rates compared with male students and non-Hispanic students. These statistics pale in comparison to the Centers for Disease Control and Prevention report that suicide rates have increased over the past two decades for children and adolescents. Of particular concern is that suicide is now the second leading cause of death in youth aged 10 to 19 years.

Through Dr Wagner's Presidential Initiative, the American Academy of Child and Adolescent Psychiatry (AACAP) is leading the effort to increase awareness, screening, and education to address depression in children and adolescents. The inspiration for this issue of *Child and Adolescent Psychiatric Clinics of North America* was to bring together the expert clinical wisdom, knowledge, and experience of AACAP members combined with a review of the current literature. By drawing upon our AACAP Committees, we have experts in each area to highlight unique characteristics and clinical considerations of depression in youth. Depression is shaped by the many important variables that reflect the diversity among children and adolescents in the United States.

We have organized the articles into three broad categories: (1) Environment/settings, where children and adolescents may reside/receive care, including the child welfare system, primary care settings, juvenile justice systems, military settings, schools, colleges, and home; (2) Diagnostic clusters, that represent comorbid clinical conditions, including autism spectrum disorder, hearing impairment, medical conditions, HIV,

Child Adolesc Psychiatric Clin N Am 28 (2019) xv–xvi
https://doi.org/10.1016/j.chc.2019.03.001
1056-4993/19/© 2019 Published by Elsevier Inc.

and substance use disorders; and (3) Ethnic and cultural identities, including African American, Latino, American Indian, and LGBT (lesbian, gay, bisexual, and transgender) children and adolescents.

Our hope is that this special issue will serve as a practical "how-to guide" to help equip child and adolescent psychiatrists and professionals who treat depressed youth to appreciate unique considerations important in the identification, assessment, course of illness, and/or treatment across our diverse spectrum of youth and populations.

Warren Y.K. Ng, MD, MPH
Division of Child and Adolescent Psychiatry
Columbia University Irving Medical Center
New York Presbyterian Hospital/
Columbia University Medical Center
635 West 165th Street, #EI 610
New York, NY 10032, USA

Karen Dineen Wagner, MD, PhD
Department of Psychiatry and Behavioral Sciences
University of Texas Medical Branch
Galveston, TX 77555, USA

E-mail addresses:
Yyn2@cumc.columbia.edu (W.Y.K. Ng)
kwagner@utmb.edu (K.D. Wagner)

Depression in Maltreated Children and Adolescents

Michael D. De Bellis, MD, MPH[a],*, Kate B. Nooner, PhD[b],
Jeanette M. Scheid, MD, PhD[c], Judith A. Cohen, MD[d]

KEYWORDS

- Depressive disorders • Maltreatment • Children • Adolescents • Suicide
- Self-injury • Selective serotonin reuptake inhibitors (SSRIs)
- Trauma-focused cognitive behavior therapy

KEY POINTS

- Child maltreatment affects 9.1 to 17.1 of every 1000 US children and adolescents. Maltreated youth are at high risk for depression but may present with more externalizing symptoms.
- Clinicians should screen their young patients for past or ongoing trauma and maltreatment.
- Maltreated youth are at high risk for treatment-resistant depression caused by comorbid posttraumatic stress disorder, which can be overlooked without a trauma-informed approach.
- Combination treatment with selective serotonin reuptake inhibitors and cognitive behavior therapy (CBT) with a trauma-informed approach should be considered for depressed maltreated youth.
- Behavioral management can be integrated with trauma-focused CBT to treat the externalizing disorders that commonly occur in maltreated depressed youth.

INTRODUCTION

Depressive disorders are common consequences of experiencing child maltreatment. Depressive disorders herein termed depression, are defined in the Diagnostic and Statistical Manual of Mental Disorders-5 (DSM-5), under the chapter "Depressive Disorders," as major depressive disorder, persistent depressive disorder (formerly dysthymia), disruptive mood dysregulation disorder, other specified depressive

[a] Healthy Childhood Brain Development and Developmental Traumatology Research Program, Department of Psychiatry and Behavioral Sciences, Duke University Medical Center, Box 104360, Durham, NC 27710, USA; [b] Department of Psychology, University of North Carolina Wilmington, 601 South College Road, TL 2074, Wilmington, NC 28409, USA; [c] Department of Psychiatry, Michigan State University, 909 Wilson Road, East Lansing, MI 48824, USA; [d] Drexel University College of Medicine, Allegheny Health Network, 4 Allegheny Center, 8th Floor, Pittsburgh, PA 15212, USA
* Corresponding author.
E-mail address: michael.debellis@duke.edu

Child Adolesc Psychiatric Clin N Am 28 (2019) 289–302
https://doi.org/10.1016/j.chc.2019.02.002
1056-4993/19/© 2019 Elsevier Inc. All rights reserved.

disorder, and unspecified depressive disorder.[1] The diagnostic criteria for a major depressive disorder did not change from the DSM fourth edition text revision (DSM-IV-TR).[2] This critical review of depression in maltreated youth includes literature from DSM-IV-TR and DSM-5. Maltreated youth may also have 3 types of depressive disorders listed under the chapters "Anxiety Disorders" in DSM-IV-TR and "Trauma- and Stressor-Related Disorders," in the DSM-5, namely adjustment disorder with depressed mood, adjustment disorder with mixed anxiety and depressed mood, and adjustment disorder with mixed disturbance of emotions and conduct.[3] Adjustments disorders do not have enough symptoms to meet other DSM diagnostic criteria and occur in response to an identified stressor. Adjustments disorders can be acute, with symptoms occurring less than 3 months, or chronic, with symptoms occurring more than 3 months.

A literature search of PubMed and PsychINFO articles published from 2000 to 2018 using keywords and MeSH terms "depression" (and DSM-5 terms for depressive disorders), "maltreatment" "emotional, physical or sexual abuse," "neglect," "childhood," "child," and "adolescence" were crossed individually with "incidence," "prevalence," "assessment," "practice parameters," "evidence-based treatment," "psychopharmacology," "psychotherapy," "medications," "suicide, and " self-injury," which were limited to the English language, were reviewed and selected for this article. Our criteria were that the articles be peer reviewed and methodologically sound. When reviews were needed to summarize important information, meta-analyses or peer-reviewed reviews published by depression or maltreatment researchers were cited.

CHILD MALTREATMENT

Child maltreatment is defined by law (The Child Abuse Prevention and Treatment Act) and investigated by Child Protective Services (CPS) as physical, sexual, or emotional abuse, and/or neglect by a caregiver that results in harm, potential for, or threat of harm to a child.[4] CPS usually codes emotional abuse or physical neglect in youth who witness interpersonal or domestic violence. According to the National Child Abuse and Neglect Data System, each year 3 million referrals are made to CPS, involving 6 million children. Of these, fewer than 700,000 youth, about 9.1 of every 1000 children, are identified as victims, with 75% classified as neglect, 16% as physical abuse, and 9% sexual abuse.[5] Perpetrators are mainly biological parents (88%), and about half of the perpetrators are female.[5] Parental factors such as substance use disorder (SUD), history of maltreatment, and depression are the strongest risk factors for abusing or neglecting a child.[5] At greatest risk are children, aged 0 to 4 years, because 80% of the 1545 maltreatment-related fatalities in 2011 resulted from neglect, physical abuse, or their combination.[6]

The actual US child abuse and neglect rates are likely higher than official reports. The National Incidence Study of Child Abuse and Neglect 4 estimated rates of child abuse and neglect by US caretakers in 2005 to 2006 to be 17.1 of every 1000 children (approximately 1.25 million children).[7] The National Incidence Study applied 2 definitional standards: a harm standard, restricted to children who were harmed by child abuse and neglect, and the endangerment standard, for children not yet harmed, but at high risk of being harmed. Most states apply only the harm standard in their official reports.

CHILD MALTREATMENT IS A MAJOR RISK FACTOR FOR YOUTH AND ADULT DEPRESSION

Maltreated children have greater rates of depression, posttraumatic stress disorder (PTSD), behavioral problems, suicidal thoughts, suicide attempts, self-injury, and

SUDs compared with nonmaltreated youth.[8] In a meta-analysis of adults with histories of child maltreatment, all forms of abuse and neglect increased the odds ratio of having depression from 2 to 3.00.[9] Emotional abuse, with an odds ratio of 3.53, most strongly increased depression risk.[9] Although the 12-month prevalence rate of depression in the United States is 7%,[1] the depression rate in maltreated individuals is estimated to be 24.7%. In the Longitudinal Studies of Child Abuse and Neglect, a study of 638 at-risk youth, emotional abuse also showed the strongest association to depression in girls, whereas emotional neglect was the strongest predictor of depression in boys.[10] Widom and colleagues[11] (2007) found that child abuse and neglect before age 11 years was associated with an increased risk for depression in young adulthood (odds ratio, 1.51) compared with those without maltreatment histories from similar sociodemographic backgrounds. Depression in abused and neglected youth had a much earlier age of onset (between ages 5 and 10 years) than depression in nonmaltreated youth.[11] A challenge for detecting depression in maltreated youth is that emotional abuse or emotional neglect may not be reported to CPS or the police. Thus, it is important for clinicians to screen their young patients for past or ongoing maltreatment. When maltreatment is identified, prompt referral to early evidence-based trauma-focused treatment (described later) may be a potent strategy for curtailing or preventing the onset of later depression in those youth for whom it is not already present.

DEPRESSED YOUTH SHOULD BE ASSESSED FOR MALTREATMENT HISTORY, TYPE OF DEPRESSION, AND THE PRESENCE OF OTHER DIAGNOSTIC AND STATISTICAL MANUAL OF MENTAL DISORDERS-5 AXIS I COMORBIDITY
Depression Definitions

Another challenge in identifying depression in maltreated youth is that core symptoms of depression are similar to the core symptoms of distress that are commonly seen in maltreated youth. Even though the symptoms overlap, it is important to account for maltreatment exposure when diagnosing and treating depressive disorders. A major depressive episode includes having depressed/irritable mood or loss of interest or pleasure, for the same 2-week period for most of the day/nearly every day, along with at least 4 of the following symptoms:

1. Significant decreased or increased appetite with weight loss, or failure to make expected weight for developmental stage or weight gain
2. Insomnia or hypersomnia early every day
3. Psychomotor agitation or retardation
4. Fatigue or loss of energy
5. Feelings of worthlessness or inappropriate guilt
6. Poor concentration or indecision
7. Recurrent thoughts of death, suicidal ideation, plan, or attempt

Core symptoms of a persistent depressive disorder (dysthymia) include having clinically significant depressed/irritable mood for 1 year or more along with at least 2 symptoms of depressive disorder or 1 symptom of depressive disorder and chronic feelings of hopelessness. Core symptoms of a disruptive mood dysregulation disorder (DMDD), include a period of 12 months or more of severe temper outbursts that are inconsistent with developmental stage and occur on average 2 to 3 times a week, along with persistent irritable mood in at least 2 settings.[1] Although there are few published studies on the incidence or prevalence of DMDD in maltreated youth, there is significant overlap of DMDD with oppositional defiant disorder (ODD) and attention-deficit/hyperactivity disorder (ADHD).[12] Some maltreatment researchers posit that DMDD is similar in clinical presentation to developmental trauma disorder, not present in the DSM-5, and may represent PTSD symptoms of reenactment and irritability.[13] There are no evidence-based treatments for either disorder, so treatment should focus on evidence-based treatments for depression along with PTSD, ODD, and ADHD, as appropriate.

ASSESSING MALTREATMENT AND TRAUMA IN YOUTH

Depressed maltreated youth should be assessed for current and past maltreatment experiences and other traumas. One method for asking about adverse experiences is to normalize the question as can be found in structured clinical interviews, which includes informing youth and parents separately that good and bad things happen to everyone and asking what each believes is the worst thing that happened in the youth's life and why. For young children, asking them to draw a picture of the best and worst things in their lives may be helpful. In maltreated youth, depression is commonly comorbid with PTSD, ODD, ADHD, separation anxiety disorder (particularly in cases of intimate partner violence toward primary caregiver) in children, as well as conduct disorder and alcohol use disorder (AUD) and SUD in adolescents. There are many structured clinical interviews (some are free of charge) and self-reports listed in **Table 1** that outline methods of asking questions about maltreatment, other adverse child experiences, and DSM-5 axis I disorders. In maltreated youth, multiple trauma exposures may be present. It is important to document the age of onset, duration, and offset of these events and identify the impact of these events on the child's emotional, cognitive, and behavioral development.

RISK FACTORS FOR DEPRESSION IN MALTREATED CHILDREN

Children of depressed parents have a 2-fold increased risk for depression and those with at least 1 parent and grandparent with depression are at highest risk.[14] Parental depression, PTSD, and SUDs increase the risk of having a child who is reported for maltreatment.[15] Other direct risk factors for depression in youth with high familial depression risk include irritability, fear behaviors, externalizing symptoms or anxiety before first depressive episode, economic disadvantage, and recent psychosocial adversity (eg, being bullied, death in family, parental conflict).[16] These risk factors for depression are commonly seen in maltreated youth.

REPORTING CHILD MALTREATMENT

When assessing the impact of potential maltreatment during a comprehensive clinical examination, it is important to first outline the limits of confidentiality. If a child or adolescent responds in the affirmative to the maltreatment or other traumatic stress questions, the clinician must follow up appropriately according to the clinical guidelines of the setting that the child is in and in full accordance with mandatory child abuse reporting laws. It is recommended that clinicians identify resources in the community to address any urgent concerns associated with trauma disclosure as part of setting up clinical services (eg, child abuse reporting lines, domestic violence shelters, emergency room access). In cases in which a clinician is mandated to report maltreatment, the youth's safety is the first concern. In most cases, clinicians can make a report in a transparent way. Reporting maltreatment after explaining the laws, the clinician's legal obligations, and the need for youth and family safety does not have to result in ending the clinician's treatment relationship with the youth and the family.

Table 1
Interviews and self-reports for assessment of diagnoses, maltreatment, and other traumatic experiences in children and adolescents

Measure	What It Assesses	Given to?	Age (y)	Where to Obtain the Measure
National Child Traumatic Stress Network Measure Review of assessment instruments	This user-friendly Web site lists a database for trauma-informed mental health screenings, assessments for clinicians to use with parents, children, and adolescents, including interviews and self-reports	Interviews and self-reports	Infancy to −18	https://www.nctsn.org/treatments-and-practices/screening-and-assessments/measure-reviews/all-measure-reviews
Diagnostic Infant and Preschool Assessment	Standardized assessment of 11 traumatic life events, PTSD, major depressive disorder, ADHD, separation anxiety disorder, and generalized anxiety disorder	Child's caregiver	Birth to 6	http://www.midss.org/sites/default/files/dipa_version_11_17_10.pdf
The Preschool Age Psychiatric Assessment	Structured interview that assesses different types of traumas and adverse life events, including various types of child abuse and neglect and the age at which each event was experienced, as well as developmentally sensitive version of PTSD and for diagnosing psychiatric disorders in preschool children	Child's caregiver	2–5	http://devepi.duhs.duke.edu/papa.html
Kiddie Schedule for Affective Disorders and Schizophrenia – Present and Lifetime Version for DSM-5	Semistructured interview that assesses 12 different types of trauma, including various types of child abuse and neglect and the age at which each event was experienced, as well as PTSD, and all major axis I disorders	Caregiver and youth as interview or computerized self-report	3–18	https://www.kennedykrieger.org/patient-care/faculty-staff/joan-kaufman

(continued on next page)

Table 1
(continued)

Measure	What It Assesses	Given to?	Age (y)	Where to Obtain the Measure
Child PTSD Symptom Scale for DSM-5	Self-report instrument or clinical interview that assesses DSM-5 symptoms for PTSD	Youth self-report or interview	7–18	https://www.ncbi.nlm.nih.gov/pubmed/28820616
UCLA PTSD Reaction Index for DSM-5	A comprehensive trauma history profile for many discrete forms of trauma, including abuse, neglect, bullying, and community violence, and the age at which each event was experienced. Includes a PTSD scale for DSM-5	Caregiver and youth as interview or self-report	7–18	https://www.reactionindex.com/index.php/
Trauma Symptom Checklist for Children	Self-report instrument that assesses PTSD and related problems, such as depressive, anxiety, and dissociative symptoms	Youth self-report	8–16	https://www.parinc.com/Products/Pkey/461
The Child and Adolescent Psychiatric Assessment	Structured interview that assesses different types of trauma and adverse life events, including various types of child abuse and neglect and the age at which each event was experienced, as well as PTSD and all major axis I disorders	Caregiver and youth interview	9–18	http://devepi.duhs.duke.edu/capa.html
Childhood Trauma overall mental health Questionnaire	Assesses childhood physical abuse, sexual abuse, emotional abuse, emotional neglect, and physical neglect	Youth self-report	12 to adulthood	http://www.pearsonclinical.com/psychology/products/100000446/childhood-trauma-questionnaire-a-retrospective-self-report-ctq.html

Abbreviation: UCLA, University of California, Los Angeles.

Youth may not disclose ongoing maltreatment until a therapeutic alliance is built, which may take place many months after treatment initiation. Educating caregivers and their youth about these systems and the urgent need for child safety usually leads to cooperation with CPS investigations and maintaining the youth and family in treatment.

ESTABLISHING THE DIAGNOSIS OF DEPRESSION AND TREATMENT PLAN

Depressed maltreated youth should be screened for symptom severity and assessed for safety pertaining to child abuse and neglect, suicide, and homicide, which could indicate the need for CPS/police involvement or a higher level of care. Clinicians can use the mood disorder sections of the interviews or depression, irritability or anxiety, self-reports, or other rating scales listed in **Table 1** to serve as a baseline that can be used to examine the effectiveness of the treatment plan. Hospitalization is a short-term stabilization strategy for youth whose level of function is severely impaired, who may be suicidal or homicidal (eg, secondary to severe irritability), who have depressive symptoms with psychosis, or would benefit from an inpatient environment because of unstable family support and inability to adhere to outpatient treatment.

Given that maltreated youth are more likely to have medical issues than nonmaltreated youth,[17] it is important for depressed youth to have a medical evaluation to rule out medical causes of depression. The American Academy of Child and Adolescent Psychiatry has a practice parameter for the assessment and treatment of children and adolescents with depressive disorders.[18] Medical disorders (eg, hypothyroidism, sleep disorders, mononucleosis, anemia, cancer, autoimmune diseases, premenstrual dysphoric disorder, chronic fatigue syndrome, vitamin deficiencies involving folic acid, and side effects of medications) should be ruled out as part of the treatment plan. If there is a history of physical abuse or head injury involving loss of consciousness, head computed tomography or MRI of the brain may be indicated to rule out an organic cause for depression. The medical evaluation can be completed as inpatient or outpatient depending on the youth's severity of depression and individual needs.

The treatment of depression is usually divided into 3 phases: acute, continuation, and maintenance.[18] The acute phase involves stabilization of dangerous behaviors, and initial evaluation, which includes an assessment of child maltreatment and other ongoing stressors, family support, family conflict, parental mental disorder, school function, and peer relationships. These factors should be assessed because they can contribute to persistence or desistence of depression and may need to be addressed in the youth's treatment. The aim of the acute phase is full remission of depression (a period of ≥ 2 weeks and < 2 months with no or few depressive symptoms) or recovery (a period of > 2 months with no depressive symptoms). Continuation treatment is required for depressed youths to secure a successful treatment response during the acute phase and prevent depression relapses. New stressors can put maltreated youth with a history of depression at high risk for relapse or recurrence of depression, including suicidal, homicidal, and self-injurious thoughts and behaviors. Maintenance treatment is used to prevent recurrences in youth who have had a more severe, recurrent, and chronic depressive disorder. Because maltreated youth are more likely to have a severe and recurrent form of depression with poor prognosis,[19] treatment planning should include all 3 phases, including psychotherapy that includes learning cognitive and behavioral strategies to manage ongoing stressors to prevent the recurrence of depression symptoms, including suicidality. **Fig. 1** represents a working guideline for the treatment of maltreated youth with depression.

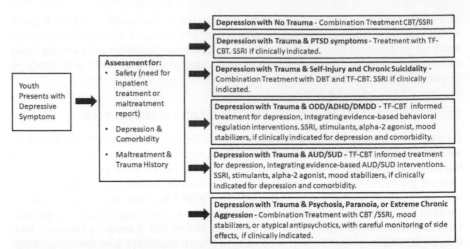

Fig. 1. Guideline for treating maltreated youth with depression. AUD, alcohol use disorder; CBT, cognitive behavioral therapy; DBT, dialectical behavior therapy; SUD, substance use disorder; TF-CBT, trauma-focused cognitive behavioral therapy.

COMBINED PSYCHOTHERAPY AND PSYCHOPHARMACOLOGY TREATMENT ARE THE EVIDENCE-BASED TREATMENTS FOR DEPRESSION IN YOUTH AND SHOULD BE THE FIRST APPROACH FOR MALTREATED DEPRESSED YOUTH

A landmark study, The Treatment for Adolescents with Depression Study (TADS), showed that, in adolescents (aged 12–17 years), combined treatment with fluoxetine (a selective serotonin reuptake inhibitor [SSRI]) and cognitive behavior therapy (CBT) with an 86% response rate, compared with 81% for fluoxetine alone and 81% for CBT alone, was judged to be superior to either treatment alone at 36 weeks after treatment initiation, and the combination treatment was also associated with decreased suicidal ideation compared with fluoxetine treatment alone.[20] Maltreated depressed youth in the TADS study showed better outcomes with combined treatment than with CBT alone.[21] According to a meta-analysis of 13 pediatric trials involving 3004 children and adolescents that examined the SSRIs fluoxetine, paroxetine, sertraline, citalopram, and escitalopram, SSRIs showed the greatest benefits within the first 4 weeks of treatment initiation and then had a smaller benefit compared with studies in adults thereafter.[22] Another meta-analysis compared 34 antidepressant trials, including 5260 children and adolescents and 14 antidepressant treatments (amitriptyline, citalopram, clomipramine, desipramine, duloxetine, escitalopram, fluoxetine, imipramine, mirtazapine, nefazodone, nortriptyline, paroxetine, sertraline, and venlafaxine) and found that only fluoxetine was statistically significantly more effective than placebo.[23] Fluoxetine was better tolerated and imipramine, venlafaxine, and duloxetine had more discontinuations because of adverse events compared with placebo.

The Treatment of SSRI-Resistant Depression in Adolescents (TORDIA) trial defined treatment-resistant depression as clinically significant depression that has not responded to acute treatment with a SSRI.[24] In this randomized controlled trial of a clinical sample of 334 patients aged 12 to 18 years with a primary diagnosis of major depressive disorder who had not responded to 2 months of SSRI treatment, patients were randomized to 12 weeks of (1) switch to a second, different SSRI (paroxetine, citalopram, or fluoxetine, 20–40 mg); (2) switch to a different SSRI plus CBT; (3) switch to venlafaxine (150–225 mg); or (4) switch to venlafaxine plus CBT. The combination of

CBT and a switch to another antidepressant resulted in a higher rate of clinical response than did a medication switch alone, and venlafaxine was not tolerated as well as other SSRIs.[24] By 24 weeks, patients in the TORDIA study, who showed remission of depression, also showed reductions in symptoms of anxiety, ADHD, disruptive behavior disorders symptoms,[25] and parent-child conflict.[26] The patients with a history of physical abuse had a lower rate of response to combination treatment in the TORDIA study, and those without maltreatment histories showed the best outcomes.[27]

There are several evidence-based therapies for the treatment of depression: CBT, whose focus is on increasing behavioral activation and decreasing negative cognitive distortions; interpersonal psychotherapy, whose focus is on shifting the patient's outlook and interaction in key relationships and interpersonal life events; and supportive therapy. All show improvement in youth depression, with a moderate effect size.[28] Data from a recent meta-analysis of 13 randomized trials of 796 children and adolescents showed that computer-based and Internet-based cognitive behavioral treatments decreased anxiety and depressive symptoms and may be an attractive treatment alternative to regular face-to-face treatment.[29] Although all of these treatments have been used with maltreated youth with depression, maltreated youth are less likely to access psychotherapy resources and have more limited computer access than nonmaltreated youth.[30]

TREATMENT OF DEPRESSED MALTREATED YOUTH WITH POSTTRAUMATIC STRESS DISORDER SYMPTOMS

Child maltreatment becomes biologically embedded in the stress systems of its victims, leading to cognitive deficits, high rates of depression, PTSD, other mental disorders, immune dysregulation, and adverse brain development.[31–33] Clinicians may consider treating depressed maltreated youth with PTSD symptoms and an identified trauma with a trial of trauma-focused CBT (TF-CBT) as a first-line treatment. TF-CBT includes psychoeducation, learning parenting skills, relaxation training, affective modulation, cognitive restructuring, and behavioral coping skills. After these skills are mastered, trauma narration and processing to correct cognitive distortions and in vivo mastery of traumatic reminders are implemented. Then conjoint child and parent sessions and safety planning skills are addressed. A critical review suggests that TF-CBT is the best evidence-based treatment of maltreated youth.[34] Behavioral management strategies can easily be integrated with TF-CBT to treat the behavioral regulation problems that commonly occur in traumatized children (ADHD, ODD) (see Ref.[35]). Information about therapist training and certification in TF-CBT is available at https://tfcbt.org. The National Child Traumatic Stress Network Learning Collaboratives (NCTSN), whose mission is "to raise the standard of care and improve access to services for traumatized children, their families and communities throughout the United States" (www.nctsn.org) is an excellent trauma-informed resource for clinicians working with maltreated youth with depression. If depression is severe, SSRIs can be offered, with careful monitoring of suicidality.

TREATMENT OF DEPRESSED MALTREATED YOUTH WITH SELF-INJURY AND SUICIDALITY

Dialectical behavior therapy (DBT), a cognitive behavioral, evidence-based, multimodal, outpatient treatment that involves individual, group treatment, and life skills coaching, is effective for reducing self-injury and suicidality as well as depression and PTSD.[36] DBT was modified for adolescents with borderline personality disorder traits and was found to be more effective than enhanced usual care in reducing self-harm, suicidal ideation, and depression.[37] DBT is a promising treatment of maltreated adolescents with depression, self-injury, and suicidality.

TREATMENT OF DEPRESSED MALTREATED YOUTH WITH EXTERNALIZING DISORDERS

There are important evidence-based interventions for disruptive behavioral disorders and for antisocial behaviors in youth with early trauma (eg, multisystemic therapy[38]). The American Academy of Child and Adolescent Psychiatry established practice parameters for the assessment and treatment of children and adolescents with ADHD,[39] ODD, and conduct disorder.[40] Many of these interventions can be integrated into TF-CBT or evidence-based treatments for depression and undertaken concurrently as part of a community treatment approach. Psychostimulants have a moderate to large effect and the alpha-2 agonist, guanfacine, a small to moderate effect on oppositional behavior, conduct problems, and aggression in youth with ADHD, with and without ODD or conduct disorder.[41] Stimulants may improve mood and decrease irritability, outbursts, and DMDD symptoms.[42] The Center for Education and Research on Mental Health Therapeutics Treatment of Maladaptive Aggression in Youth consensus guidelines include the possibility of using second-generation antipsychotic medications for psychosis or severe aggression only after a comprehensive assessment, treatment as indicated for underlying disorders, in combination with evidence-based behavioral interventions and with regular monitoring and planned taper/discontinuation as soon as feasible.[43] Intensive case management may be necessary to address significant behavioral symptoms.

TREATMENT OF DEPRESSED MALTREATED YOUTH WITH ALCOHOL AND SUBSTANCE USE DISORDERS

Maltreatment is a strong risk factor for developing AUD and SUD in adolescents and adults.[44,45] Depression in maltreated youth is highly comorbid with AUD and SUD. It is important to ask about tobacco, alcohol, marijuana, and other drug use as described in the assessments outlined in **Table 1**. Adolescents may "self-medicate" symptoms (eg, sad/irritable mood, insomnia) of depression with substances. Toxicology tests are indicated in an assessment of depression if the clinician is concerned about AUD/SUD. The American Academy of Child and Adolescent Psychiatry has a practice parameter for the assessment and treatment of child and adolescents with substance use disorders.[46] This practice parameter has detailed descriptions on the types of formal screening tools that can be helpful in AUD/SUD assessment. These recommendations for the formal evaluation and the ongoing assessment of SUD include toxicologic tests of bodily fluids, such as urine, to detect the presence of specific substances. Toxicologic tests may assist in making a differential diagnosis because some substances (eg, cannabis, alcohol) may cause depressive symptoms and, once an individual is sober, the depression may remit. According to this practice parameter, treatment of AUD/SUD must be evidence based, should be done in the least restrictive setting that is safe and effective, should involve family/caregivers and family therapy, should be comprehensive (eg, including treatment of comorbid disorders, educational/vocational issues, or addressing legal issues), and may involve medications to treat cravings or the underlying depression that may have led to AUD/SUD.

Seeking Safety is an evidence-based treatment model that emphasizes safety, integration of trauma and AUD/SUD issues, coping skills, and hope, and consistently shows positive outcomes in adolescents and adults with interpersonal trauma histories.[47] If a depressed adolescent has these problems, then referral for this evidence-based treatment is appropriate. Further information can be sought at www.seekingsafety.org. A modified version of TF-CBT, Risk Reduction through Family Therapy, has been shown in a small randomized controlled trial to significantly reduce substance abuse and trauma symptoms in traumatized youth with significant substance use.[48]

FACTORS TO EXPLORE IF EVIDENCE-BASED TREATMENTS ARE NOT ALLEVIATING DEPRESSION IN MALTREATED YOUTH

Caregivers and youth may complain about ineffectiveness of medications that were previously effective. It is always important to reevaluate the target symptoms and differential diagnosis when this occurs. There are several possible reasons for treatment resistance:

1. Noncompliance with drug regimen as prescribed
2. Unrealistic expectations of what a medication will and will not do to change mood and behaviors
3. New onset of maltreatment or increase in chronic stressors that may lead to increased depression
4. Significant side effects, such as akathisia or sleepiness
5. A medical issue
6. Growth spurts/increased drug metabolism during adolescence may require dose increase
7. The need to change to another medication, drug class, or type of CBT may be indicated
8. PTSD/trauma symptoms that have not been addressed or that emerge during treatment

SUMMARY

This article outlines approaches for the treatment of depression in maltreated children and adolescents. At the time of this writing, combination treatment with SSRIs and CBT with a trauma-informed approach should be considered for depressed maltreated youth. Behavioral management can be integrated with TF-CBT to treat the externalizing disorders that commonly occur in maltreated depressed youth. However, randomized clinical trials of depressed maltreated youth are needed to make progress and help guide maltreated youth to recovery.

REFERENCES

1. American Psychiatric Association. Depressive disorders. In: Diagnostic and statistical manual of mental disorders: fifth edition. Arlington (VA): American Psychiatric Publishing; 2013. p. 155–88.
2. American Psychiatric Association. Mood disorders. In: Diagnostic and statistical manual of mental disorders: fourth edition text revision. Washington, DC: American Psychiatric Press; 2000. p. 345–428.
3. American Psychiatric Association. Trauma- and stressor-related disorders. In: Diagnostic and statistical manual of mental disorders: fifth edition. Arlington (VA): American Psychiatric Publishing; 2013. p. 265–90.
4. Leeb RT, Paulozzzi L, Melanson C, et al. Child maltreatment surveillance: uniform definitions for public Health and recommended data elements. Atlanta (GA): Centers for Disease Control and Prevention; 2008.

5. Petersen A, Joseph J, Feit M. Committee on child maltreatment research policy and practice for the next decade phase II board on children youth and families Institute of Medicine National Research Council new directions in child abuse and neglect research. Washington, DC: National Academy of Sciences The National Academies Press; 2013.

6. GAO (Government Accountability Office). Child maltreatment: strengthening national data on child fatalities could aid in prevention. Washington, DC: GAO; 2011.

7. Sedlak AJ, Mettenburg J, Basena M, et al. Fourth national incidence study of children abuse and neglect (NIS-4): report to congress. Washington, DC: U.S. Department of Health and Human Services, Administration for Children and Families; 2010.

8. Gilbert R, Widom CP, Browne K, et al. Burden and consequences of child maltreatment in high-income countries. Lancet 2009;373:68–81.

9. Mandelli L, Petrelli C, Serretti A. The role of specific early trauma in adult depression: a meta-analysis of published literature. Childhood trauma and adult depression. Eur Psychiatry 2015;30:665–80.

10. Paul E, Eckenrode J. Childhood psychological maltreatment subtypes and adolescent depressive symptoms. Child Abuse Negl 2015;47:38–47.

11. Widom CS, DuMont K, Czaja SJ. A prospective investigation of major depressive disorder and comorbidity in abused and neglected children grown up. Arch Gen Psychiatry 2007;64(1):49–56.

12. Freeman AJ, Youngstrom EA, Youngstrom JK, et al. Disruptive mood dysregulation disorder in a community mental health clinic: prevalence, comorbidity and correlates. J Child Adolesc Psychopharmacol 2016;26(2):123–30.

13. Ford JD, Spinazzola J, van der Kolk B, et al. Toward an empirically based developmental trauma disorder diagnosis for children: factor structure, item characteristics, reliability, and validity of the developmental trauma disorder semi-structured interview. J Clin Psychiatry 2018;79(5):17m11675.

14. Weissman MM, Berry OO, Warner V, et al. A 30-year study of 3 generations at high risk and low risk for depression. JAMA Psychiatry 2016;73(9):970–7.

15. De Bellis M, Broussard E, Wexler S, et al. Psychiatric co-morbidity in caregivers and children involved in maltreatment: a pilot research study with policy implications. Child Abuse Negl 2001;25:923–44.

16. Rice F, Sellers R, Hammerton G, et al. Antecedents of new-onset major depressive disorder in children and adolescents at high familial risk. JAMA Psychiatry 2017;74(2):153–60.

17. Smith DK, Johnson AB, Pears KC, et al. Child maltreatment and foster care: unpacking the effects of prenatal and postnatal parental substance use. Child Maltreat 2007;12:150.

18. Birmaher B, Brent D, Bernet W, et al. Practice parameter for the assessment and treatment of children and adolescents with depressive disorders. J Am Acad Child Adolesc Psychiatry 2007;46(11):1503–26.

19. Nanni V, Uher R, Danese A. Childhood maltreatment predicts unfavorable course of illness and treatment outcome in depression: a meta-analysis. Am J Psychiatry 2012;169:141–51.

20. The TADS Team. The treatment for adolescents with depression study (TADS) long-term effectiveness and safety outcomes. Arch Gen Psychiatry 2007; 64(10):1132–44.

21. Lewis CC, Simons AD, Nguyen LJ, et al. Impact of childhood trauma on treatment outcome in the treatment for adolescents with depression study (TADS). J Am Acad Child Adolesc Psychiatry 2010;49(2):132–40.

22. Varigonda AL, Jakubovski E, Taylor MJ, et al. Systematic review and meta-analysis: early treatment responses of selective serotonin reuptake inhibitors in pediatric major depressive disorder. J Am Acad Child Adolesc Psychiatry 2015;54(7):557–64.

23. Cipriani A, Furukawa TA, Salanti G, et al. Comparative efficacy and acceptability of 21 antidepressant drugs for the acute treatment of adults with major depressive disorder: a systematic review and network meta-analysis. Lancet 2018; 391(10128):1357–66.

24. Brent D, Emslie G, Clarke G, et al. Switching to another SSRI or to venlafaxine with or without cognitive behavioral therapy for adolescents with SSRI-resistant depression: the TORDIA randomized controlled trial. JAMA 2008;299(8):901–13.

25. Hilton RC, Rengasamy M, Mansoor B, et al. Impact of treatments for depression on comorbid anxiety, attentional, and behavioral symptoms in adolescents with selective serotonin reuptake inhibitor-resistant depression. J Am Acad Child Adolesc Psychiatry 2013;52(5):482–92.

26. Rengasamy M, Mansoor BM, Hilton R, et al. The bi-directional relationship between parent-child conflict and treatment outcome in treatment-resistant adolescent depression. J Am Acad Child Adolesc Psychiatry 2013;52(4):370–7.

27. Shamseddeen W, Asarnow JR, Clarke G, et al. Impact of physical and sexual abuse on treatment response in the treatment of resistant depression in adolescent study (TORDIA). J Am Acad Child Adolesc Psychiatry 2011;50(3):293–301.

28. Weisz JR, McCarty CA, Valeri SM. Effects of psychotherapy for depression in children and adolescents: a meta-analysis. Psychol Bull 2006;132(1):132–49.

29. Ebert DD, Zarski AC, Christensen H, et al. Internet and computer-based cognitive behavioral therapy for anxiety and depression in youth: a meta-analysis of randomized controlled outcome trials. PLoS One 2015;10(3):e0119895.

30. Fang X, Brown DS, Florence CS, et al. The economic burden of child maltreatment in the United States and implications for prevention. Child Abuse Negl 2012;36(2):156–65.

31. De Bellis MD, Hooper SR, Chen SD, et al. Posterior structural brain volumes differ in maltreated youth with and without chronic posttraumatic stress disorder. Dev Psychopathol 2015;27:1555–76.

32. De Bellis MD, Zisk A. The biological effects of childhood trauma. In: Cozza SJ, Cohen JA, Dougherty JG, editors. Child and adolescent psychiatric clinics of North America: disaster and trauma, vol. 23. Philadelphia: Elsevier; 2014. p. 185–222.

33. Morey RA, Haswell CC, Hooper SR, et al. Amygdala, Hippocampus, and ventral medial prefrontal cortex volumes differ in maltreated youth with and without chronic posttraumatic stress disorder. Neuropsychopharmacology 2016;41: 791–801.

34. Leenarts LE, Diehle J, Doreleijers TA, et al. Evidence-based treatments for children with trauma-related psychopathology as a result of childhood maltreatment: a systematic review. Eur Child Adolesc Psychiatry 2013;22(5):269–83.

35. Cohen JA, Berliner L, Mannarino A. Trauma focused CBT for children with co-occurring trauma and behavior problems. Child Abuse Negl 2010;34(4):215–24.

36. Harned MS, Korslund KE, Linehan MM. A pilot randomized controlled trial of dialectical behavior therapy with and without the dialectical behavior therapy

prolonged exposure protocol for suicidal and self-injuring women with borderline personality disorder and PTSD. Behav Res Ther 2014;55:7–17.

37. Mehlum L, Tormoen AJ, Ramberg M, et al. Dialectical behavior therapy for adolescents with repeated suicidal and self-harming behavior: a randomized trial. J Am Acad Child Adolesc Psychiatry 2014;53(10):1082–91.

38. Curtis NM, Ronan KR, Borduin CM. Multisystemic treatment: a meta-analysis of outcome studies. J Fam Psychol 2004;18(3):411–9.

39. Dulcan M. Practice parameters for the assessment and treatment of children, adolescents, and adults with attention-deficit/hyperactivity disorder. American Academy of Child and Adolescent Psychiatry. J Am Acad Child Adolesc Psychiatry 1997;36(10 Suppl):85s–121s.

40. Steiner H. Practice parameters for the assessment and treatment of children and adolescents with conduct disorder. American Academy of Child and Adolescent Psychiatry. J Am Acad Child Adolesc Psychiatry 1997;36(10 Suppl):122s–39s.

41. Pringsheim T, Hirsch L, Gardner D, et al. The pharmacological management of oppositional behaviour, conduct problems, and aggression in children and adolescents with attention-deficit hyperactivity disorder, oppositional defiant disorder, and conduct disorder: a systematic review and meta-analysis. Part 1: psychostimulants, alpha-2 agonists, and atomoxetine. Can J Psychiatry 2015; 60(2):42–51.

42. Baweja R, Belin PJ, Humphrey HH, et al. The effectiveness and tolerability of central nervous system stimulants in school-age children with attention-deficit/ hyperactivity disorder and disruptive mood dysregulation disorder across home and school. J Child Adolesc Psychopharmacol 2016;26(2):154–63.

43. Rosato N, Correll CU, Pappadopulos E, et al. Treatment of maladaptive aggression in youth: CERT guidelines II. Treatments and ongoing management. Pediatrics 2012;129(6):e1577–86.

44. Carliner H, Gary D, McLaughlin KA, et al. Trauma exposure and externalizing disorders in adolescents: results from the National Comorbidity Survey Adolescent Supplement. J Am Acad Child Adolesc Psychiatry 2017;56(9):755–64.

45. De Bellis MD. Developmental traumatology: a contributory mechanism for alcohol and substance use disorders. Psychoneuroendocrinology 2001;27:155–70.

46. Bukstein OG, Work Group on Quality Issues. Practice parameter for the assessment and treatment of children and adolescents with substance use disorders. J Am Acad Child Adolesc Psychiatry 2005;44(6):609–21.

47. Najavits LM, Hien D. Helping vulnerable populations: a comprehensive review of the treatment outcome literature on substance use disorder and PTSD. J Clin Psychol 2013;69(5):433–79.

48. Danielson CK, McCart M, Walsh K, et al. Reducing substance use risk and mental health problems among sexually assaulted adolescents: a pilot randomized controlled trial. J Fam Psychol 2012;26:628–35.

Depression in Children and Adolescents Involved in the Child Welfare System

Michael W. Naylor, MD[a],*, Sarah M. Wakefield, MD[b],
Wynne Morgan, MD[c], Alka Aneja, MD[d]

KEYWORDS

- Child welfare system • Foster care • Child maltreatment • Depression • Treatment

KEY POINTS

- Child maltreatment is associated with psychopathology in children and adolescents, including major depression, suicidal behavior, and nonsuicidal self-injurious behavior.
- Child maltreatment is associated with a more severe and chronic course of depression with poor treatment response compared with patients with depression with no history of maltreatment.
- Involvement with the child welfare system presents an additional risk for the development of psychopathology, independent of maltreatment.
- Trauma-focused cognitive behavioral therapy has been shown to be effective in the treatment of trauma-related symptoms and to relieve symptoms of depression.
- Successful treatment of youth in the child welfare system requires the clinician to collaborate with other care providers and stakeholders to help plan and implement youth care.

INTRODUCTION

Child maltreatment presents a significant public health challenge. Exposure to childhood adversity has been linked to an array of adverse health outcomes in adulthood,[1] and is strongly associated with the onset of psychiatric illness during adolescence.[2,3]

Child maltreatment is common. In 2016, there was an estimated 4,100,000 reports of child maltreatment involving 7,400,000 children nationally. Approximately 55.1 per

Disclosure Statement: None.
[a] Department of Psychiatry, University of Illinois at Chicago, Institute for Juvenile Research, 1747 West Roosevelt Road, M/C 747, Room 155, Chicago, IL 60608, USA; [b] School of Medicine, Texas Tech University Health Sciences Center, Texas Tech University, 3601 4th Street, STOP 8103, Lubbock, TX 79430, USA; [c] Division of Child and Adolescent Psychiatry, Department of Psychiatry, University of Massachusetts Medical School, 55 Lake Avenue North, Worcester, MA 01655, USA; [d] Department of Psychiatry, Fremont Hospital, 39001 Sundale Drive, Fremont, CA 94538, USA
* Corresponding author.
E-mail address: mnaylor@uic.edu

Child Adolesc Psychiatric Clin N Am 28 (2019) 303–314
https://doi.org/10.1016/j.chc.2019.02.001
1056-4993/19/© 2019 Elsevier Inc. All rights reserved.

1000 children experienced maltreatment. Nearly 75% of victims were neglected, 18.2% were physically abused, and 8.5% were sexually abused.[4] A prospective cohort study of a nationally representative probability sample of adolescents documented a high prevalence of self-reported child maltreatment. Supervision neglect was the most common (41.5%), followed by physical assaults by parents or caregivers (28.4%), physical neglect (11.8%), and contact sexual abuse by 4.5%.[5]

An extensive body of literature documents the association between child maltreatment and depression. Adolescents and adults with a history of physical and sexual abuse are at an increased risk for lifetime major depression compared with those not maltreated.[6,7] Child maltreatment is a risk factor even for patients whose first episode of depression presents later in life.[8]

Age of exposure to child maltreatment affects the development of depression, with early childhood being a time of unique vulnerability.[9] There is a "dosage effect" in that youth who experienced more types of maltreatment or a series of abusive episodes, as opposed to a single incident, endorsed greater severity of depression, anxiety, hopelessness, and suicidal ideation.[7,10–12]

Childhood maltreatment is associated with poor outcomes in patients with depression who have more severe depression, psychotic subtype, recurrent and chronic depression, decreased rates of remission of depression and high rates of suicidal behavior.[13–15]

Child maltreatment also confers an increased risk of suicidal thoughts and behaviors in adolescents, even after controlling for depression severity. These findings are consistent across gender, racial, and ethnic lines.[16] A history of child maltreatment is associated with an earlier age of onset of suicidal ideation and behavior.[17]

A history of child maltreatment has a deleterious effect on response to treatment. Adolescents with a history of sexual or physical abuse are less responsive to cognitive behavioral therapy (CBT) for depression than patients without.[18,19] Childhood maltreatment is associated with a lower probability of response to antidepressant pharmacotherapy in depressed adults.[20]

Involvement with the child welfare system presents an additional risk for the development of psychopathology, independent of maltreatment. By definition, most children involved in the child welfare system have experienced child maltreatment. Various risk factors have been implicated in children's involvement in the child welfare system, including caregiver substance abuse and depression, caregiver history of child abuse, lack of social supports for the caregiver, and impaired child development.[21] In addition, children in the child welfare system are considerably more likely than other children to experience parental incarceration, and are more likely than children living in poverty to be exposed to adverse childhood experiences.[22]

Poverty is a powerful risk factor for both child maltreatment and involvement in the child welfare system. Poverty can predispose to child abuse and neglect through parental stress. The incidence of child maltreatment is nearly 6 times higher for children in low socioeconomic status families compared with other children. The incidence of physical and sexual abuse is 3 times higher, and the incidence of physical neglect nearly 9 times higher, in poor families. Furthermore, children placed in foster care are largely from economically disadvantaged families. In 2011, 12.9 per 1000 children in the overall population were in child welfare agency-initiated out-of-home placement. The rate of out-of-home placement was considerably higher (nearly 6 of every 100 children) for children from poor families.[23]

The increased risk of mental health issues is present at a child's first contact with the child welfare system. Youth investigated for possible child maltreatment demonstrate high levels of psychopathology. In one study, 48% of children demonstrated emotional and behavioral problems severe enough to warrant referral to mental health services.[24] A second study found high rates of depression (9%), suicidality (13.9%), anxiety (13.5%), and attention-deficit/hyperactivity disorder. Girls were more likely to report depression than boys.[25]

Rates of mental illness and depression are even higher for children whose maltreatment has been substantiated and are in the custody of the child welfare system. A meta-analysis of 8 studies of children in the child welfare system found that 49% of foster children were identified as having a current mental illness and 11% with depressive disorders.[26] Rates of psychiatric disorders are higher in older adolescents. McMillen and colleagues[11] found that 61% of older youth in foster care had at least one psychiatric disorder during their lifetime. The prevalence of major depression was 3 times higher than rates from a community sample.

The adverse impact of involvement with the child welfare system persists even after foster children leave foster care. Compared with peers in the general population, adolescent and young adult alumni of the child welfare system were more likely to be depressed, to have been hospitalized for suicide attempts, and to be hospitalized for serious psychiatric illnesses including depression. Adolescents and young adults who had been in long-term foster care had the worst outcomes.[27,28]

Factors specific to the child welfare experience, associated with the development of emotional and behavioral disorders in children in the foster care system, include multiple and sudden placement moves and childcare provider alienation.[29] Placement instability has been associated with both short- and long-term mental and behavioral symptoms, independent of maltreatment characteristics.[30] An authoritarian parenting style is associated with internalizing problems in foster children.[31]

Type of placement determines the rate of emotional and behavioral disturbances in children involved with the child welfare system. Children placed in kinship care have greater placement stability, fewer behavior and emotional problems, and enhanced well-being than those placed in nonkinship foster care.[32,33] Children in foster care do better than those in institutional settings.[34]

Although diagnostic criteria for depressive disorder are unchanged for children and adolescents who have experienced child maltreatment, care must be taken not to over diagnose depression in this population. As described by Griffin and colleagues,[35] several symptoms of child traumatic stress overlap with those of depression, including self-injurious behaviors in response to trauma-related stimuli, social withdrawal, affective numbing, and impaired sleep.

Causes of Depression in Children in the Foster Care System

As McLaughlin[36] has pointed out, it can be challenging to assimilate the data regarding the specific causes of these difficulties because of the variation in definitions used in recent research. Perinatal exposure to substance use, maternal stress and mental illness symptoms; exposure to maltreatment and placement instability are risk factors for the future development of depression for children involved in the child welfare system and will be the subject of greater exploration.

Perinatal exposure to stress

Children typically come into contact with the child welfare system owing to concerns of abuse or neglect by their primary caretakers. Caretakers who abuse or neglect a child may be suffering from mental health symptoms, and youth in foster care may have higher rates of exposure to mental illness and substance use, often beginning in utero. Brain development is most rapid during the fetal period.[37] Maternal prenatal stress, including that due to depression during pregnancy, adversely affects fetal development and is an established risk factor for preterm birth and low birth weight.[38] Preterm birth and low birth weight have been associated with neurocognitive, socio-emotional, and behavioral difficulties.[39] Mothers with a history of prenatal depression and anxiety are 1.5 to 2 times more likely to have a child with behavioral difficulties.[40] Bornstein and colleagues[41] reported that preschool-aged children with lower levels of socioemotional development had more internalizing and externalizing behaviors at ages 10 and 14 years.

There are several postulated mechanisms for the disruption of neonatal development by maternal stress. Welberg and colleagues[42] and Wyrwoll and colleagues[43] have demonstrated that maternal stress is correlated with reduced enzymatic activity of the placenta increasing fetal exposure to maternal stress hormones, in turn resulting in a lifelong risk for anxiety. Increased exposure to cortisol in utero may alter the development of the hypothalamic pituitary adrenal axis in the developing fetus.[44] Maternal prenatal stress has also been associated with restriction in uterine blood supply,[43] resulting in changes in the normal patterns and volume of circulation in the fetal brain.[45] In addition, maternal stress is associated with a higher risk of pre-eclampsia[46,47] and accompanying increases of placental corticotropin-releasing hormone. Increased levels of corticotropin-releasing hormone are associated with both preterm delivery and a negative effect on hypothalamic pituitary adrenal axis development, risk factors for future difficulty with socioemotional, and behavioral functioning.[48]

The prenatal environment and early attachment patterns are independent predictors of future socioemotional development in children. Although prenatal exposure to maternal stress can expose a child to early developmental risk, the quality of the attachment relationship after birth can predict future psychosocial function.[49] Parenting stress is associated with emotional and behavioral disorders in children as young as 3 years of age, especially in children with insecure attachment relationships with the primary caregiver.[50] This risk seems to be mitigated by a secure attachment relationship between the primary caregiver and child.

Maltreatment

Poly-victimization, or exposure to multiple types and frequent events of maltreatment, is the norm, not the exception, for youth involved in the child welfare system.[51] Greater severity of maltreatment predicts greater number of mental and behavioral symptoms in foster care youth.[52] It may be that the frequency, duration, severity, and exposure to different types of maltreatment differentiates maltreated children and adolescents involved in the child welfare system from maltreated youth not engaged in the child welfare system.[53]

As noted, maltreatment has long been associated with maladaptive effects on development in children. Green and colleagues[54] demonstrated that 45% of child psychiatric disorders are the likely result of adverse experiences in childhood. Prevention of these sequelae is precisely the goal of the child welfare system. Maltreatment has been linked with deficits in many areas of neurobiological and socioemotional development, including high rates of cognitive, motor, and language delays.[55,56] More specifically, it is important to screen children engaged in the welfare system for depression because maltreatment is associated with future development of depressive disorders.[57]

The neurobiological underpinnings of the link between maltreatment and depression are unclear and deserve additional study. Depression may be linked to difficulties in the processing of rewards and threats with reduced reward sensitivity.[58] Maltreatment may affect the development of these neurobiological pathways. McEwen[59] introduced the concept of allostatic loading as an explanation for a link between stress and future maladaptive response. Allostasis is the body's way of adapting to current stress and maintaining homeostasis. In the short term, homeostasis is achieved through alteration of stress hormones, including adrenaline and cortisol, but comes at a future cost of "overload" to the body's stress response system.

Genetic polymorphism and epigenetic modifications have been found to interact with trauma, affecting the risk of depression especially at critical neurodevelopmental periods.[60] Several studies have found that abuse during these critical neurodevelopmental periods can affect brain circuitry, endocrinologic function, immune system, and the physiologic reaction to stress.[61,62]

Placement issues

The most unique stressors for children involved in the child welfare system are those related to placement. Stressors may include separation from nonabusive supports, including siblings, teachers, and school counselors, and also the familiar neighborhood.

Instability of placement, the quality of placement, and uncertainty related to future placement or reunification may affect a child's future socioemotional function. McGuire and colleagues[63] reported that "placement stability is critical for mental health of youth in foster care, regardless of type, severity, or frequency of their maltreatment experience." Placement instability, defined as moves that do not result in a child's permanent placement,[64] is typical of a child's experience in the child welfare system.[65] Changes in placement are made for a variety of reasons, but are typically related to behavioral or medical problems outside the skill range of the placement.[66,67] The number of placement changes varies across different settings. Rubin and colleagues[68] reported that about one-third of youth in foster care have 3 or more placement changes. Pecora and colleagues[69] found that one-third of foster children reported 8 or more changes, whereas McGuire and colleagues[63] reported the average number of placement changes was 9. Placement instability contributes to depressive, anxiety, and aggressive symptoms in youth involved in the child welfare system.[70] These symptoms increase over time for youth in out-of-home placement compared with youth who remain in their home of origin.[71]

Treatment

Trauma-focused CBT (TF-CBT), consisting of 9 components: psychoeducation, relaxation skills, affective modulation skills, cognitive coping skills, trauma narration and processing, in vivo mastery of trauma reminders, conjoint youth-parent sessions, and enhancing safety and future development delivered through weekly sessions (typically 12–16 sessions) to children and their caregivers (when available), has been studied extensively and is the primary psychotherapeutic intervention for children and adolescents with symptoms referable to traumatic stress because of child maltreatment. It has been shown to be more effective than treatment-as-usual and wait-list controls in reducing symptoms of posttraumatic stress disorder (PTSD), anxiety, hyperarousal and depression.[72] With modifications, the interventions are effective for preschool-aged children with a history of maltreatment.[73,74] TF-CBT has been shown to be effective in community-based clinics for intimate partner violence[75] and in residential treatment facilities for adjudicated youth.[76] Therapeutic benefits were found to persist after 1 year, with some symptoms continuing to improve. A higher baseline severity of internalizing and depressive symptoms was predictive of children who continued to meet diagnostic criteria for PTSD at the 12-month follow-up.[77] Preliminary data suggest that TF-CBT can be delivered remotely via tele-medicine without deleterious impact on effectiveness.[78]

In a Cochran review, Gillies found that children and adolescents who received psychological therapies (CBT, eye movement desensitization and reprocessing therapy, narrative therapy, supportive therapy) after a trauma were less likely to be diagnosed with PTSD, and had fewer symptoms of PTSD up to a month after treatment, compared with those who received no treatment, highlighting the importance for youth in the child welfare system to have access to therapeutic interventions. Of the therapeutic modalities compared, CBT showed moderate evidence that it may be more effective in reducing PTSD symptoms at 1 month, although no therapies showed evidence of reduced symptoms past a month.[79] Significantly, CBT for depression seemed to be less effective for patients with depression with a history of physical and sexual abuse.[18,19,80]

Multiple treatments are available for child welfare involved children and families. Providers can search for specific interventions and their respective evidence bases through the California Evidence-Based Clearinghouse for Child Welfare (CEBC). The CEBC was established to help identify, select, and implement evidence-based child welfare practices to improve child and family well-being and increase permanency. The CEBC Program Registry provides information on evidence-based and non-evidence-based child welfare-related practices. The CEBC rates these practices on a 5-point scale ranging from "Well-Supported by Research Evidence" to "Concerning Practice" that potentially present a risk of harm to clients served, based on the available research evidence.[81]

Pharmacotherapy
Very little research has been done to examine the effectiveness of pharmacotherapy in the treatment of depression of children with a history of maltreatment. Seedat and colleagues[82] conducted a 12-week open label study of a fixed dose of citalopram in 8 adolescents with PTSD. They reported a statistically significant decrease in severity of PTSD, with improvement in re-experiencing, hyperarousal, and avoidance, but no improvement in self-reported symptoms of depression. In a second study, Seedat and colleagues[83] compared the response of 24 children and adolescents with 14 adults with PTSD with an 8-week open trial of citalopram. Both groups demonstrated significant reduction in severity of PTSD and Clinical Global Impressions (CGI) ratings. Adolescents had a significantly greater improvement in hyperarousal symptoms. Although there was significant comorbidity with major depression in both groups, the investigators did not study the impact of citalopram on depression severity. A double-blind placebo-controlled study of children and adolescents with PTSD randomized to sertraline (n = 67) or placebo (n = 62) failed to show an advantage for sertraline over placebo in mean change in total PTSD symptoms severity, CGI improvement score, or change in depression severity, as measured by the CDRS-R. Older adolescents showed greater improvement than younger adolescents.[84] In a small placebo-controlled study examining the benefit of adding sertraline to TF-CBT, Cohen and colleagues[85] found that all patients showed significant improvement in PTSD and anxiety symptoms, and total psychopathology measures over time, but there were no significant differences between patients receiving TF-CBT and sertraline and those receiving TF-CBT and placebo on any of these measures. Patients on sertraline showed greater improvement in Children's Global Assessment Scale scores than those receiving placebo.

SUMMARY

Youth involved with the child welfare system are often involved in other child-serving systems, such as the criminal justice system, and special educational programs through their schools. Clinicians working with foster children must understand their role vis-à-vis these other child-serving systems and collaborate with care providers and other stakeholders to help plan and implement a youth's care, and to obtain information from various sources on their functioning and response to services. Clinicians should monitor the youth's functioning in the various areas of their lives, including school, peer relationships, and functioning at home and in the community, with the goal of enhancing placement permanence.[86,87]

REFERENCES

1. Felitti VJ, Anda RF, Nordenberg D, et al. Relationship of childhood abuse and household dysfunction to many of the leading causes of death in adults. The adverse childhood experiences (ACE) study. Am J Prev Med 1998;14:245–58.
2. McLaughlin KA, Green JG, Gruber MJ, et al. Childhood adversities and first onset of psychiatric disorders in a national sample of US adolescents. Arch Gen Psychiatry 2012;69:1151–60.
3. Edwards VJ, Holden GW, Felitti VJ, et al. Relationship between multiple forms of childhood maltreatment and adult mental health in community respondents: results from the adverse childhood experiences study. Am J Psychiatry 2003; 160:1453–60.
4. U.S. Department of Health and Human Services, Administration for Children and Families, Administration on Children, Youth and Families. Children's Bureau. Child Maltreatment; 2016. Available at: https://www.acf.hhs.gov/sites/default/files/cb/cm2016.pdf. Accessed October 18, 2018.
5. Hussey JM, Chang JJ, Kotch JB. Child maltreatment in the United States: prevalence, risk factors, and adolescent health consequences. Pediatrics 2006;118: 933–42.
6. Widom CS, DuMont K, Czaja SJ. A prospective investigation of major depressive disorder and comorbidity in abused and neglected children grown up. Arch Gen Psychiatry 2007;64:49–56.
7. Pillay AL, Schoubben-Hesk S. Depression, anxiety, and hopelessness in sexually abused adolescent girls. Psychol Rep 2001;88:727–33.
8. Comijs HC, van Exel E, van der Mast RC, et al. Childhood abuse in late-life depression. J Affect Disord 2013;147:241–6.
9. Dunn EC, Nishimi K, Gomez SH, et al. Developmental timing of trauma exposure and emotion dysregulation in adulthood: are there sensitive periods when trauma is most harmful? J Affect Disord 2018;227:869–77.
10. Miller AB, Jenness JL, Oppenheimer CW, et al. Childhood emotional maltreatment as a robust predictor of suicidal ideation: a 3-year multi-wave, prospective investigation. J Abnorm Child Psychol 2017;45:105–16.
11. McMillen JC, Zima BT, Scott LD Jr, et al. Prevalence of psychiatric disorders among older youths in the foster care system. J Am Acad Child Adolesc Psychiatry 2005;44:88–95.
12. Danielson CK, de Arellano MA, Kilpatrick DG, et al. Child maltreatment in depressed adolescents: differences in symptomatology based on history of abuse. Child Maltreat 2005;10:37–48.
13. Holshausen K, Bowie CR, Harkness KL. The relation of childhood maltreatment to psychotic symptoms in adolescents and young adults with depression. J Clin Child Adolesc Psychol 2016;45:241–7.
14. Gaudiano BA, Zimmerman M. The relationship between childhood trauma history and the psychotic subtype of major depression. Acta Psychiatr Scand 2010;121: 462–70.

15. Nanni V, Uher R, Danese A. Childhood maltreatment predicts unfavorable course of illness and treatment outcome in depression: a meta-analysis. Am J Psychiatry 2012;169:141–51.

16. King CA, Merchant CR. Social and interpersonal factors relating to adolescent suicidality: a review of the literature. Arch Suicide Res 2008;12:181–96.

17. Dunn EC, McLaughlin KA, Slopen N, et al. Developmental timing of child maltreatment and symptoms of depression and suicidal ideation in young adulthood: results from the national longitudinal study of adolescent health. Depress Anxiety 2013;30:955–64.

18. Shamseddeen W, Asarnow JR, Clarke G, et al. Impact of physical and sexual abuse on treatment response in the treatment of resistant depression in adolescent study (TORDIA). J Am Acad Child Adolesc Psychiatry 2011;50:293–301.

19. Barbe RP, Bridge JA, Birmaher B, et al. Lifetime history of sexual abuse, clinical presentation, and outcome in a clinical trial for adolescent depression. J Clin Psychiatry 2004;65:77–83.

20. Klein DN, Arnow BA, Barkin JL, et al. Early adversity in chronic depression: clinical correlates and response to pharmacotherapy. Depress Anxiety 2009;26: 701–10.

21. English DJ, Thompson R, White CR. Predicting risk of entry into foster care from early childhood experiences: a survival analysis using LONGSCAN data. Child Abuse Negl 2015;45:57–67.

22. Turney K, Wildeman C. Adverse childhood experiences among children placed in and adopted from foster care: evidence from a nationally representative survey. Child Abuse Negl 2017;64:117–29.

23. Pelton LH. The continuing role of material factors in child maltreatment and placement. Child Abuse Negl 2015;41:30–9.

24. Burns BJ, Phillips SD, Wagner HR, et al. Mental health need and access to mental health services by youths involved in child welfare: a national survey. J Am Acad Child Adolesc Psychiatry 2004;43:960–70.

25. Heneghan A, Stein REK, Hurlburt MS, et al. Mental health problems in teens investigated by U.S. child welfare agencies. J Adolesc Health 2013;52:634–40.

26. Bronsard G, Alessandrini M, Fond G, et al. The prevalence of mental disorders among children and adolescents in the child welfare system: a systematic review and meta-analysis. Medicine 2016;95:e2622.

27. Vinnerljung B, Hjern A, Lindblad F. Suicide attempts and severe psychiatric morbidity among former child welfare clients-a national cohort study. J Child Psychol Psychiatry 2006;47:723–33.

28. Dregan A, Brown J, Armstrong D. Do adult emotional and behavioural outcomes vary as a function of diverse childhood experiences of the public care system? Psychol Med 2011;41:2213–20.

29. Hillen T, Gafson L. Why good placements matter: pre-placement and placement risk factors associated with mental health disorders in pre-school children in foster care. Clin Child Psychol Psychiatry 2015;20:486–99.

30. Proctor LJ, Skriner LC, Roesch S, et al. Trajectories of behavioral adjustment following early placement in foster care: predicting stability and change over 8 years. J Am Acad Child Adolesc Psychiatry 2010;49:464–73.

31. Fuentes MJ, Salas MD, Bernedo IM, et al. Impact of the parenting style of foster parents on the behaviour problems of foster children. Child Care Health Dev 2015;41:704–11.

32. Rubin DM, Downes KJ, O'Reilly AL, et al. Impact of kinship care on behavioral well-being for children in out-of-home care. Arch Pediatr Adolesc Med 2008; 162:550–6.

33. Winokur M, Holtan A, Batchelder KE. Kinship care for the safety, permanency, and well-being of children removed from the home for maltreatment. Cochrane Database Syst Rev 2014;(1):CD006546.

34. McLaughlin KA, Zeanah CH, Fox NA, et al. Attachment security as a mechanism linking foster care placement to improved mental health outcomes in previously institutionalized children. J Child Psychol Psychiatry 2012;53:46–55.

35. Griffin G, McClelland G, Holzberg M, et al. Addressing the impact of trauma before diagnosing mental illness in child welfare. Child Welfare 2011;90:69–89.

36. McLaughlin KA. Future direction in childhood adversity and youth psychopathology. J Clin Child Adolesc Psychol 2016;45:361–82.

37. Joseph R. Fetal brain behavior and cognitive development. Dev Rev 2000;20: 81–98.

38. Bussieres E-L, Tarabulsy GM, Pearson J, et al. Maternal prenatal stress and infant birth weight and gestational age: a meta-analysis of prospective studies. Dev Rev 2015;36:179–99.

39. Grote NI, Bridge JA, Gavin AR, et al. A meta-analysis of depression during pregnancy and the risk of preterm birth, low birth weight, and intrauterine growth restriction. Arch Gen Psychiatry 2010;67:1012–24.

40. Madigan S, Oatley H, Racine N, et al. A meta-analysis of maternal prenatal depression and anxiety on child socioemotional development. J Am Acad Child Adolesc Psychiatry 2018;57:645–57.

41. Bornstein MH, Hahn C-S, Haynes OM. Social competence, externalizing, and internalizing behavioral adjustment from early childhood through early adolescence. Dev Psychopathol 2010;22:717–35.

42. Welberg LAM, Thrivikraman KV, Plotsky PM. Chronic maternal stress inhibits the capacity to up-regulate placental 11B-hydroxysteroid dehydrogenase type 2 activity. J Endocrinol 2005;186:R7–12.

43. Wyrwoll CS, Homes MC, Seckl JR. 11beta-hydroxysteroid dehydrogenases and the brain: from zero to hero, a decade of progress. Front Neuroendocrinol 2011;32:265–86.

44. O'Donnell K, O'Connor T, Glover V. Prenatal stress and neurodevelopment of the child: focus on the HPA axis and role of the placenta. Dev Neurosci 2009;31: 346–51.

45. Sjostrom K, Valentin L, Thelin T, et al. Maternal anxiety in late pregnancy and fetal hemodynamics. Eur J Obstet Gynecol Reprod Biol 1997;74:149–55.

46. Landsbergis PA, Hatch MC. Psychosocial work stress and pregnancy induced hypertension. Epidemiology 1996;7:346–51.

47. Hobel CJ, Dunkel-Schetter C, Roesch SC, et al. Maternal plasma corticotropin-releasing hormone associated with stress at 20 weeks' gestation in pregnancies ending in pre-term delivery. Am J Obstet Gynecol 1999;180(Suppl 2):S257–63.

48. Hostinar CE, Gunnar MR. Future directions in the study of social relationships as regulators of the HPA axis across development. J Clin Child Adolesc Psychol 2013;42:564–75.

49. McGoron L, Gleason MM, Smyke AT, et al. Recovering from early deprivation: attachment mediates effects of caregiving on psychopathology. J Am Acad Child Adolesc Psychiatry 2012;51:683–93.

50. Tharner A, Luijk MPCM, van IJzendoorn MH, et al. Infant attachment, parenting stress, and child emotional and behavioral problems at age 3 years. Parenting 2012;12:261–81.

51. Turner HA, Finkelhor D, Ormrod R. Poly-victimization in a national sample of children and youth. Am J Prev Med 2010;38:323–30.

52. Jackson Y, Gabrielli J, Fleming K, et al. Untangling the relative contribution of maltreatment severity and frequency to type of behavioral outcome in foster youth. Child Abuse Negl 2014;38:1147–59.

53. Hambrick EP, Oppenheim-Weller S, N'zi AM, et al. Mental health interventions for children in foster care: a systematic review. Child Youth Serv Rev 2016;70:65–77.

54. Green JG, McLaughlin KA, Berglund P, et al. Childhood adversities and adult psychopathology in the national comorbidity survey replication (NCS-R) I: associations with first onset of DSM-IV disorders. Arch Gen Psychiatry 2010;62: 113–23.

55. Pears KC, Kim HK, Fisher PA. Psychosocial and cognitive functioning of children with specific profiles of maltreatment. Child Abuse Negl 2008;32:958–71.

56. Cicchetti D. Socioemotional, personality, and biological development: illustrations from a multilevel developmental psychopathology perspective on child maltreatment. Annu Rev Psychol 2016;67:187–211.

57. Danese A, Moffitt TE, Harrington H, et al. Adverse childhood experiences and adult risk factors of age-related disease: depression, inflammation, and clustering of metabolic risk markers. Arch Pediatr Adolesc Med 2009;163:1135–43.

58. Insel T, Cuthbert B, Garvey M, et al. Research domain criteria (RDoC): toward a new classification framework for research on mental disorders. Am J Psychiatry 2010;167:748–51.

59. McEwen BS. Allostasis and allostatic load Implications for neuropsychopharmacology. Neuropsychopharmacology 2000;22:108–24.

60. Williams LM, Gatt JM, Schofield PR, et al. 'Negativity bias' in risk for depression and anxiety: brain-body fear circuitry correlates, 5-HTT-LPR and early life stress. Neuroimage 2009;47:804–14.

61. McGee RA, Wolfe DA, Yuen SA, et al. The measurement of maltreatment: a comparison of approaches. Child Abuse Negl 1995;19:233–49.

62. Kaffman A, Meaney MJ. Neurodevelopmental sequelae of postnatal maternal care in rodents: clinical and research implications of molecular insights. J Child Psychol Psychiatry 2007;48:224–44.

63. McGuire A, Cho B, Huffhines L, et al. The relation between dimensions of maltreatment, placement instability, and mental health among youth in foster care. Child Abuse Negl 2018;86:10–21.

64. Fisher PA, Mannering AM, Van Scoyoc A, et al. A translational neuroscience perspective on the importance of reducing placement instability among foster children. Child Welfare 2013;92:9–36.

65. Farmer EMZ, Wagner HR, Burns BJ, et al. Treatment foster care in a system of care: sequences and correlates of residential placements. J Child Fam Stud 2003;12:11–25.

66. James S. Why do foster care placements disrupt? An investigation of reasons for placement change in foster care. Soc Serv Rev 2004;78:601–27.

67. Seltzer RR, Johnson SB, Minkovitz CS. Medical complexity and placement outcomes for children in foster care. Child Youth Serv Rev 2017;83:285–93.

68. Rubin DM, Alessandrini EA, Feudtner C, et al. Placement stability and mental health costs for children in foster care. Pediatrics 2004;113:1336–41.

69. Pecora PJ, Kessler RC, Williams J. Findings from the Northwest foster care alumni study. Seattle (WA): Casey Family Programs; 2015.

70. Newton RR, Litrownik AJ, Landsverk JA. Children and youth in foster care: disentangling the relationship between problem behaviors and number of placements. Child Abuse Negl 2000;24(10):1363–74.

71. Lawrence CR, Carlson EA, Egeland B. The impact of foster care on development. Dev Psychopathol 2006;18:57–76.

72. Gillies D, Taylor F, Gray C, et al. Psychological therapies for the treatment of post traumatic stress disorder in children and adolescents. Evid Based Child Health 2013;8:1004–116.

73. Cohen JA, Mannarino AP. A treatment outcome study for sexually abused pre-school children: initial findings. J Am Acad Child Adolesc Psychiatry 1996;35: 42–50.

74. Scheeringa MS, Weems CF, Cohen JA, et al. Trauma-focused cognitive-behavioral therapy for posttraumatic stress disorder in three-through six year-old children: a randomized clinical trial. J Child Psychol Psychiatry 2011;52: 853–60.

75. Cohen JA, Mannarino AP, Iyengar S. Community treatment of posttraumatic stress disorder for children exposed to intimate partner violence: a randomized controlled trial. Arch Pediatr Adolesc Med 2011;165:16–21.

76. Cohen JA, Mannarino AP, Jankowski K, et al. A randomized implementation study of trauma-focused cognitive behavioral therapy for adjudicated teens in residential treatment facilities. Child Maltreat 2016;21:156–67.

77. Mannarino AP, Cohen JA, Deblinger E, et al. Trauma-focused cognitive-behavioral therapy for children: sustained impact of treatment 6 and 12 months later. Child Maltreat 2012;17:231–41.

78. Stewart RW, Orengo-Aguayo RE, Cohen JA, et al. A pilot study of trauma-focused cognitive-behavioral therapy delivered via telehealth technology. Child Maltreat 2017;22:324–33.

79. Gillies D, Maiocchi L, Bhandari AP, et al. Psychological therapies for children and adolescents exposed to trauma. Cochrane Database Syst Rev 2016;(10):CD012371.

80. Lewis CC, Simons AD, Nguyen LJ, et al. Impact of childhood trauma on treatment outcome in the treatment for adolescents with depression study (TADS). J Am Acad Child Adolesc Psychiatry 2010;49:132–40.

81. California Evidence-Based Clearinghouse for Child Welfare (CEBC). Available at: http://www.cebc4cw.org/. Accessed November 12, 2018.

82. Seedat S, Lockhat R, Kaminer D, et al. An open trial of citalopram in adolescents with post-traumatic stress disorder. Int Clin Psychopharmacol 2001;16:21–5.

83. Seedat S, Stein DJ, Ziervogel C, et al. Comparison of response to a selective serotonin reuptake inhibitor in children, adolescents, and adults with posttraumatic stress disorder. J Child Adolesc Psychopharmacol 2002;12:37–46.

84. Robb AS, Cueva JE, Sporn J, et al. Sertraline treatment of children and adolescents with posttraumatic stress disorder: a double-blind, placebo-controlled trial. J Child Adolesc Psychopharmacol 2010;20:463–71.

85. Cohen JA, Mannarino AP, Perel JM, et al. A pilot randomized controlled trial of combined trauma-focused CBT and sertraline for childhood PTSD symptoms. J Am Acad Child Adolesc Psychiatry 2007;46:811–9.

86. American Academy of Child and Adolescent Psychiatry. A guide for community serving child agencies on psychoatropic medications for child & adolescents 2012. Available at: https://www.aacap.org/App_Themes/AACAP/docs/clinical_

practice_center/systems_of_care/Psychopharm_in_SOC_Feb_2012.pdf.   Accessed November 19, 2018.
87. Lee T, Fouras G, Brown R. Practice parameter for the assessment and management of youth involved with the child welfare system. J Am Acad Child Adolesc Psychiatry 2015;54:502–17.

Collaborative and Integrated Care for Adolescent Depression

Ian Kodish, MD, PhD[a], Laura Richardson, MD, MPH[b],
Abigail Schlesinger, MD[c],*

KEYWORDS

- Collaborative care • Integrated care • Adolescent depression
- Child and adolescent psychiatry

KEY POINTS

- There is a growing evidence-base supporting the provision of integrated care for adolescent depression in primary care.
- Psychiatrists can partner with pediatric primary care providers to improve access to high-quality treatment for adolescent depression.
- Various forms of collaborative models exist, offering creative opportunities for integrating mental health care into a range of pediatrics practice settings.

Although depression is a prevalent pediatric condition, fewer than half of youth age 12 to 17 with major depressive disorder (MDD) receive any treatment.[1] Subsyndromal depressive symptoms are also common, and associated with significant impairment and risk.[2] Unfortunately, the number and distribution of child and adolescent psychiatrists are not adequate to fully meet the needs of adolescent youth.[3,4] Therefore, new approaches are required to help improve the ability of all youth to receive appropriate interventions for depression.

Pediatric primary care providers (PCPs) are well placed to recognize adolescent depressive symptoms. Most children and adolescents in the United States have access to a PCP,[5] and PCPs are often the first professionals that families turn to with concerns about behavior and mood. To improve the ability to recognize depressive

Disclosure Statement: No disclosures.
[a] Department of Psychiatry and Behavioral Sciences, University of Washington School of Medicine, 4800 Sand Point Way Northeast, O/A 5.154, Seattle, WA 98105, USA; [b] Department of Pediatrics, University of Washington School of Medicine, Seattle Children's Research Institute, M/S CSB-200, PO Box 5371, Seattle, WA 98105, USA; [c] UPMC Western Psychiatric Hospital, UPMC Children's Hospital of Pittsburgh, University of Pittsburgh School of Medicine, 11279 Perry Highway, Suite 204, Wexford, PA 15090, USA
* Corresponding author.
E-mail address: schlesingerab@upmc.edu

Child Adolesc Psychiatric Clin N Am 28 (2019) 315–325
https://doi.org/10.1016/j.chc.2019.02.003
childpsych.theclinics.com
1056-4993/19/© 2019 Elsevier Inc. All rights reserved.

illness, in 2009 the US Preventive Services Task Force first recommended primary care depression screening in adolescents 12 and older.[6] The Guidelines for Adolescent Depression in Primary Care (GLAD-PC) further recommends that pediatric PCPs, when indicated, additionally provide access to evidence-based interventions for depressed adolescents, as well as implement appropriate safety strategies for acute concerns.[7,8] Unfortunately, many pediatric primary care clinics do not have systems to implement evidence-based treatments for adolescent depression,[7] and are unlikely to report feeling prepared to provide psychopharmacologic treatments.[9] GLAD-PC therefore recommends that pediatricians pursue more training in depression/behavioral health as well as redesign their practice structure to better support the critical provision of behavioral health care.

Child and adolescent psychiatrists interested in improving access to evidence-based care for adolescent depression can support their primary care partners in implementing these clinical refinements. Through enhanced partnerships, child and adolescent psychiatrists can improve the ability of primary care physicians to provide family-centered, youth-driven, culturally competent care within pediatric practices. To forge effective collaborations, child and adolescent psychiatrists should become informed of the evidence-base for integrated models of care for adolescent depression. This article will help providers acquire this knowledge by reviewing the following:

1. Types of integrated care models
2. The evidence-base for the collaborative approaches
3. Potential methods to optimize primary-care–based models

THE CONTINUUM OF INTEGRATED CARE MODELS

Many terms have been used to describe integrated physical-behavioral health care models. A continuum of integrated care exists, from coordinated off-site care to fully integrated models of collaboration. There are several methods by which behavioral and physical health treatment can be integrated, including by location, systems of care, medical record sharing, and coordination of treatment planning. Heath and colleagues[10] described a continuum of care with an increasing number of shared processes, from coordinated, to colocated, to integrated. In a fully integrated model, the patient would experience one care plan in a seamless process of coordinated providers capable of effectively recognizing and treating depressive symptoms.

Although integrating behavioral health treatment approaches into medical settings offers promise to address the need for improved identification and management of youth with depression, evidence demonstrating improved outcomes remains somewhat limited. Nevertheless, several studies have revealed important benefits of various collaborative models, including significant improvements in clinical severity and quality-of-life (QoL) measures (standardized subjective assessments of personal well-being), as well as enhanced engagement, enabling more youth to receive appropriate treatment modalities. We review findings from studies examining the impact of various models of collaborative care for adolescent depression, beginning with the most fully integrated approaches.

INTEGRATED CARE

One of the most studied forms of fully integrated care is the "Collaborative Care" model. "Collaborative Care" refers to a system of primary care services performed collectively by a care coordinator, a primary care provider, and a collaborative psychiatrist. A care coordinator provides evidence-based nonmedication interventions, offers proactive follow-up for all patients with depressive symptoms, and uses a registry to systematically track response to treatment.[11] PCPs take the responsibility for prescribing medication, when appropriate, and a collaborating psychiatrist routinely meets with the care coordinator for registry review to make recommendations for patients not responding to interventions. Collaborative care models are team-driven, population-focused, measurement-guided, and evidence-based.[11]

The most compelling evidence for the effectiveness of collaborative care models to improve management of depressed youth comes from randomized controlled trials (RCTs) examining the clinical impact of providing more robust and tailored treatments for depressed youth within a primary care clinic setting. Highly significant improvements were observed in a model using a depression care manager to enhance treatment engagement, provide care coordination, and deliver evidence-based brief cognitive behavioral therapy on-site.[12] Care managers consisted of master's level clinicians who initially provided psychoeducation and then elicited the patients' perspectives on symptom impairments and specific preferences in management, subsequently linking them to treatment with antidepressant medication, brief cognitive behavioral therapy (CBT), or both. All patients received symptom monitoring to assess response to their treatment of choice. Care managers also participated in weekly supervision with a psychiatrist, a psychologist, and the pediatrician. Treatments were advanced according to a stepped-care algorithm, and clinical outcomes were compared with a control group engaged in enhanced usual care (UC) over the course of 12 months. Youth who received the collaborative intervention showed significantly greater adherence to evidence-based treatments (86% to 26%). More importantly, adolescents in the intervention group were more likely to respond to treatment (68% vs 39%), achieve remission (50% vs 21%), and also reported a higher level of satisfaction with care.[12] Active outreach efforts, interventions to engage parents as active supports in the care delivery, and maintaining frequent contact were thought to account for these robust effects.

The Youth in Primary Care Study was an RCT led by Asarnow and colleagues[13] that used care managers to support pediatricians in assessment and symptom management. Choice of treatment modality was driven by the preference of the patient and clinician using a randomized encouragement design.[13] Care managers were also trained to deliver manualized CBT using various therapeutic approaches, and clinical outcomes were measured after 6 months in comparison with UC. Although results showed concerningly low rates of mental health treatment engagement among both groups (32.1% vs 17.2%), outcome measures at 6 months revealed significant improvements on measures of depression, higher mental health–related QoL scores, and greater overall satisfaction with mental health care. Subsequent examination selectively comparing outcomes of depressed youth who had engaged in evidence-based treatments revealed that collaborative management reduced the risk of severe depression after 6 months of treatment from 45.2% to 10.9%, regardless of initial severity of symptoms.[14]

Longer-term benefits were also seen at 12 and 18 months after intervention. Although the primary outcome measures did not maintain clinical significance, indirect intervention effects were seen, with lower rates of severe depression and depressive symptoms, and improved mental health–related QoL.[15] These important benefits were felt to be due to sustained improvements from initial treatment impacts, enhancing the ability of youth to manage severe depression symptoms. In addition, although treatment engagement under UC conditions is understood to decline with increasing age in the collaborative intervention condition, this decline was slower and nonsignificant.[16] Even among those adolescents who initially voiced preference for watchful waiting over active treatment, the clinical intervention was associated with similar treatment engagement rates over 6 months as those initially seeking active treatment.

Collaborative models may therefore be particularly useful to address the lack of engagement in the adolescent and young adult population by fostering a more open and empowering patient-provider relationship. Supporting access to treatment for depressed youths through primary care is likely to pay important clinical dividends beyond the period of active intervention, stressing the importance of active efforts to enhance screening and engagement early in the course of illness while continuing to engage older adolescent populations that are at greater risk of suboptimal care. A recent retrospective study examined the effectiveness of an enhanced collaborative care program within clinical practice–based pediatric settings for adolescents with elevated scores on the Patient Health Questionnaire-9.[17] Nurse care managers coordinated care and tracked symptoms, while using motivational interviewing and establishing behavioral activation goals to enhance engagement. Adolescents who did not enter the collaborative intervention (UC) were referred to community providers, and PCPs could attend weekly integrated behavioral health huddles as well as contact the nurse care managers for consultation. Nonrandomized youth receiving the practice-based collaborative intervention demonstrated improved rates of both remission (28% compared with 19%) and response (43% compared with 28%) when compared with UC, consistent with other studies revealing modest to moderate benefit. The less pronounced treatment effects compared with Richardson and colleagues[12] may be driven by the nature of real-world implementation compared with a trial setting with recruited study participants, or the fact that CBT therapy was delivered by a referred provider instead of on-site by dedicated care managers.

Other models of care have prioritized integrating evidence-based behavioral therapy approaches for youth with significant anxiety symptoms as a means of enhancing treatment engagement. A recent study assessed the effectiveness of brief behavioral therapy (BBT) and assisted referral to care for youths in multiple pediatrics clinics who met full or probable criteria for common psychiatric diagnoses in children.[18] Youths in the BBT group were provided weekly 45-minute sessions delivered in the clinic by master's level clinicians, and subsequently showed significantly higher rates of clinical improvement and overall improved functioning. Although the population was dominated by youth with primary anxiety symptoms (61.6%) and only 5.9% exhibited clinically significant depression without concurrent anxiety, comorbidity was common (32.4%). Interestingly, although the comparison group was still supported with robust referral services that successfully linked youth to treatment, it did not produce the clinical outcome comparable to the BBT intervention. Although the intervention was similarly beneficial for overall clinical improvement even when youth struggled with comorbid depression, the intervention was not effective for specifically improving Children's Depression Rating Scale–Revised (CDRS-R) scores, suggesting that although anxiety symptoms may respond to brief behaviorally focused treatments, depressive symptoms may require more extensive or tailored treatment interventions in addition to active efforts to engage in treatment beyond offering referrals.

The feasibility of collaborative care often requires more robust staffing and treatment modalities than currently exist in routine care. In addition, patients diagnosed with MDD as children are thought to have lifetime general health care expenditures double those of their peers,[19] yet the fiscal benefits of collaborative models are challenging to assess because of many potentially costly indirect effects of unmanaged depression. The cost of collaborative models to manage adolescents with depression in primary care settings was recently examined in a randomized clinical trial evaluating the impact of a collaborative intervention on measures of health care expenditures and quality-adjusted life-years from baseline to 12 months.[20] Findings revealed the collaborative treatment intervention to be only marginally more expensive than treatment as usual. Yet the benefits of improved clinical effectiveness resulted in overall cost-effectiveness, primarily from QoL years gained from improved functioning. This difference was significant, even by the most conservative threshold used to estimate reimbursements.

Other means to maximize the value of collaborative interventions may come from addressing more specific patterns of care utilization that might drive health care costs among depressed youth. In a study by Wright and colleagues,[21] adolescents who screened positive for moderate to severe depression had higher health care expenditures than those with mild to moderate depression (49% higher) as well as those who screened negative for depression (247% higher). Costs were found to be elevated across all types of care expenditures, including outpatient care, emergency care, inpatient mental health care, and inpatient medical care, as well as for medications and diagnostic tests. It is thought that some of the increased costs among both adolescent and adult populations with depression and chronic disease are due to greater utilization for somatic symptoms, such as headache and fatigue, in addition to higher mental health care expenses.[22]

Colocated Models

Colocated models of care exist on a continuum between coordinated and integrated models. In these models, behavioral health and physical health providers share space, and may share medical records. Colocated models have exhibited some benefits in engagement, including higher attendance at first session of a positive parenting program[23] and higher overall rates of care for mental health problems.[24] Evidence for improved outcomes, however, is lacking, and some findings suggest that colocation may not even meaningfully improve coordination of care. A survey of pediatricians found that on-site mental health providers were used by approximately one-third of practitioners, yet interestingly, these pediatricians did not exhibit any increase in the frequency of comanaging patients with mental health providers, nor any differences on the likelihood of identifying, treating, or referring children with common mental health diagnoses.[25] These findings highlight the importance of developing strategies for collaboration when setting up colocated arrangements, weaving mental health care into treatment approaches as a core aspect of primary care management.

Coordinated Models

Coordinated models of care may involve primary care screening, care coordinators, or care navigators but do not require colocation of or frequent communication between behavioral health and physical health providers. These models can provide consultation and training, psychiatric phone consultation, and psychiatric telepsychiatry visits. Improved access to psychiatric consultation and systematic clinical case reviews to more effectively address complex symptoms may help reduce the "clinical inertia" commonly seen in clinical management. Several consultation models using coordinated phone or video conferencing with child and adolescent psychiatrists have demonstrated benefits on behavioral health care when managed by PCPs.[26,27] For instance, adult patients who had their PCP engage in case reviews with psychiatry consultants were found to exhibit significantly improved clinical outcomes at 6 months,[28] and among patients not achieving significant improvement by 8 weeks of treatment, case review greatly enhanced the likelihood of being prescribed a new depression medication to more actively target persisting symptoms.[29] Similarly, phone consultation with psychiatry providers revealed improvements in the rate of use of selective serotonin reuptake inhibitors when considered to be clinically indicated for depressed youth directly managed by primary care physicians.[30] Recent studies have revealed that such services can also shape prescribing patterns among PCPs, as evidenced by reductions in the use of antipsychotics from a child and adolescent psychiatry consultative service designed to limit the potential negative long-term impacts of these medicines that carry risks of untoward side effects.[31]

Surveys of pediatricians engaged in a telepsychiatry behavioral health consultation service revealed a perception of improved patient care for youth with mental illness, improved comfort and confidence at caring for youth with mental illness, greater comfort prescribing psychiatric medicines, and improved access to health care for youth.[26] Pediatricians participating in a telephone consultation program adherent with the principles of Extension for Community Healthcare Outcomes framework showed improved self-efficacy and treatment practices in relation to identifying and treating children and adolescents with autism spectrum disorder.[27] Interestingly, in studies evaluating the initial Massachusetts state psychiatry phone consultation program, phone consultation alone was sufficient for PCPs to manage 42% of youth who would otherwise be referred to specialty services, and approximately 15% of patients who went on to receive a psychiatric evaluation were able to be subsequently managed by the PCP after just 1 visit.[32] These findings highlight the potential for video or phone consultative models to not only optimize the prescribing patterns of pediatricians but also to improve their own sense of comfort in effectively managing these challenging psychiatric symptoms.

High-Risk Populations

Because depressed youth often go without treatment even when quality care is accessible, efforts to engage high-risk populations should also be a priority of health care providers. Treatment outcomes for depression among minority populations are particularly concerning, with much lower rates of seeking treatment for major depression and less fidelity to recommended treatments in large clinical trials,[33] highlighting the need for culturally tailored strategies within collaborative care models. Initial findings do offer promise that collaborative care management can bridge this gap and reduce outcome disparities, even after adjusting for demographic and clinical covariates.[34]

Using family support specialists to address the challenges with engaging youth at higher risk of experiencing disparities in mental health treatments has also shown some promise. One model used collaborative practice care team to integrate child mental health specialists into pediatrics huddles, facilitate access to mental health notes, and actively include pediatricians in the postevaluation recommendations to the family. Family support specialists were also part of the care team and felt to be critical to elucidate family history, psychosocial vulnerabilities, and current stressors impacting the symptom presentation, allowing for more tailored approaches to management. Children receiving this robust collaborative practice intervention were 4 times as likely to access psychiatric evaluations and 7 times as likely to participate in follow-up appointments.[35]

Augmenting Integrated Care Models

Collaborative models have also increasingly examined technological approaches to implementing behavioral health care in primary care settings, including those targeting depression management in youth. Mobile health symptom tracking technology is an attractive option due to the increasing accessibility of phone apps, and provide an efficient means of not only engaging youth in attending to their symptoms, but also revealing longitudinal symptom patterns. Simple symptom trackers using mobile technology have been associated with significant improvements in patients' self-reported emotion regulation skills and emotional self-awareness ratings, yet did not translate into clinical improvements in depression severity.[36] Because youth with depression also commonly exhibit other signs of emotional and behavioral impairments, such as irritability, distractibility, and behavioral agitation, collaborative approaches that address externalizing symptoms may also play an important role in the clinical management of depression. One study found that screening paired with access to a phone-based parenting intervention was associated with a reduction in aggressive behaviors and attentional impairments in young children who tested positive on a brief psychosocial screen (regardless of diagnosis),[37] whereas others have revealed benefits for management of children with oppositional defiance disorder.[38] Although these studies do not directly address major depression disorder, they provide insight in the potential of parenting interventions in younger populations. Kolko and colleagues[39] also showed improvement in oppositional behaviors in youth up to age 12 with an intervention that included care management, predominantly with parents and pediatricians, and psychiatric recommendations for treatment of attention-deficit/hyperactivity disorder.

Another small RCT for youth with elevated CDRS-R depression scores examined the effectiveness of a CBT computer game compared with traditional counseling approaches. Results showed comparable efficacy at reducing depressive symptoms in adolescents, even in higher-risk populations not participating in mainstream education.[40] The program design was also tailored to improve engagement, with more visually appealing graphic interfaces instead of text. Although participants did not report a change in QoL or hopelessness, significant improvements were seen on CDRS-R and Reynolds Adolescent Depression Scale after 5 weeks compared with waitlist controls, and improvements were maintained after 10-week follow-up. These findings suggest that if used, even impersonal CBT approaches may be engaging and highly valuable in the management of adolescent depression, enhancing insight and building resiliency.

One study examined the impact a computer-based intervention for depression in pediatrics clinics by comparing strategies that physicians could use to engage patients in care. Some were offered brief motivational interviewing (MI) (5–10 minutes), and others received an even more circumscribed recommendation composed of brief advice (1–2 minutes). Although patients who received MI did reveal some reduction in subsequent depressive episodes, both groups showed similarly high engagement, which likely led to the similar treatment response after 12 weeks.[41] Remarkably, the clinical benefits of the computer-based intervention persisted for both groups after 1 year, including significant reduction in self-harm and suicidality measures.[42]

Several studies have also examined the indirect impact of provider trainings on mental health treatments. Communication skills training designed to increase engagement in behavioral health care was shown to enhance parent-rated functioning in minority youth, a population that has traditionally been more challenging to engage in mental health services.[43] Other trainings primarily focused on addressing substance use in youth and found positive results from training providers in screening and brief motivational approaches was effective to reduce substance misuse, increase readiness to change their use patterns, and decreasing the consequences of misuse.[44,45]

Recommendations for Child and Adolescent Psychiatrists

Psychiatrists are well placed to work with pediatric providers to help transform the system by providing education, phone consultation, formal and informal consultation systems, and/or providing formal support of a care coordinator/embedded therapist.

The fiscal sustainability of collaborative care models remains to be seen, although child and adolescent psychiatrists have a role in helping to advocate for implementation in real-world settings. Medicare coverage now provides reimbursement for collaborative care codes, allowing the members of the collaborative care team to be reimbursed for management of the population and "indirect services," such as case discussion and telephone support. Unfortunately, the use of these codes can be complex, and the uptake of the codes by Medicaid and private payers has not been robust. Therefore, the ability of primary care practices to provide collaborative care models with high fidelity to the collaborative care model has been limited to systems that are able to provide alternative funding structures.[23] In the interim, individual pediatric practices and systems continue to pursue relationships with behavioral health providers in attempts to improve collaboration, coordination, and quality of care.

Child and adolescent psychiatrists who are interested in working in integrated physical-behavioral health models of care should first educate themselves about the burgeoning field of integrated care. The American Academy of Pediatrics has a number of resources to support their physicians, as well as a recent book entitled *Mental Health Care of Children and Adolescents: A Guide for Primary Care Clinicians*, edited by Jane Foy.[46] This book includes an extensive list of resources ranging from screening instruments to interventions. IntegratedCareforKids.org is a Web site provided by the Academy of Child and Adolescent Psychiatry designed to serve as a resource for professionals interested in integrated physical/behavioral health care, and PALforkids.org is multistate-sponsored and grant-funded consultation program based in Washington specifically designed to support PCPs in behavioral health care management. Both sites have academic, programmatic, advocacy and clinical resources and are updated at least yearly.

SUMMARY

As health care systems move from fee for service to broader population-based health strategies, it is imperative that child and adolescent psychiatrists and pediatric PCPs work together to support models that improve access to care and clinical outcomes for adolescents with depression. Implementation of such models will require that pediatricians, child and adolescent psychiatrists, and other behavioral health providers develop new skills and evolve practice processes to engage youth with evidence-based care approaches. With the improvement of reimbursement and enhanced collaboration among the network of care providers, we can help bend the curve so that depression and suicide are no longer the major causes of morbidity and mortality in adolescence.[47]

REFERENCES

1. Substance Abuse and Mental Health Services Administration. Key substance use and mental health indicators in the United States: results from the 2016 national survey on drug use and health (HHS publication No. SMA 17-5044, NSDUH series H-52). Rockville (MD): Center for Behavioral Health Statistics and Quality, Substance Abuse and Mental Health Services Administration; 2017. Available at: https://www.samhsa.gov/data/.

2. Uchida M, Fitzgerald M, Woodworth H, et al. Subsyndromal manifestations of depression in children predict the development of major depression. J Pediatr 2018;201:252–8.

3. Kim WJ, American Academy of Child and Adolescent Psychiatry Task Force on Workforce Needs. Child and adolescent psychiatry workforce: a critical shortage and national challenge. Acad Psychiatry 2003;27(4):277–82.
4. Available at: https://www.aacap.org/aacap/resources_for_primary_care/workforce_issues.aspx. Accessed on December 18, 2019.
5. Mulye TP, Park MJ, Nelson CD, et al. Trends in adolescent and young adult health in the United States. J Adolesc Health 2009;45(1):8–24.
6. Available at: https://www.uspreventiveservicestaskforce.org/Page/Document/RecommendationStatementFinal/depression-in-children-and-adolescents-screening1. Accessed on October 23, 2018.
7. Zuckerbrot RA, Cheung A, Jensen PS, et al, GLAD-PC Steering Group. Guidelines for adolescent depression in primary care (GLAD-PC): part I. Practice preparation, identification, assessment, and initial management. Pediatrics 2018. https://doi.org/10.1542/peds.2017-4081 [pii:e20174081].
8. Cheung AH, Zuckerbrot RA, Jensen PS, et al, GLAD-PC Steering Group. Guidelines for adolescent depression in primary care (GLAD-PC): part II. Treatment and ongoing management. Pediatrics 2018. https://doi.org/10.1542/peds.2017-4082 [pii:e20174082].
9. Freed GL, Dunham KM, Switalski KE, et al. Recently trained general pediatricians: perspectives on residency training and scope of practice. Pediatrics 2009;123(Supplement 1):S38–43.
10. Heath B, Wise Romero P, Reynolds K. A review and proposed standard framework for levels of integrated healthcare. Washington, DC: SAMHSA-HRSA Center for Integrated Health Solutions; 2013.
11. Gerrity M. Integrating primary care into behavioral health settings: what works. Available at: http://www.integration.samhsa.gov/integrated-care-models/Integrating-Primary-Care-Report.pdf. Accessed October 18, 2018.
12. Richardson LP, Ludman E, McCauley E, et al. Collaborative care for adolescents with depression in primary care: a randomized clinical trial. JAMA 2014;312(8):809–16.
13. Asarnow JR, Jaycox LH, Duan N, et al. Effectiveness of a quality improvement intervention for adolescent depression in primary care clinics: a randomized controlled trial. JAMA 2005;293(3):311–9.
14. Wells KB, Tang L, Carlson GA, et al. Treatment of youth depression in primary care under usual practice conditions: observational findings from Youth Partners in Care. J Child Adolesc Psychopharmacol 2012;22(1):80–90.
15. Asarnow JR, Jaycox LH, Tang L, et al. Long-term benefits of short-term quality improvement interventions for depressed youths in primary care. Am J Psychiatry 2009;166(9):1002–10.
16. Rapp AM, Chavira DA, Sugar CA, et al. Integrated primary medical-behavioral health care for adolescent and young adult depression: predictors of service use in the youth partners in care trial. J Pediatr Psychol 2017;42(9):1051–64.
17. Shippee ND, Mattson A, Brennan R, et al. Effectiveness in regular practice of collaborative care for depression among adolescents: a retrospective cohort study. Psychiatr Serv 2018;69(5):536–41.
18. Weersing VR, Brent DA, Rozenman MS, et al. Brief behavioral therapy for pediatric anxiety and depression in primary care: a randomized clinical trial. JAMA Psychiatry 2017;74(6):571–8.
19. Knapp M, McCrone P, Fombonne E, et al. The Maudsley long-term follow-up of child and adolescent depression: 3. Impact of comorbid conduct disorder on service use and costs in adulthood. Br J Psychiatry 2002;180:19–23.

20. Wright DR, Haaland WL, Ludman E, et al. The costs and cost-effectiveness of collaborative care for adolescents with depression in primary care settings: a randomized clinical trial. JAMA Pediatr 2016;170(11):1048–54.

21. Wright DR, Katon WJ, Ludman E, et al. Association of adolescent depressive symptoms with health care utilization and payer-incurred expenditures. Acad Pediatr 2016;16(1):82–9.

22. Richardson LP, Russo JE, Lozano P, et al. The effect of comorbid anxiety and depressive disorders on health care utilization and costs among adolescents with asthma. Gen Hosp Psychiatry 2008;30(5):398–406.

23. Wildman BG, Langkamp DL. Impact of location and availability of behavioral health services for children. J Clin Psychol Med Settings 2012;19(4):393–400.

24. Kolko DJ, Perrin E. The integration of behavioral health interventions in children's health care: services, science, and suggestions. J Clin Child Adolesc Psychol 2014;43(2):216–28.

25. McCue Horwitz S, Storfer-Isser A, Kerker BD, et al. Do on-site mental health professionals change pediatricians' responses to children's mental health problems? Acad Pediatr 2016;16(7):676–83.

26. Malas N, Klein E, Tengelitsch E, et al. Exploring the telepsychiatry experience: primary care provider perception of the Michigan child collaborative care (MC3) program. Psychosomatics 2018. https://doi.org/10.1016/j.psym.2018.06.005.

27. Mazurek MO, Curran A, Burnette C, et al. ECHO autism STAT: accelerating early access to autism diagnosis. J Autism Dev Disord 2018. https://doi.org/10.1007/s10803-018-3696-5.

28. Bao Y, Druss BG, Jung HY, et al. Unpacking collaborative care for depression: examining two essential tasks for implementation. Psychiatr Serv 2016;67(4):418–24.

29. Sowa NA, Jeng P, Bauer AM, et al. Psychiatric case review and treatment intensification in collaborative care management for depression in primary care. Psychiatr Serv 2018;69(5):549–54.

30. Hilt RJ, Chaudhari M, Bell JF, et al. Side effects from use of one or more psychiatric medications in a population-based sample of children and adolescents. J Child Adolesc Psychopharmacol 2014;24(2):83–9.

31. Barclay RP, Penfold RB, Sullivan D, et al. Decrease in statewide antipsychotic prescribing after implementation of child and adolescent psychiatry consultation services. Health Serv Res 2017;52(2):561–78.

32. Aupont O, Doerfler L, Connor DF, et al. A collaborative care model to improve access to pediatric mental health services. Adm Policy Ment Health 2013;40(4):264–73.

33. Howland RH. Sequenced treatment alternatives to relieve depression (STAR*D). Part 2: study outcomes. J Psychosoc Nurs Ment Health Serv 2008;46(10):21–4.

34. Lagomasino IT, Dwight-Johnson M, Green JM, et al. Effectiveness of collaborative care for depression in public-sector primary care clinics serving Latinos. Psychiatr Serv 2017;68(4):353–9.

35. Grimes KE, Creedon TB, Webster CR, et al. Enhanced child psychiatry access and engagement via integrated care: a collaborative practice model with pediatrics. Psychiatr Serv 2018;69(9):986–92.

36. Reid SC, Kauer SD, Hearps SJ, et al. A mobile phone application for the assessment and management of youth mental health problems in primary care: a randomised controlled trial. BMC Fam Pract 2011;12:131.

37. Borowsky IW, Mozayeny S, Stuenkel K, et al. Effects of a primary care-based intervention on violent behavior and injury in children. Pediatrics 2004;114(4): e392–9.
38. Lavigne JV, Lebailly SA, Gouze KR, et al. Treating oppositional defiant disorder in primary care: a comparison of three models. J Pediatr Psychol 2008;33(5): 449–61.
39. Kolko DJ, Campo JV, Kilbourne A, et al. Collaborative care outcomes for pediatric behavioral health problems: a cluster randomized trial. Pediatrics 2014;133(4): e981–92.
40. Merry SN, Stasiak K, Shepherd M, et al. The effectiveness of SPARX, a computerised self help intervention for adolescents seeking help for depression: randomised controlled non-inferiority trial. BMJ 2012;344:e2598.
41. Van Voorhees BW, Fogel J, Reinecke MA, et al. Randomized clinical trial of an Internet-based depression prevention program for adolescents (Project CATCH-IT) in primary care: 12-week outcomes. J Dev Behav Pediatr 2009; 30(1):23–37.
42. Saulsberry A, Marko-Holguin M, Blomeke K, et al. Randomized clinical trial of a primary care internet-based intervention to prevent adolescent depression: one-year outcomes. J Can Acad Child Adolesc Psychiatry 2013;22(2):106–17.
43. Wissow LS, Gadomski A, Roter D, et al. Improving child and parent mental health in primary care: a cluster-randomized trial of communication skills training. Pediatrics 2008;121(2):266–75.
44. Hides L, Carroll S, Scott R, et al. Quik fix: a randomized controlled trial of an enhanced brief motivational interviewing intervention for alcohol/cannabis and psychological distress in young people. Psychother Psychosom 2013;82(2): 122–4.
45. D'Amico EJ, Miles JN, Stern SA, et al. Brief motivational interviewing for teens at risk of substance use consequences: a randomized pilot study in a primary care clinic. J Subst Abuse Treat 2008;35(1):53–61.
46. Foy J, editor. Mental health care of children and adolescents: a guide for primary care clinicians. Itasa (IL): American Academy of Pediatrics; 2018.
47. Heron M. Deaths: leading causes for 2015. Natl Vital Stat Rep 2017;66(5):1–76.

Depression in Justice-involved Youth

Sarah Mallard Wakefield, MD[a],*, Regina Baronia, MD[b], Stephanie Brennan, MD[c]

KEYWORDS

- Juvenile justice • Justice-involved youth • Depression • Treatment

KEY POINTS

- Justice-involved youth experience high rates of child maltreatment and involvement in the child welfare system.
- Justice-involved youth experience high rates of mental disorder, including major depression.
- Successful treatment of justice-involved youth requires early screening and referral for evidence-based services.
- Multisystemic therapy and cognitive behavior therapies, among others, offer effective strategies for decreasing mental disorder along with recidivism for justice-involved youth.
- Juvenile mental health courts provide oversight for screening, referral, and consistency in care.

INTRODUCTION

In 2017, law enforcement nationwide made 809,700 arrests of persons younger than 18 years.[1] According to the National Center for Juvenile Justice Juvenile Court Statistics, in 2016, 79% of justice-involved youth were 10 to 15 years of age.[2] Exceedingly high rates of mental health diagnoses are consistently found when justice-involved youth are surveyed worldwide,[3–9] with up to 100% of youth reporting criteria consistent with at least 1 mental health diagnosis.[8] Multiple mental health diagnoses are common for justice-involved youth. Drerup and colleagues[10] identified criteria for 1 mental health diagnosis in 92% of boys and 97% of girls. Thirty-four percent of boys and 60% of girls met criteria for 3 or more mental health diagnoses.

Disclosures: None.
[a] Department of Psychiatry, School of Medicine, Texas Tech University Health Sciences Center, 3601 4th Street, STOP 8103, Lubbock, TX 79430, USA; [b] Department of Psychiatry, Texas Tech University Health Sciences Center, 3601 4th Street, STOP 8103, Lubbock, TX 79430, USA; [c] Department of Pediatrics, Texas Tech University Health Sciences Center, 3601 4th Street, STOP 9406, Lubbock, TX 79430, USA
* Corresponding author.
E-mail address: sarah.wakefield@ttuhsc.edu

Child Adolesc Psychiatric Clin N Am 28 (2019) 327–336
https://doi.org/10.1016/j.chc.2019.02.010
1056-4993/19/© 2019 Elsevier Inc. All rights reserved.

childpsych.theclinics.com

In the National Comorbidity Survey Adolescent Supplement, 10,123 youth aged 13 to 17 years were studied from 2001 to 2004.[11] Youth with any psychiatric disorder were more likely to commit a crime, including violent crime, than youth without a psychiatric diagnosis.[11] Additional studies have also shown that a mental health diagnosis increased the likelihood of juvenile justice involvement, especially in the absence of an effective caregiver,[12] and that a lifetime diagnosis of depression is predictive of future juvenile justice involvement.[13]

The rate of diagnoses seems to increase with increasing involvement in the juvenile justice system.[14] Youth processed in adult courts have higher prevalence of psychiatric disorders than incarcerated adults.[15] Mental health diagnosis has been correlated with an 80% increased rate of recidivism compared with individuals without a mental health diagnosis,[12] and, for justice-involved youth, symptoms of mental illness have been found to persist into adulthood.[16]

It may make sense that justice-involved youth have higher rates of mental health diagnoses when considering diagnoses of conduct disorder and oppositional defiant disorder. However, justice-involved youth also have a higher prevalence of depression than what is expected in the general population. A study of 350 youth involved in family court, juvenile detention, residential facilities, and juvenile court found that 49.4% of youth met criteria for depressive disorder.[17] These symptoms are common in justice-involved youth and are typically present on first arrest. Burke and colleagues[3] found that 74% of first-time juvenile offenders met criteria for a mental health disorder, and female youth in the justice system have higher rates of depression than justice-involved youth boys.[6,18,19] Thoughts of suicide and suicidal behaviors are common in justice-involved youth and increase with greater contact with the justice system. Stokes and colleagues[20] identified a history of depression, sexual abuse, and other trauma as the most common predictors of suicidal thoughts and behaviors in justice-involved youth.

CAUSES OF DEPRESSION IN JUSTICE-INVOLVED YOUTH

It is more the rule than the exception that justice-involved youth are also youth involved in the child welfare system. For all youth who came before the juvenile court in Washington's King County, 67% had prior contact with the child welfare system. The percentage increased to 89% for youth with 3 or more contacts with the juvenile court.[21] In Los Angeles County, the number who had at least 1 referral to the child welfare system for maltreatment increased to 83%. Seventy percent of these youth were referred to the child welfare system before age 10 years, and 43% before age 5 years.[22] Youth who come in contact with the justice system have had 5 child welfare referrals on average.[22,23]

Justice-involved youth have astoundingly high rates of abuse history compared with the general population.[3,24–26] More than 67% of boys and more than 75% of girls report physical abuse, and more than 10% of boys and 40% of girls report sexual abuse.[24] Justice-involved youth with histories of trauma experience an average of 5 distinct traumas, most of which are experienced in the first 5 years of life.[25]

A history of abuse in justice-involved youth has been associated with nearly every type of psychiatric disorder.[24] Justice-involved youth who have experienced trauma present with both internalizing and externalizing symptoms,[25] and maltreatment has proved a strong direct correlate with depression for this population.[27] In a study of 350 youth involved in family court, juvenile detention, residential facilities, and juvenile court, 94% reported a history of 1 or more traumas, and 45.7% of the overall population met criteria for posttraumatic stress disorder (PTSD).[17] The average number of traumas reported by these youth was 5.4, which correlated with an 8-fold increase in PTSD diagnosis, a 7-fold increase in a depressive disorder diagnosis, and a 6-fold increase in history of substance abuse compared with those youth with history of only 1 traumatic event.

Justice-involved female youth seem to have a higher rate of major depressive disorder over time compared with boys,[28] although similar rates of trauma exposure exist between girls and boys. Girls report significantly higher rates of sexual abuse,[25] up to 6 times the sexual abuse and severe physical abuse rates reported by boys.[24] Female youth also report higher rates of posttraumatic symptoms compared with boys.[6,18,19] For girls, sexual abuse is associated with every psychiatric diagnosis[24] but is particularly associated with PTSD, depressive disorders, increased likelihood of suicidal behaviors, running away, and substance abuse.[29] Surveys of 186 juvenile justice–involved girls indicated that a history of physical and emotional abuse also predicted depressive symptoms.[30]

For boys, maltreatment has been associated with every psychiatric diagnosis except anxiety disorders.[24] Jencks and Leibowitz[31] studied predictors of depression in male youth charged with a sexual offense and found that depressed affect was most strongly predicted by history of emotional abuse and exposure to multiple traumas. Traumatic brain injury (TBI) is more common in youth involved in the juvenile justice system than in youth in the general population, but justice-involved male youth are more likely to report a history of TBI than girls involved in the juvenile justice system.[16] A history of trauma predicts future symptoms of mental illness for black, white, and Hispanic justice-involved youth.[32] There are no significant differences in rates of depression based on ethnicity.[19]

Despite their traumatized past, only about 20% of justice-involved youth accessed mental health services over a 3-year period. A diagnosis of oppositional defiant disorder was most likely to precipitate contact with mental health services. Justice-involved youth meeting criteria for depression, anxiety disorders, and attention-deficit/hyperactivity disorder were less likely to have accessed mental health services.[3] Eighty-five percent of justice-involved youth reported at least 1 barrier to accessing mental health services. Most frequent barriers included the belief that the problem would resolve on its own, uncertainty of where to find help, difficulty in accessing help, fear of others' perceptions, and cost.[33] Brady and colleagues[34] (2014) outlined "structurally embedded stressors" in school, community, and home environments, in addition to inadequate resources, as a cause for systems to focus on child behavior rather than on depressive symptoms. This approach may lead to the impulse to punish rather than treat children who present with externalizing symptoms.

Family and social modeling may also mitigate or exacerbate depressive symptoms for justice-involved youth. Family support has been shown to reduce reports of depressive symptoms.[30] Even nonparent family members, especially siblings and extended family, are important emotional supports for teens.[35] Children receiving mental health services in the community are more likely to become justice-involved if their living situations are disrupted.[36] As the number of living transitions increase, they have more significant justice involvement. Delinquency in adolescents with depression has also been associated with affiliation with other justice-involved youth and lack of prosocial involvement.[37]

ASSESSMENT AND INTERVENTION

Justice-involved youth have high rates of mental illness symptoms. Most symptoms are present on first arrest, and symptoms likely contribute to the behaviors that led to arrest. Effective care for these youth lies in an overall system of early identification, accurate assessment, and evidence-based intervention. This system has been correlated with reduced symptom burden as well as reduced recidivism.[38]

On the continuum of prevention and treatment strategies, the first step is to prevent youth from becoming involved in the justice system. Schools and primary care clinicians are on the front lines for these children where they can screen for trauma early and often. When a youth is referred for assessment within the special education system, to their primary care clinician, or for a mental health evaluation, better interventions are needed than just recognizing externalizing symptoms. Clinicians must work to peel back the layers with effective screening and evaluation to expose the true cause of the youth's behaviors.

Children living in communities with high rates of "structurally embedded stressors"[34] should be targets of prevention programs. Although many exist, there are 2 specific community-based programs, 1 targeting female youth and 1 targeting boys, and these have been correlated with improvement in symptoms of children with high-risk behaviors. The Girls Advocacy Project (GAP) is a 6-month strengths-based program set in the female youth's natural community environment.[39] GAP was found to be significantly associated with greater resilience, and decreased engagement in violence, crime, and substance abuse. In addition, GAP was associated with decreased depression, anxiety, and anger symptoms. The Stop Now and Plan (SNAP) program is an education and skill-building intervention for boys 6 to 11 years of age with antisocial behaviors.[40] SNAP showed reduction in aggression, externalizing behaviors, depression, and number of other future criminal charges.

Dembo and colleagues[41] studied health risk behavior among 777 newly justice-involved youth, both male and female, and suggested that grouping newly incarcerated youth based on lower, higher, and highest health risk would allow for best use of limited resources. Dembo and colleagues[41] found high rates of depression among newly arrested youth, consistent with current literature, and cited a "critical need" for "front end, juvenile justice intake facilities to provide behavioral and public health screening, with treatment follow up on newly arrested youth." History of trauma exposure, abuse, and polyvictimization are all linked to higher rates of behavioral and mental health symptoms[42] and should be included in early screening efforts at first contact with the justice system. Youth should also be screened for a history of TBI,[16] gang involvement,[43] substance abuse, and mental health symptoms. The Massachusetts Youth Screening Instrument-Second Version (MAYSI-2) seems to be a useful screening tool for justice-involved youth.[6] The MAYSI-2 is a brief screening tool that can be administered by law enforcement officials without professional training to assess immediate mental health needs of children 12 to 17 years of age.[44] The MAYSI-2 screens for current suicidal ideation, substance abuse, as well as symptoms that may correlate with a mental health diagnosis and warrant referral for more comprehensive mental health assessment and treatment.

Once identified, linking justice-involved youth with mental health services has shown improvement in overall mental health symptoms, including decreased depressive, anxiety, and psychotic symptoms, and improved family function, school function, and frequency of dangerous behaviors toward others.[45] Recidivism decreased from 72% to 29% when services were received for longer than just 1 month.

Several interventions have shown efficacy in studies targeting justice-involved youth. Multisystemic therapy (MST) has decades of research supporting use in youth and families at high risk of justice involvement and as an alternative to incarceration for those who have already made contact.[46] MST is a family and community-based intervention through which the youth and family unit receive therapeutic interventions and social supports in their immediate communities.[47] When held to the standard of the original model, MST has shown efficacy in reducing recidivism at a cost saving to the system at large.[48] Sheidow and colleagues[49] adapted MST for "emerging adults" (MST-EA) with serious mental illness and justice system involvement and published a pilot study of 57 subjects who met this description. MST-EA was correlated with improvement in mental health symptoms and decrease in recidivism at discharge.

Other interventions with diagnosis-specific indications, such as cognitive behavior therapy (CBT), would be expected to decrease symptoms in justice-involved youth with that diagnosis. CBT is also correlated with lower recidivism rates for justice-involved youth when delivered in either the community or residential setting.[50–57] A meta-analysis suggested that CBT, even when delivered in a group setting, is correlated with a reduction in depressive symptoms in justice-involved youth.[58] Aggression replacement therapy (ART) is a 10-week CBT program that is listed as an effective program by the Office of Juvenile Justice and Delinquency Prevention.[59] ART has shown both reduced recidivism and cost savings when delivered competently to justice-involved youth.[60] Dialectical behavioral therapy (DBT) uses a CBT framework and focuses on improving self-regulating skills to deal with difficult situations.[61] When delivered in a comprehensive system-wide fashion, DBT is associated with large cost savings compared with youth detention.[62] Olafson and colleagues[63] found significant reduction in posttraumatic stress, depression, and anger symptoms following trauma-focused group treatment in juvenile justice residential facilities using the Trauma and Grief Component Therapy for Adolescents and Think Trauma intervention training for all staff at the residential facility.

Multidimensional treatment foster care (MTFC) is an intensive therapeutic intervention used instead of and to reduce placement in residential treatment centers.[64] Youth are placed in foster care with highly trained foster parents who deliver a consistent therapeutic environment of positive reinforcement; appropriate supervision; and clear, consistent, nonviolent limit setting. MTFC is correlated with reduction in delinquent behaviors in addition to reduction in depressive symptoms and suicidal thoughts compared with youth in congregate care.[65,66] MTFC seems to have the most dramatic effect for youth with the highest severity of depressive symptoms,[66] with benefits lasting into adulthood.[65]

Juvenile mental health courts (JMHCs) are an increasingly popular method for linking justice-involved youth with mental health services. JMHC is a regularly scheduled special docket, typically with a less formal interaction style, and age-appropriate screening and assessment for mental health needs.[67] Youth are involved in JMHCs for 1 year on average. The first JMHC was established in 1998 in Pennsylvania and courts continue to increase in number around the country. At the time of this publication, at least 41 such courts are in existence in 15 states. JMHCs vary in design. About half of the current courts allow all youth with a diagnosed mental health disorder to participate, and most include youth with both misdemeanor and felony charges. JMHCs assess youth for mental health needs and facilitate access to mental health services through a closely supervised probation program including individual outpatient treatment, family therapy, and case management.[68] Despite varying design, most current JMHCs share some characteristics, including team-based approach to case review, specialized probation officers trained in mental health, system-wide accountability, graduated incentives, and sanctions.[67]

SUMMARY

The relationship of juvenile justice involvement and mental health diagnosis is complex. It is clear that justice-involved youth are at exceedingly high risk of trauma exposure; multisystem involvement; and mental health distress, including depression.[17] Justice-involved youth carry with them both a high symptom burden and a high cost to society.[10] Both could be reduced through evidence-based prevention, screening, and treatment strategies. Prevention strategies should be targeted toward communities and families with high risk of justice involvement. Screening for trauma and mental health symptoms should be part of typical school practice and primary care visits with subsequent access to community health and mental health services.[11] Routine mental health screening and assessment of adolescents entering juvenile justice should be universal.[10] Great care should be taken to support families of justice-involved youth through family-focused programs within the youth's community when safe. Youth in residential facilities should have access to family support,[35] and families should engage in training modules focused on promoting successful youth reentry. Disruptions in treatment programs, clinical care providers, and effective medication should be limited as much as possible as youth move through the juvenile justice system. JMHCs can be an effective mechanism for advocacy, increasing access to care and improving family involvement in care.

Effective treatment of mental disorders may reduce future justice involvement, whereas lack of treatment increases the likelihood of justice involvement into adulthood.[69] Multiple effective programs exist to improve the lives of justice-involved youth and subsequently decrease the cost to society of detaining and adjudicating these youth within the juvenile justice system. These youth, who carry such a high burden of adverse childhood experiences, benefit from and deserve clinical thoughtfulness, attention, and effective care.

REFERENCES

1. Office of juvenile justice and delinquency prevention statistical briefing book. Available at: https://www.ojjdp.gov/ojstatbb/crime/qa05101.asp?qaDate=2017. Accessed January 20, 2019.
2. Hockenberry S, Puzzanchera C. Juvenile court statistics 2016. Pittsburgh (PA): National Center for Juvenile Justice; 2018.
3. Burke JD, Mulvey EP, Schubert CA. Prevalence of mental health problems and service use among first-time juvenile offenders. J Child Fam Stud 2015;24(12): 3774–81.
4. Ghazali SR, Chen YY, Aziz HA. Childhood maltreatment and symptoms of PTSD and depression among delinquent adolescents in Malaysia. J Child Adolesc Trauma 2018;11(2):151–8.
5. Poyraz Fındık OT, Rodopman Arman A, Erturk Altınel N, et al. Psychiatric evaluation of juvenile delinquents under probation in the context of recidivism. Psychiatr Clin Psychopharmacology 2018. https://doi.org/10.1080/24750573.2018. 1505282.
6. Van Damme L, Grisso T, Vermeiren R, et al. Massachusetts Youth Screening Instrument for mental health needs of youths in residential welfare/justice institutions: identifying gender differences across countries and settings. J Forensic Psychiatr Psychol 2016;27(5):645–64.
7. Lemos I, Faísca L. Psychosocial adversity, delinquent pathway and internalizing psychopathology in juvenile male offenders. Int J Law Psychiatry 2015;42-43: 49–57.

8. Gretton HM, Clift RJW. The mental health needs of incarcerated youth in British Columbia, Canada. Int J Law Psychiatry 2011;34(2):109–15.

9. Maniadaki K, Kakouros E. Social and mental health profiles of young male offenders in detention in Greece. Crim Behav Ment Health 2008;18(4):207–15. Cited 17 times.

10. Drerup LC, Croysdale A, Hoffmann NG. Patterns of behavioral health conditions among adolescents in a juvenile justice system. Prof Psychol Res Pract 2008; 39(2):122–8. Cited 19 times.

11. Coker KL, Smith PH, Westphal A, et al. Crime and psychiatric disorders among youth in the US population: an analysis of the national comorbidity survey-adolescent supplement. J Am Acad Child Adolesc Psychiatry 2014; 53(8):888–98.

12. Yampolskaya S, Chuang E. Effects of mental health disorders on the risk of juvenile justice system involvement and recidivism among children placed in out-of-home care. Am J Orthopsychiatry 2012;82(4):585–93.

13. Mallet CA, Dare PS, Seck MM. Predicting juvenile delinquency: the nexus of childhood maltreatment, depression and bipolar disorder. Crim Behav Ment Health 2009;19(4):235–46.

14. Kinner SA, Degenhardt L, Coffey C, et al. Complex health needs in the youth justice system: a survey of community-based and custodial offenders. J Adolesc Health 2014;54(5):521–6.

15. Washburn JJ, Teplin LA, Voss LS, et al. Psychiatric disorders among detained youths: a comparison of youths processed in juvenile court and adult criminal court. Psychiatr Serv 2008;59(9):965–73.

16. Vaughn MG, Salas-Wright CP, Delisi M, et al. Prevalence and correlates of psychiatric disorders among former juvenile detainees in the United States. Compr Psychiatry 2015;59:107–16.

17. Rosenberg HJ, Vance JE, Rosenberg SD, et al. Trauma exposure, psychiatric disorders, and resiliency in juvenile-justice-involved youth. Psychol Trauma 2014; 6(4):430–7.

18. Conrad SM, Queenan R, Brown LK, et al. Psychiatric symptoms, substance use, trauma, and sexual risk: a brief report of gender differences in marijuana-using juvenile offenders. J Child Adolesc Subst Abuse 2017;26(6):433–6.

19. Vincent GM, Grisso T, Terry A, et al. Sex and race differences in mental health symptoms in juvenile justice: the MAYSI-2 national meta-analysis. J Am Acad Child Adolesc Psychiatry 2008;47(3):282–90.

20. Stokes ML, McCoy KP, Abram KM, et al. Suicidal ideation and behavior in youth in the juvenile justice system: a review of the literature. J Correct Health Care 2015; 21(3):222–42.

21. Halemba G, Siegel G. Doorways to delinquency: multi-system involvement of delinquent youth in King County (Seattle, WA). Pittsburgh (PA): National Center for Juvenile Justice; 2011.

22. McCroskey J, Herz D, Putnam-Hornstein E. Crossover youth: Los Angeles county probation youth with previous referrals to child protective services. Children's data network. Available at: http://foster-ed.org/crossover-youth-los-angeles-county-probation-youth-with-previous-referrals-to-child-protective-services/. Accessed January 30, 2019.

23. Hobbs AM, Peterson J. Youth re-entering Lancaster County after commitment to a state youth rehabilitation center. Omaha (NE): Juvenile Justice Institute University of Nebraska at Omaha; 2012. Available at: https://www.unomaha.edu/college-of-public-affairs-and-community-service/juvenile-justice-institute/reports-and-publications/index.php. Accessed January 30, 2019.

24. King DC, Abram KM, Romero EG, et al. Childhood maltreatment and psychiatric disorders among detained youths. Psychiatr Serv 2011;62(12):1430–8.
25. Dierkhising CB, Ko SJ, Woods-Jaeger B, et al. Trauma histories among justice-involved youth: findings from the national child traumatic stress network. Eur J Psychotraumatol 2013;4(1):20274.
26. Abram KM, Washburn JJ, Teplin LA, et al. Posttraumatic stress disorder and psychiatric comorbidity among detained youths. Psychiatr Serv 2007;58(10):1311–6.
27. Wanklyn SG, Day DM, Hart TA, et al. Cumulative childhood maltreatment and depression among incarcerated youth: impulsivity and hopelessness as potential intervening variables. Child Maltreat 2012;17(4):306–17.
28. Teplin LA, Welty LJ, Abram KM, et al. Prevalence and persistence of psychiatric disorders in youth after detention: a prospective longitudinal study. Arch Gen Psychiatry 2012;69(10):1031–43.
29. Tossone K, Wheeler M, Butcher F, et al. The role of sexual abuse in trauma symptoms, delinquent and suicidal behaviors, and criminal justice outcomes among females in a juvenile justice diversion program. Violence Against Women 2018; 24(8):973–93.
30. Goodkind S, Ruffolo MC, Bybee D, et al. Coping as a mediator of the effects of stressors and supports on depression among girls in juvenile justice. Youth Violence Juv Justice 2009;7(2):100–18.
31. Jencks JW, Leibowitz GS. The impact of types and extent of trauma on depressive affect among male juvenile sexual offenders. Int J Offender Ther Comp Criminol 2018;62(5):1143–63.
32. Caldwell-Gunes RM, Romero VI, Silver NC. The relationship between trauma and mental health issues among African American, white, and Hispanic male juvenile offenders. Am J Forensic Psychol 2015;33(2):21–38.
33. Abram KM, Paskar LD, Washburn JJ, et al. Perceived barriers to mental health services among youths in detention. J Am Acad Child Adolesc Psychiatry 2008;47(3):301–8.
34. Brady SS, Winston W, Gockley SE. Stress-related externalizing behavior among African American youth: How could policy and practice transform risk into resilience? J Soc Issues 2014;70(2):315–41.
35. Johnson JE, Esposito-Smythers C, Miranda R, et al. Gender, social support, and depression in criminal justice-involved adolescents. Int J Offender Ther Comp Criminol 2011;55(7):1096–109. Cited 15 times.
36. Graves KN, Frabutt JM, Shelton TL. Factors associated with mental health and juvenile justice involvement among children with severe emotional disturbance. Youth Violence and Juvenile Justice 2007;5(2):147–67. Cited 20 times.
37. Mellin EA, Fang H-N. Exploration of the pathways to delinquency for female adolescents with depression: implications for cross-systems collaboration and counseling. J Addict Offender Couns 2010;30(2):58–72. Cited 1 time.
38. Underwood LA, Washington A. Mental illness and juvenile offenders. Int J Environ Res Public Health 2016;13(2):1–14.
39. Javdani S, Allen NE. An ecological model for intervention for juvenile justice-involved girls: development and preliminary prospective evaluation. Fem Criminol 2016;11(2):135–62.
40. Burke JD, Loeber R. The effectiveness of the stop now and plan (snap) program for boys at risk for violence and delinquency. Prev Sci 2014;16(2):242–53.
41. Dembo R, Faber J, Cristiano J, et al. Health risk behavior among justice involved male and female youth: exploratory, multi-group latent class analysis. Subst Use Misuse 2017;52(13):1751–64.

42. Ford JD, Grasso DJ, Hawke J, et al. Poly-victimization among juvenile justice-involved youths. Child Abuse Negl 2013;37(10):788–800.

43. King KM, Voisin DR, Diclemente RJ. The relationship between male gang involvement and psychosocial risks for their female juvenile justice partners with non-gang involvement histories. J Child Fam Stud 2015;24(9):2555–9.

44. MAYSI 2. In National youth screening and assessment partners. Available at: http://www.nysap.us/MAYSI2.html. Accessed January 30, 2019.

45. Lyons JS, Griffin G, Quintenz S, et al. Clinical and forensic outcomes from the Illinois mental health juvenile justice initiative. Psychiatr Serv 2003;54(12):1629–34.

46. Henggeler SW, Melton GB, Smith LA. Family preservation using multisystemic therapy: an effective alternative to incarcerating serious juvenile offenders. J Consult Clin Psychol 1992;60(6):953–61.

47. Henggeler SW. Multisystemic therapy: an overview of clinical procedures, outcomes, and policy implications. Child Psychol Psychiatr Rev 1999;4(1):2–10.

48. Henggeler SW, Melton GB, Brondino MJ, et al. Multisystemic therapy with violent and chronic juvenile offenders and their families: the role of treatment fidelity in successful dissemination. J Consult Clin Psychol 1997;65(5):821–33.

49. Sheidow AJ, McCart MR, Davis M. Multisystemic therapy for emerging adults with serious mental illness and justice involvement. Cogn Behav Pract 2016;23(3): 356–67.

50. Andrews DA, Zinger I, Hoge RD, et al. Does correctional treatment work?: a clinically relevant and psychologically informed meta-analysis. Criminology 1990; 28(3):369–404.

51. Izzo RL, Ross RR. Meta-analysis of rehabilitation programs for juvenile delinquents: a brief report. Crim Justice Behav 1990;17(1):134–42.

52. Lipsey MW. Juvenile delinquency treatment: a meta-analysis inquiry into the variability of effects. In: Cook TD, Cooper H, Cordray DS, et al, editors. Meta-analysis for explanation: a casebook. New York: Russell Sage; 1992. p. 83–127.

53. Lipsey MW, Chapman G, Landenberger NA. Cognitive-behavioral programs for offenders. Ann Am Acad Polit Soc Sci 2001;578:144–57.

54. Lipsey MW, Landenberger NA. Cognitive-behavioral interventions. In: Welsh BC, Farrington DP, editors. Preventing crime: what works for children, offenders, victims and places. New York: Springer; 2006. p. 57–71.

55. Lipsey MW, Landenberger NA, Wilson SJ. Effects of cognitive-behavioral programs for criminal offenders. Nashville (TN): Center for Evaluation Research and Methodology, Vanderbilt Institute for Public Policy Studies; 2007.

56. Pearson FS, Lipton DS, Cleland CM, et al. The effects of behavioral/cognitive-behavioral programs on recidivism. Crime Delinquen 2002;48(3):476–96.

57. Wilson DB, Bouffard LA, Mackenzie DL. A quantitative review of structured, group-oriented, cognitive-behavioral programs for offenders. J Crim Justice Behav 2005;32(2):172–204.

58. Townsend E, Walker D-M, Sargeant S, et al. Systematic review and meta-analysis of interventions relevant for young offenders with mood disorders, anxiety disorders, or self-harm. J Adolesc 2010;33(1):9–20.

59. Office of Juvenile Justice and Delinquency Prevention Model Programs Guide. Available at: https://www.ojjdp.gov/mpg/Topic/Details/79. Accessed January 30, 2019.

60. Barnoski R. Outcome evaluation of Washington State's research-based programs for juvenile offenders. Olympia (WA): Washington State Institute for Public Policy; 2004.

61. Whitbeck B. A review of research and literature addressing evidence-based and promising practices for gang-affiliated and violent youth in juvenile institutions and detention centers. JRA literature review. 2010. Report 2.23. Available at: https://www.altsa.dshs.wa.gov/sites/default/files/SESA/rda/documents/research-2-23.pdf. Accessed January 30, 2019.

62. Aos S, Lieb R, Mayfield J, et al. Benefits and costs of prevention and early intervention programs for youth. Olympia (WA): Washington State Institute for Public Policy; 2004.

63. Olafson E, Boat BW, Putnam KT, et al. Implementing trauma and grief component therapy for adolescents and think trauma for traumatized youth in secure juvenile justice settings. J Interpers Violence 2018;33(16):2537–57.

64. Fisher PA, Gilliam KS. Multidimensional treatment foster care: an alternative to residential treatment for high risk children and adolescents. Interv Psicosoc 2012;21(2):195–203.

65. Kerr DCR, Degarmo DS, Leve LD, et al. Juvenile justice girls' depressive symptoms and suicidal ideation 9 years after multidimensional treatment foster care. J Consult Clin Psychol 2014;82(4):684–93.

66. Harold GT, Kerr DCR, van Ryzin M, et al. Depressive symptom trajectories among girls in the juvenile justice system: 24-month outcomes of an RCT of multidimensional treatment foster care. Prev Sci 2013;14(5):437–46.

67. Callahan L, Steadman HJ, Gerus L. Seven common characteristics of juvenile mental health courts. Delmar (NY): Policy Research Associates; 2013.

68. Callahan L, Cocozza J, Steadman HJ, et al. A national survey of US juvenile mental health courts. Psychiatr Serv 2012;63(2):130–4.

69. Jurma AM, Tocea C, Iancu O, et al. Psychopathological symptoms in adolescents with delinquent behavior. Rom J Leg Med 2014;22(3):193–8.

Children of Military Families

Rachel M. Sullivan, MD[a],*, Stephen J. Cozza, MD[b],
Joseph G. Dougherty, MD[c]

KEYWORDS

- Military dependents • Parental illness and injury • Deployment cycle
- Military culture • TRICARE • Military One Source • War • Isolation

KEY POINTS

- Military children with depression face special challenges and difficulties due to many unique and difficult aspects of military life.
- Military children with depression have access to insurance and special resources and programs put in place to serve this population.
- There are unique aspects of military culture that impact the stability of the family, including frequent parental travel/absences, parental illness and injury, frequent moves, social isolation, and distance from family and social support.

INTRODUCTION

It would be an understatement to say that military life is hard on families, and not just because of separation during deployments. Having a parent who is a soldier, sailor, or marine means that the parent's time is at the disposal of his or her command at all times. Military members tend to work very long hours with low pay. In order to support career progression, the military expects service members to move on average every 2 to 5 years, depending on their specific job and the needs of the military. Also, many jobs require frequent travel and time away from home even when the service member parent is not deployed. In addition, parents are unable to rely on grandparents, friends, or other family members when they have been moved to a location without that support network in place (**Fig. 1**).

There are special considerations when treating depression in children of military families. The main differences are due to stressors unique to this population, as well

Disclaimer: The views expressed by the authors are their own and may not reflect the official policy or position of the Department of the Army, Department of Defense, or the US Government.

[a] Department of Behavioral Health, Tripler Army Medical Center, 1 Jarrett White Rd, Honolulu, HI 96859, USA; [b] Center for the Study of Traumatic Stress, Department of Psychiatry, Uniformed Services University, 4301 Jones Bridge Road, Bethesda, MD 20814-4799, USA; [c] Child and Adolescent Psychiatry Fellowship, Walter Reed National Military Medical Center, 4494 North Palmer Road, Bethesda, MD 20889, USA
* Corresponding author.
E-mail address: rmrsullivan@gmail.com

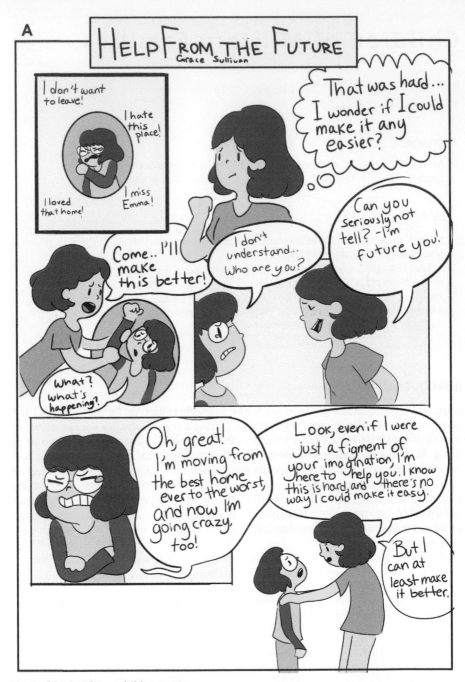

Fig. 1. (*A*, *B*) Military child, age 12.

their ability to access some resources not available to other populations. This article gives an overview of the history and evolving efforts to care for depressed children in military populations, covers cultural and military-specific stressors that these children face, discusses systems of care in place to meet their needs, and introduces some additional resources that care teams treating this population may find helpful.

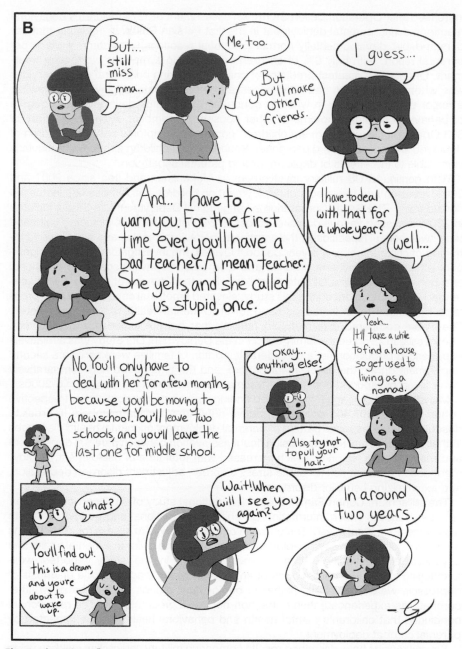

Fig. 1. *(continued)*

History

The study of military families has been a source of interest to researchers for decades, with the dynamics between returning parents and their children studied after the First World War,[1] and behavioral patterns in children and adolescents assessed in the post-Vietnam era.[2] Research on the impact of deployment on children and families increased after Operation Desert Storm. An assessment of 1274 children's behavioral reactions during parental deployment in the first Persian Gulf War[3] revealed that understandable, developmentally normal emotional reactions were commonplace per parental report, with only 6% of children experiencing symptoms warranting treatment. Of note, the greatest predictor of children requiring behavioral health services was whether counseling had been accessed before parental deployment. Likewise, a major predictive factor in whether concerning symptoms developed was degree of behavioral health symptoms of other household members. A separate study of 383 Operation Desert Storm era children[4] compared symptoms between children of deployed and non-deployed personnel. Younger-aged children appeared particularly vulnerable to the effects of deployment and parental separation.[4]

With continued US military involvement in Afghanistan and Iraq since 2001 and 2003, research into the effects of deployment on children and families has increased considerably. The RAND Corporation's Longitudinal Deployment Life Study, initiated in 2009, assessed various domains across 2724 military families, including child and teen "well-being" (specifically, the emotional, behavioral, social, and academic functioning of children), over a 3-year period.[5] Overall, the investigators found no significant effects of deployment on child and teen outcomes with regards to emotional and behavioral domains. Of note, in children less than the age of 11 years who contended with deployment during this study, elevated emotional conduct and peer problems in addition to an increased need for child mental health services were noted. They were compared with matched families that did not experience deployment. The investigators noted the family cohort in the Deployment Life Study was a relatively experienced population (ie, a considerable portion of families were serving a second deployment during the assessment period), and the time period had comparatively lower levels of reported deployment trauma compared with the early to mid-2000s.

Mansfield and colleagues[6] described findings from a nonrandomized, retrospective cohort study of 307,402 children of active-duty Army service members in order to describe a dose-response pattern of parental deployment on mental health diagnoses in their children. They reported a significant association between parental deployment and mental health histories, which increased with total time of deployment. Deployment added greatest risk for acute stress disorder, adjustment disorder, depression, and externalizing behavior disorders.[6]

The Millennium Cohort Family Study[7] is a national study of 9872 service member/ spouse dyads, in which information on children's emotional and behavioral health was gathered and assessed. The purpose of this study was to assess for associations between a military members' deployment experience and children's mental health and psychosocial functioning. Although most parents in the study reported well-functioning children, a child's odds of any mental health diagnosis or a diagnosis of depression were significantly higher in deployment groups (regardless of whether combat was experienced) than in the non-deployed group studies. The researchers concluded that children's mental health and behavioral health can be impacted by parental combat deployment.[7]

Several reports have described results comparing military and civilian children using data collected from 2011 through 2013 as part of the California Healthy Kids Survey.[8] Cederbaum and colleagues[9] reported that military-connected adolescents (7th, 9th, and 11th grade children with parents or siblings in the military) were more likely to report depressive symptoms and suicidal ideation, compared with civilian controls, and that service family member deployment was associated with greater risk. Similarly, Sullivan and colleagues[8] reported that military-connected youth were at higher risk for substance use and for carrying a weapon to school, compared with their civilian counterparts. However, these studies included limitations, such as their cross-sectional design (disallowing drawing conclusions regarding causation), student self-reporting, and their California student-only sample, which may limit generalizability of findings.

A variety of smaller studies has been carried out with families serving in the post-9-11 period, assessing for behavioral trends. Some studies have shown that the total number of months deployed during the previous 3 years was related to the degree of stress in the children's lives.[10] Children aged 3 to 5 years old with a deployed parent were more likely to experience behavioral symptoms compared with those not contending with deployment, namely, both internalizing and externalizing symptoms.[11] Likewise, poor emotional health of the non-deployed caretaker was associated with increased emotional difficulty in youth as well as poorer academic and social functioning during both the deployment periods and the reintegration.[10] A study of inpatient psychiatric hospitalization data indicated a slightly increased likelihood of admission in children aged 9 to 17 years old contending with the deployment of a parent, compared with non-deployed families.[12] An association was noted between length of deployment and admission.

Taken together, existing studies provide some indication that military children may be at risk of elevated mental health conditions, particularly when facing parental (or sibling) combat deployments; however, findings vary. To date, no population-based, methodologically rigorous prevalence studies of mental disorders in military children exist that could examine the effects of military family life on children's mental health and functioning. Future research is required.[13]

CULTURE AND MILITARY-SPECIFIC STRESSORS
Moves

Moving, commonly referred to as a "permanent change of station," is an inherent part of the military lifestyle. Regardless of service branch, the typical length of duty assignments for US-based militarily families is 3 years, although exceptions are commonplace, based on factors such as location or type of duty (eg, military schooling, specialized training).[14] Frequent moves over the course of a military career leads to children frequently negotiating new social environments and schools on a recurrent basis. In 1 study, geographic moves did not significantly correlate with anxiety or depression in those studied.[15] Although military children, when viewed as a whole, are a heterogeneous group, they tend to be viewed as resilient.[16,17] They face frequent relocations, uncertainty regarding future assignments, or potential separation from a parent due to military obligations. Of note, a positive association between family relocation and increased mental health care utilization by children and adolescents was observed.[12]

Parental Deployments and the Deployment Cycle

Of all military obligations faced by families, deployment, an inherent part of military service, can play a significant role in the well-being of military children.[15] Deployment can be viewed through the construct of the 5-stage "Deployment Cycle."[16,18] This model divides the deployment timeline into distinct phases, each containing inherent stressors and emotional challenges to be addressed and mastered by family members. *Pre-deployment* is a preparatory stage, characterized by an emphasis on training for the pending mission. Enhanced cohesion in the military unit may develop as deployment nears, while stress, confusion, or worry may be experienced in the home setting. Focusing on memorable moments and shared experiences among family members, in anticipation of pending separation, is commonplace. Parents may delay discussion of deployment timelines with young children given their limitations in their understanding of time. *Deployment* may be characterized by mixed emotions, with unpredictability regarding both the frequency of communication with family and the geographic separation from family. *Sustainment* is characterized by drawing from new sources of support on the home front, solidification of new routines, and managing changes and potential crises without a shared approach, which may have been commonplace before deployment. *Redeployment* is characterized by the anticipation and preparation for reunion. *Post-deployment* is notable for potentially realigning of roles, negotiating or adapting to new rules and expectations among family members. Children may experience conflicted emotions, perceived displays of loyalty, or variable responses to discipline related to their returning parents.

It has been suggested that the deployment cycle precipitates various stressors, which can be viewed as normative (mild to moderate), tolerable (moderate to severe), or toxic (chronic, in the context of inadequate supports).[19] Children, depending on age or developmental level, may exhibit varying behaviors as they adapt to stressors while moving through the deployment cycle. Changes in eating patterns, tantrums, regressed behaviors, or "accidents" are understandable responses when toddlers are stressed or overwhelmed. Somatic symptoms, isolating, or acting out may reflect a school-aged child's difficulty contending with a deployed parent. Adolescents may isolate themselves from the non-deployed parent, reflecting anger or apathy toward others if overwhelmed.

Parental Relationship Dynamics

Because of the constantly shifting lifestyle, high work demands, frequent separations, and the relatively young population, struggling marital relationships are common in the military. The struggling marital relationship is especially evident during times when deployments are common.[20] Remarriage, blended families with children from both marriages, and parents separated from their children due to custody challenges are commonly seen in child psychiatry clinics that treat military families.

In addition, it will come as no surprise to those who treat this population that parental stress impacts the children in these families.[21] Because moving, long separations, long work hours, and isolation from social supports are common in the inherently stressful military life, these stressors can impact the marriages of military members, causing or uncovering latent depression and stress in children. Parents with limited relationship skills, unhealthy attachment styles, or other potential challenges may find their ability to maintain a healthy marriage challenging. They may find that a relationship that might otherwise have remained intact was strained under the weight of military service. In addition, dual military couples with both members serving experience more strain, because this increases the likelihood that there will be more frequent and longer periods of separation.

Special Challenges for Learning Disabilities, Homeschooling

Military families residing overseas, or outside the continental United States, use schools operated and managed by the Department of Defense (DoD) Educational Activity (DoDEA). Schools are located in Guam, in Puerto Rico, and in 11 foreign countries. In addition to offering traditional education, limited special education services can be accessed with Individualized Education Program or 504 Plans used to meet a child's educational challenges. In overseas locations where DoDEA schools are not present, students may attend a host nation school (through the Non-DoD Schools Program), enroll in the DoD "Virtual High School," or participate in homeschooling.

Overseas Challenges

In 2016, 12% of the military's 1.2 million Active Duty members were stationed overseas (DOD, 2016). Although offering a variety of unique professional and personal opportunities to service members and their families, an overseas assignment can present some unique challenges to children. Access to various services commonplace in the United States may be limited, depending on location. Childcare on military posts or garrisons is typically accessed in Child Development Centers, which can provide services from infancy through the preschool years. Medical and behavioral health services are typically accessed at the colocated or regional military medical clinic or hospital, although subspecialty services may need to be accessed in the host nation's medical system.

In order to mitigate the likelihood of family members with particular medical or behavioral health needs being assigned to locations with limited resources, a screening process exists in the DoD. The Exceptional Family Member Program screens and enrolls children and spouses of Service Members with specific health care needs, to ensure availability of services at future military assignments. If, while stationed overseas, a medical or behavioral health matter develops the capacity of which exceeds available services, provisions may be made to expedite a return of the military family to the United States, in order to access necessary care.

Disruptions in Benefits

Parental military status impacts the degree to which their children are eligible for medical care. While on Active Duty, beneficiaries receive access to comprehensive medical and behavioral health services, through TRICARE, the military health insurance plan. Children of active duty members are eligible for coverage until the age of 21, or 23 if enrolled in college. If a service member completes their service obligation and departs the military before reaching retirement eligibility, dependent children are no longer eligible for TRICARE coverage. If a service member is administratively separated from the service, dependent children are no longer eligible for medical care. If a service member is medically retired from service, his or her beneficiaries remain eligible for medical services through TRICARE until the age of 21 or 23.

STRESSORS: PARENTAL ILLNESS, INJURY, AND DEATH

Military children face multiple unique experiences as part of their parents' military service that result in both opportunities and challenges. However, certain circumstances are likely to create added risk for elevated distress as well as depressive and anxiety symptoms. The impact of combat-related parental physical injury, illness, and death on military children has been reviewed in depth elsewhere; however, highlights of the effects of these stressors on children's mental health are summarized in this article.[22–26]

More than 50,000 service members sustained moderate to severe physical injuries in Iraq and Afghanistan since the start of combat operations in 2001, including extremity wounds (54%), abdominal (11%), head and neck (11%), facial (10%), thoracic (6%), ocular (3%), and auricular (3%) injuries that resulted in amputation, blindness, deafness, or other chronic functional impairments.[27] Children within families affected by combat injury often must contend with threats to the health and safety of their wounded service parents, relocations to military treatment centers at great distances from their homes, exposures to the potentially confusing or frightening sights within the hospital setting, medical discharge from the military, loss of military communities, friends, or resources, as well as relocations to new communities that may have little understanding of the experiences that combat-injured families have faced. Physical injuries may impact the physical, psychological, or cognitive functioning of service members, compromising their parenting and directly impacting their children's ability to adapt.

Hisle-Gorman and colleagues[28] conducted a retrospective cohort study examining the physical and mental health care utilization of military children aged 3 to 8 years from 2005 to 2007, comparing 3 groups of children: those whose parents were non-deployed; those whose parents deployed and returned without injury; and those whose parents deployed and returned with injury. They found that children of injured service members had 9% and 82% higher mental health utilization than their deployed/noninjured and non-deployed counterparts, respectively. In addition, children of injured parents also had 7% and 24% higher rates of physical health visits for new injuries than deployed/noninjured and non-deployed children, respectively. Children of injured parents were also more likely than the other groups to have health care visits related to child maltreatment; 21% higher than deployed/noninjured, and 200% higher than non-deployed children. Taken together, these findings identify heighted risk for military children affected by parent injury for a variety of negative physical and mental health effects.

Traumatic brain injury (TBI) (resulting from combat and other duty- or non-duty-related accidents) appears to have unique and caustic effects within the close relationships of those affected. TBI results in unique neuropsychiatric sequelae, such as personality changes, loss of control, emotional reactivity and irritability, and apathy or lack of energy that has particularly noxious effects on interpersonal relationships, including those with children. TBI has been associated with compromised parenting, increased externalizing behavior in children, as well as emotional and posttraumatic symptoms in children.[29] Other studies have identified feelings of loss, isolation, and loneliness among children of TBI-affected parents.[30,31] Children of TBI or other physically injured parents are often required to partake in caregiving responsibilities, adding further stress and emotional burden. Moderate or severe TBI often leads to long-term neuropsychiatric impairment, placing tremendous burden on young families with children, especially those with lesser financial or social support.[32]

In addition to physical injuries, combat exposure has also been associated with greater service member risk of posttraumatic stress disorder (PTSD), depression, anxiety disorder, and substance abuse.[33] The prevalence of PTSD among veterans of the recent wars in Iraq and Afghanistan is estimated to be 5% to 15%, suggesting that as many as 400,000 veterans may have been affected.[34] PTSD has consistently been associated with negative effects within families, including poorer marital satisfaction, impaired family functioning, and increased family distress and violence.[35] Children are invariably affected by parental PTSD, depending on age, developmental level, and temperament. Younger children and those with preexisting medical, mental health, or developmental conditions are likely to be more highly impacted. For example, Rosenheck and Nathan[36] reported distress, depression, poor self-esteem, aggression, impaired social relationships, and academic difficulties in a study of children of Vietnam veterans with PTSD.

Nearly 16,000 military service members died while on active duty in the decade following September 11, 2001 from accidents (34%), combat (32%), suicides (15%), illnesses (15%), homicides (3%), and terrorism (<1%).[23] These military duty–related deaths resulted in 12,641 young (mean age = 10.3 years) children bereaved of their military service parents (typically fathers), and most from sudden and violent means, which adds risk for negative mental health outcomes. Although there are no current reports of the effects of parental deaths on military children, death of parents has been associated with a range of negative mental health outcomes (eg, depression, anxiety, posttraumatic symptoms) in the general population of parentally bereaved children in the United States.[37-39] The effect of parental death appears to be most negatively impactful to young children, which is particularly relevant to the military community because 50% of military children are under the age of 5 years. The death of a parent may result in greater stress for military children, because such deaths typically result in loss of military housing, moves from military communities, loss of military identity, and possible loss of friends, schools, and other sources of support.

SYSTEMS OF CARE AND PREVENTIVE PROGRAMS

One of the most significant benefits of being a military child is universal coverage with the military's insurance, TRICARE. However, insurance coverage does not always equal access to care due to the increasing shortage of child and adolescent behavioral health services in the United States. Despite this nationwide shortage, the military medical system is dedicated to providing adequate and timely care. Providing care is especially challenging in remote locations with few or any child psychiatrists in the referral area. A needs assessment in 2006 (Michael Faran, unpublished data, 2006) showed a severe, unmet need. In response, both governmental and nongovernmental systems of care have been designed and implemented to serve this highly vulnerable population.

The Child and Family Behavioral Health System

The Child and Family Behavioral Health System is a system of care designed to assist Army families with the goal of maximizing limited resources for the children of military members. It was designed as a consultative model, using child therapists and psychiatrists as consultants to primary care so that children may receive timely and appropriate care even in remote locations. These experts educate pediatric primary care providers in depression treatment and provide consultation via a child psychiatrist available by phone to primary care providers in each geographic region. When necessary, direct subspecialty care is provided for the sickest patients who exhibit a wide variety of behavioral and psychiatric challenges. In addition, some locations may have psychologists, social workers, or psychiatrists embedded within pediatric clinics.

School-Based Behavioral Health

School behavioral health services are generally provided by licensed clinical social workers or psychologists at on-post schools, with some programs reaching out to off-post schools as well. This program delivers behavioral health care in the child's school environment, improving outcomes by improving access to care, decreasing school disruption, and decreasing the burden on families to find services. In addition, most programs also include consultation to school staff when it comes to school milieu problems (ie, bullying), classroom dynamics problems, or concerns regarding individual students. With parental permission, the school-based providers assess a child individually and in the school setting. This assessment, along with the input and collaboration of school staff, can be invaluable in identifying and supporting depressed students.

Government, Nongovernment, and Partner Organizations

There are many government, nonprofit, and other partner organizations that donate their time and efforts to supporting military families. Other programs that are affiliated with the military that provide resources include Army Community Services, The FOCUS (Families Overcoming Under Stress) Project, Military One Source, and the

Military and Family Life Counseling (MFLC) Program. Each program serves a unique role in supporting military children and their families and can provide resources, counseling, education, and support to families in transition or during times of struggle.

One interesting example is the Sesame Workshop's Military Families Initiatives, which partnered with the military's Psychological Health Center of Excellence and PBS to create original content in support of the children of military families. Another successful initiative is through the program Give an Hour. This nonprofit organization has created a national network of mental health care providers who give an hour of their time each week to help members of the military and their families cope with the "unseen wounds" associated with military service. With more than 5000 members and growing, these caring professionals can provide tens of millions of dollars in free mental health services each year. One additional example is the Military Family Association, which supports health care access for military children and sponsors therapeutic and recreational camps and outings, family retreats, and educational support for military children. Another noteworthy program, the Zero to Three Program, supports the health and development of infants, toddlers, and their families.

SUMMARY

Military families experience unique cultural contexts that contribute as stressors and challenges for depressed military children and youth. This article provides a brief overview of the history of military family care, an understanding of ongoing efforts to provide effective and timely care for these children, and an understanding of the unique stressors and challenges that the depressed military child faces. Military life is hard on families; isolation from support, separation due to military demands on the service member, frequent moves and school changes, deployments, parental danger and injury, as well as living in foreign countries are just some of the challenges that can cause a depressed military child to struggle even more than one might already expect due to their diagnosis. In addition, one must be mindful of the cultural expectations of a military member and family, the strain that military life can have on a marriage, and the possible disruption of benefits when leaving the military. In response to these stressors and challenges, the DoD is dedicated to providing robust services for the unique needs of military children and their families. If the treating child and adolescent psychiatrist is able to identify and use programs such as FOCUS, Military One Source, the MFLC program, and partnerships with nonmilitary organizations, then they can help bridge the gap between the needs of the depressed military child and basic community resources that may be inadequate or not specifically tailored to this unique population.

REFERENCES

1. Lester P, Flake E. How wartime military service affects children and families. Future Child 2013;23(2):121–44.
2. Lagrone DM. The military family syndrome. Am J Psychiatry 1978;135(9):1040–3.
3. Rosen LN. Children's reactions to the desert storm deployment: initial findings from a survey of Army families. Mil Med 1993;158:465–9.
4. Jensen PD. Children's response to parental separation during Operations Desert Storm. J Am Acad Child Adolesc Psychiatry 1996;35:433–41.
5. Meadows SO, Tanielian T, Karney B, et al. The deployment life study. Longitudinal analysis of military families across the deployment cycle. Rand Health Q 2017; 6(2):7.

6. Mansfield AJ, Kaufman JS, Engel CC, et al. Deployment and mental health diagnoses among children of US Army personnel. Arch Pediatr Adolesc Med 2011; 165(11):999–1005.

7. Fairbank JA, Briggs EC, Lee RC, et al. Mental health of children of deployed and nondeployed military service members: the Millennium Cohort Family Study. J Dev Behav Pediatr 2018;39(9):683–92.

8. Sullivan K, Capp G, Gilreath TD, et al. Substance abuse and other adverse outcomes for military-connected youth in California: results from a large-scale normative population survey. JAMA Pediatr 2015;169(10):922–8.

9. Cederbaum JA, Gilreath TD, Benbenishty R, et al. Well-being and suicidal ideation of secondary school students from military families. J Adolesc Health 2014; 54(6):672–7.

10. Chandra A, Lara-Cinisomo S, Jaycox LH, et al. Children on the homefront: the experience of children from military families. Pediatrics 2010;125(1):16–25.

11. Chartrand M, Frank DA, White LF, et al. Effect of parent's wartime deployment on the behavior of young children in military families. Arch Pediatr Adolesc Med 2008;162(11):1009–14.

12. Millegan J, Engel C, Liu X, et al. Parental Iraq/Afghanistan deployment and child psychiatric hospitalization in the US military. Gen Hosp Psychiatry 2013;35(5): 556–60.

13. Committee on the Assessment of the Readjustment Needs of Military Personnel, Veterans, and Their Families; board on the Health of Select Populations, Institute of Medicine. Returning home from Iraq and Afghanistan: assessment of readjustment needs of veterans, service members, and their families. Washington (DC): National Academies Press (US); 2013.

14. Palmer CA. Theory of risk and resilience factors in military families. Mil Psychol 2008;20(3):213–30.

15. Johnson NH, Vidal C, Lilly FRW. Absence of a link between childhood parental military service on depression and anxiety disorders among children. Mil Med 2018;183(9/10):e502–8.

16. Esposito-Smythers C. Military youth and the deployment cycle: emotional health consequences and recommendations for interventions. J Fam Psychol 2011; 25(4):497–507.

17. Easterbrooks MA, Ginsberg K, Lerner RM. Resilience among military youth. Future Child 2013;23(2):9–120.

18. Pincus SH, et al. The emotional cycle of deployment: a military family perspective. US Army Medical Department Journal 2001;139–45.

19. Lemmon KL, Chartrand MM. Caring for America's children: military youth in a time of war. Pediatr Rev 2009;30:e42–8.

20. Riviere LA, Merrill JC, Thomas JL, et al. 2003-2009 marital functioning trends among U.S. enlisted soldiers following combat deployments. Mil Med 2012; 177(10):1169–77.

21. Gewirtz AH, Erbes CR, Polusny MA, et al. Helping military families through the deployment process: strategies to support parenting. Prof Psychol Res Pr 2011;42(1):56–62.

22. Cozza SJ, Lerner RM, editors. Military children and families, the future of children, (monograph). Princeton (NJ): Princeton-Brookings; 2013.

23. Cozza SJ, Fisher JE, Zhou J, et al. Bereaved military dependent spouses and children: those left behind in a decade of war (2001-2011). Mil Med 2017;182: e1684–90.

24. Cozza SJ, Cohen JA, Dougherty JG. Disaster and trauma. Child Adolesc Psychiatr Clin N Am 2014;23(2):xiii–xvi.
25. Holmes AK, Rauch PK, Cozza SJ. When a parent is injured or killed in combat. Future Child 2013;23(2):143–62.
26. Van Ost SL, Leskin GA, Doud TD, et al. Children and families of ill and injured service members and veterans. In: Care of military service members, veterans, and their families. Washington, DC: American Psychiatric Press; 2014.
27. Owens BD, Kragh JF Jr, Wenke JC, et al. Combat wounds in operation Iraqi freedom and operation enduring freedom. J Trauma 2008;64:295–9.
28. Hisle-Gorman E, Harrington D, Nylund CM, et al. Impact of parents' wartime military deployment and injury on young children's safety and mental health. J Am Acad Child Adolesc Psychiatry 2015;54(4):294–301.
29. Pessar LF, Coad ML, Linn RT, et al. The effects of parental traumatic brain injury on the behaviour of parents and children. Brain Inj 1993;7:231–40.
30. Butera-Prinzi F, Perlesz A. Through children's eyes: children's experience of living with a parent with an acquired brain injury. Brain Inj 2004;18(1):83–101.
31. Charles N, Butera-Prinzi F, Perlesz A. Families living with acquired brain injury: a multiple family group experience. NeuroRehabilitation 2007;22:61–76.
32. Verhaeghe S, Defloor T, Grypdonck M. Stress and coping among families of patients with traumatic brain injury: a review of the literature. J Clin Nurs 2005;14: 1004–12.
33. Hoge CW, Auchterlonie JL, Milliken CS. Mental health problems, use of mental health services, and attrition from military service after returning from deployment to Iraq or Afghanistan. JAMA 2006;295:1023–32.
34. Tanielian TL, Jaycox L. Invisible wounds of war: psychological and cognitive injuries, their consequences, and services to assist recovery, vol. 720. Santa Monica (CA): Rand Corporation; 2008.
35. Galovski T, Lyons JA. Psychological sequelae of combat violence: a review of the impact of PTSD on the veteran's family and possible interventions. Aggress Violent Behav 2004;9:477–501.
36. Rosenheck R, Nathan P. Secondary traumatization in children of Vietnam veterans. Hosp Community Psychiatry 1985;36:538–9.
37. Currier JM, Holland JM, Neimeyer RA. The effectiveness of bereavement interventions with children: a meta-analytic review of controlled outcome research. J Clin Child Adolesc Psychol 2007;36:253–9.
38. Finkelstein H. The long-term effects of early parent death: a review. J Clin Psychol 1988;44:3–9.
39. Reinherz HZ, Giaconia RM, Hauf AM, et al. General and specific childhood risk factors for depression and drug disorders by early adulthood. J Am Acad Child Adolesc Psychiatry 2000;39:223–31.

Youth Depression in School Settings

Assessment, Interventions, and Prevention

Shashank V. Joshi, MD[a,b,]*, Nadia Jassim, BS, MFA[a], Nithya Mani, MD[b]

KEYWORDS

- Depression in schools • School-based mental health • Suicide prevention
- Well-being promotion • Depression prevention in schools

KEY POINTS

- School settings are where youth spend a significant amount of their waking hours and are ideal places for intervening when a depressive disorder is present.
- Depressive disorders have a high incidence in the school population. This can affect learning, social interactions, and classroom engagement.
- Educators can be the eyes and ears and serve as expert consultants for the clinician, who can in turn be the expert consultant to help educators engage effectively with all students, especially those affected by depression.
- Depressive symptoms usually manifest across home, social, and educational settings, and the range of interventions is often much broader in schools, where staff and school clinicians can help to implement instructional and behavioral strategies.
- Depression prevention programs and interventions that cultivate student and teacher well-being are part of emerging best practices in the school-based literature.

INTRODUCTION

For child and adolescent psychiatrists caring for youth with depressive disorders, educational settings are crucial environments to understand, and where possible, to actively engage.[1–4] Depressive disorders have a high incidence in the school population (about 27% of heterosexual youth and 63% of LGBT youth report feeling sad or hopeless for at least 2 weeks in a row in 2016).[5] This can affect learning, social interactions, and classroom engagement. Teachers and other school staff can be key

Disclosure Statement: The authors report no financial conflicts regarding the content in this article.
[a] School Mental Health Team, Division of Child and Adolescent Psychiatry, Lucile Packard Children's Hospital @ Stanford, Stanford University School of Medicine, 401 Quarry Road, Stanford, CA 94305-5719, USA; [b] Lucile Packard Children's Hospital @ Stanford, Stanford University School of Medicine, 401 Quarry Road, Stanford, CA 94305-5719, USA
* Corresponding author. 401 Quarry Road, Stanford, CA 94305-5719.
E-mail address: svjoshi@stanford.edu

partners to help both clinicians and parents comprehend the social, educational, and cultural context where depressive symptoms may be present. Several interventions have been developed to help affected youth gain better access to the school curriculum, despite their depressive symptoms. Furthermore, prevention programs that focus on mental health promotion have shown promise in improving subjective well-being among youth.[3,6] As clinicians strive to understand the ecological and contextual factors in a student's life, careful attention should be paid to the *supporting alliance* among parents, teachers, and clinicians,[3] such that members of each of these groups can be resources for one another to best support youth affected by all mood conditions.[4] The supporting alliance is a concept that is based on the therapeutic alliance in mental health and applies to relationships among trusted adults in a young person's life. As mainstreaming in public schools has become more common, teachers are engaging with an ever-diversifying set of students. Mainstreaming requires that partnerships with parents, therapists, and other important adult figures be enhanced. If these relationships are strong and communication is easy and regular, teacher attrition and burnout can be prevented.[2,3]

Affected students are entitled to several educational interventions through both formal (legal) and informal mechanisms. Unfortunately, youth with depressive disorders are at high risk for school problems, including poor attendance, underachievement, and dropping out. When in the midst of a depressive episode, these students can find it especially hard to pay attention, think clearly, solve problems, recall information, or engage in group learning activities, let alone follow classroom rules.[4,7]

Previous work[8] has highlighted how depressive disorders can cause at least 3 types of problems for youth in school settings: those caused by the core symptoms themselves (eg, difficulty concentrating), those caused by secondary factors (eg, peer issues), and those associated with the treatment itself (eg, medication side effects or missed school with attending appointments). Youth with any mood condition may struggle with learning issues, and educators should strive to be aware of the additional layers of impaired concentration, reduced motivation, and emotional upheavals that mood conditions can create.[4,8]

Table 1 lists common issues seen in the classroom due to core symptoms of mood disorders; **Table 2** lists secondary factors that can contribute to problems in the classroom, and **Table 3** lists problems associated with treatment.[4,8]

Several online, social media, and book resources are available for both adults and peers who care for these youth as well as for the affected youth themselves, and these are listed at the end of this article for further reference (**Box 1**).

ASSESSMENT IN SCHOOL SETTINGS
Assessment

Identifying children at risk and diagnosing depression in the school setting can present unique challenges. For school-aged children, irritability or loss of interest can be the first signs of a depressive disorder. For teens, sad mood, sleep issues, weight changes, and thinking problems may be the predominant presenting symptoms.[9,10] For those who might appear quieter or withdrawn, these symptoms do not typically lead to disruptive behavior, and so these students may be overlooked.[9] Furthermore, students may feel isolated or stigmatized, making it harder for them to ask for help.

Given the difficulty in identifying students who are struggling, routine screening can be an effective and helpful tool.[11] Although there may be concerns about the feasibility of screening every student, studies using school nurses show general acceptability of

Table 1	
Common problems caused by the core symptoms of a depressive disorder	
Mood changes	• Extremes in mood (sad, angry, anxious) can be especially difficult to manage in school and can severely disrupt the learning process and experience of affected youth
Loss of interest	• May result in a lack of engagement in school activities • Negative cycle may ensue: not completing work leads to lower grades, which can lead to lower self-worth, loss of motivation, and withdrawal/absenteeism—leading the student to fall behind and feel so overwhelmed they cannot take the first step toward reengagement
Fatigue	• Sadness or sleep difficulties during depressive episodes can lead to fatigue and decreased school engagement
Concentration difficulties	• Especially frustrating for youth who would otherwise excel academically • Inability to focus and think clearly may be due to their depression or to a medication side effect
Agitation or tuning out	• Can be associated with a constant feeling of having to move (pacing, tapping fingers or feet, restless legs) and be disruptive to peers; tuning out can make a student feel as if they are going "in slow motion"

Reprinted with permission from A Clinical Handbook for the Diagnosis and Treatment of Pediatric Onset Mood Disorders, (Copyright ©2019). American Psychiatric Association. All Rights Reserved.

this practice.[12,13] A key consideration before screening is ensuring an adequate referral system exists for those found to need further assessment. Many screening tests are available and have been shown effective; ease of use and availability will likely determine widespread utilization (**Table 4**).

Once a student has been identified as having symptoms of depression, assessment by a mental health professional is essential to more fully evaluate and appropriately refer or treat the student. Despite its wide use, unstructured diagnostic interviews

Table 2	
Problems caused by secondary factors	
Peer problems	• Among the most devastating and long lasting to youth in school settings • Associated with social isolation and withdrawal • As peer networks are ever-changing and sometimes fragile, turning down invitations for play dates or hanging out can result in no further invitations from a specific peer • Lost opportunities to play are also lost opportunities to learn and build social skills; affected students may fall further behind socially and be included less often by peer groups • Helping students to make social contacts with healthy and resilient peers with similar interests can help enhance mental health and build community
Other secondary problems	• Social isolation due to depressive disorders has downstream effects, for example, if a student spends the morning worrying about who to play with at recess, they will not be focused on the teacher's lessons • A student might act up just to avoid stressful times of day, for example, being sent to the office or detention may seem easier than facing one's social fears • School staff, parents, and clinicians need to be creative in efforts to understand problems like these in order to address them properly

Reprinted with permission from A Clinical Handbook for the Diagnosis and Treatment of Pediatric Onset Mood Disorders, (Copyright ©2019). American Psychiatric Association. All Rights Reserved.

Table 3 Problems caused by treatment	
Medication side effects	• Range from nuisances to significant challenges • Side effects may be embarrassing (eg, falling asleep due to sedative effects) or uncomfortable (feeling thirsty, having dry mouth, or being dizzy and nauseous) • Medication titrations can be associated with headaches or drowsiness, further interfering with schoolwork
Other problems associated with treatment	• Once-daily dosing is ideal, but not always possible • School-administered medications may present challenges (school nurse availability, stigma regarding the need to leave class for medicine, logistical challenges [must obtain an "extra medication bottle" for school]) • Missing school activities for therapy/other appointments can cause a student who is already struggling to have even more problems

Reprinted with permission from A Clinical Handbook for the Diagnosis and Treatment of Pediatric Onset Mood Disorders, (Copyright ©2019). American Psychiatric Association. All Rights Reserved.

do not always correlate to standardized interviews.[21] Therefore, the gold standard for postscreening assessment would be a semistructured interview in conjunction with a broadband scale and caregiver interviews.[19] Although time intensive, this is the ideal way to elicit information about the student's symptoms, psychosocial environment, and subjective history. Trauma-informed assessments will ensure that posttraumatic stress disorder symptoms masking as depression will not be missed.[22]

Table 4
Screening instruments useful for assessing youth depression symptoms

Instrument	Description	Advantages
Quick Inventory of Depressive Symptoms self-report (QIDS-SR)	16-item scale; self-report	Suitable for use in adolescents; reliable in identifying symptoms of depression[14]
Patient Health Questionnaire (PHQ-9M)	9-item scale; self-report modified for adolescents	Good validity as a screener over the QIDS but may not have the same level or validity in tracking depressive symptoms[15]
Patient Health Questionnaire (PHQ-2)	2-item scale adapted from PHQ-9	Brief. Has sensitivity of 96% and specificity of 82% for detecting those who meet criteria for probable depression on PHQ-9[16]
Center for Epidemiologic Studies–Depression	20-item scale self-report	Widely used, suitable for adolescents; high internal consistency.[17] However, not as effective in studying well-being[18]
(Beck Depression Inventory for Youth)	20-item scale rating scale	High internal consistency; validity and reliability have been established for depression[19]
Kessler-10 and Kessler-6	10-item scale of psychological distress with a 6-item scale embedded	Good precision for assessing psychological distress; can differentiate anxiety from depression[20]

Classroom Interventions

Classroom interventions by mental health professionals are not done individually, but rather should incorporate the school staff and use an already fostered relationship. As consultants, mental health professionals should follow the 3R's of school consultation as outlined by Bostic and Rauch.[23] First, one must pay close attention to the relationships that need to be built. For consultation to be effective, a trusting partnership must be fostered between the larger social system in a student's life, including parents, therapists, and school staff.[3] Second, recognition of the human motivation, specifically the motives and concerns that may hinder promotion of depression awareness in schools, is imperative. In order to make an intervention, it is important for a mental health provider to use their understanding of staff motivation to collaborate and align with multiple professionals who have different but potentially overlapping goals.[24] Last, a consultant should support the staff in generating responses to difficult events or situations. Providing staff with new skills to support and teach affected students, finding common goals to unite students, parents, and staff, and helping to identify a path to achieve these goals are necessary to empower those within the school to feel comfortable with these interventions.[4] In addition, mental health professionals can be an important resource in helping parents advocate for their child to get the school accommodations they need through an appropriate individualized education plan (IEP), 504 Plan, or other classroom interventions. In order to develop this relationship, it is essential to spend individual time with the parents as part of the consultation to address any concerns they may have.[4]

Table 5 highlights the educational implications and classroom strategies for students who struggle with Depressive Disorders.

Table 5	
Educational manifestations of depressive disorders and classroom strategies	
Educational Manifestations	Instructional Strategies and Classroom Accommodations
Fluctuations in mood, energy, and motivation that may be seasonal or cyclical	During times of low mood, energy, and motivation, reduce academic workload and demands; adjust accordingly when mood, energy, and motivation increase
Difficulty concentrating or completing assignments	Provide students with books on tape or recorded instructions when concentration is low
Difficulty understanding complex instructions; challenges reading long written passages of text	Break assignments into smaller sections and monitor student progress, checking comprehension periodically
Difficulty with prompt arrival and "readiness to learn" in the early morning due to difficulty sleeping	Accommodate late arrivals by arranging for separate workspace if needed; ensure that IEP or 504 Plan accounts for this, especially relevant during medication changes
Easily frustrated and prone to sadness, embarrassment, or anger	Identify a place where student can go for privacy until they can regain control
Difficulty with social skills, boundaries, and peer relationships	Seat student next to peers whom the student feels would be helpful to their classroom functioning, with changes made as needed

(continued on next page)

Table 5 (continued)	
Fluctuations in cognitive and physical abilities and presence of side effects, especially with medication changes	Adjust the homework and in-class work to prevent overload; adjust for need for frequent hydration and bathroom breaks
Impaired planning, organizing, and abstract reasoning	Provide skills training with occupational therapist, school psychologist, or learning specialist to improve these
Prone to heightened sensitivity to perceived criticism and may react emotionally over seemingly small things	Create a plan for self-calming strategies (journaling, listening to music, drawing, walking out of class/running classroom errands at designated intervals)
May experience high levels of anxiety that interfere with their ability to logically assess a situation; difficulty or shame/self-doubt in communicating educational needs	Have a "lead school staff" whom the student knows and trusts the most: a guidance counselor, administrator, teacher, or other staff member who could be honest with the student to assist during times of high distress and be the single point of communication
Marked decreases in interest in school work and activities; especially problematic for group assignments	Group student with peers whom the student feels is helpful to their classroom functioning, with changes made as needed
Fluctuations in cognitive and physical abilities and presence of side effects, especially with medication changes	Adjust the homework and in-class load to prevent the student from becoming overwhelmed; adjust for need for frequent hydration and bathroom breaks
Grades may drop significantly due to lack of interest, loss of motivation, or excessive absences	Adjust expectations accordingly and meet with student, parent, and guidance counselor regularly to review progress; be flexible and realistic about educational goals (school failures and unmet expectations can exacerbate depressive symptoms)
Prone to "all-or-none" thinking (all bad or all good)	Keep a record of accomplishments to show to student at low points

Data from Refs.[5,25,26]

TREATMENT IN SCHOOL SETTINGS

A systematic review of depression prevention and treatment programs[27] found support for prevention and early intervention programs in schools, most of which are based on cognitive behavioral therapy (CBT). Indicated approaches appear to produce the strongest results, with universal and selective trials also having positive effects. An example of a time-limited individual treatment with strong evidence for use in school populations is interpersonal therapy, adapted for adolescents (IPT-A).[28] In a study that spanned 5 school health clinics in New York City, adolescents treated with IPT-A showed greater symptom reduction and improvement in overall functioning compared with treatment as usual. The core components of IPT-A include 3 phases of treatment delivered over 12 weeks. The adapted-for-teens version differs from adult IPT in that it is shorter (12 weeks vs 16–20 weeks), adds a parent component, and focuses less on the sick role. The treatment manual is clear and concise, and focuses on current interpersonal issues that are most important to adolescents, including grief, interpersonal disputes, role transitions, and interpersonal deficits.

PREVENTION STRATEGIES

Several programs have shown promise as preventative in the development of depression.

Examples of school-based depression prevention programs have been summarized nicely in a review by Calear.[9] The investigator suggests important factors to be considered before implementing a depression prevention program in schools, such as consideration of target audience (universal prevention directed to all students; indicated prevention directed to students with elevated symptoms of depression, or selected prevention directed only at students identified as being at high-risk of developing depression); program scheduling, support and protocols for referrals, and the assurance of full buy-in from school administrative leaders. Specific programs that are aimed at preventing depression and increasing mental health awareness are listed in **Table 6** and include the RAP-Kiwi, MoodGYM, Penn Resiliency Program, IPT-AST, Stress Inoculation Training, Brain Driver Education, and Positive Action programs. Other approaches with growing empirical support focus on mindfulness and resilience. Several scholarly reviews highlight how these programs can be implemented for children, adolescents, and young adults.[37–40]

An example of a best practices universal prevention classroom curriculum is Break Free From Depression (BFFD).[41] The goal of BFFD is to raise student awareness and knowledge about depression and to highlight risk factors working against help-seeking behaviors for the students themselves or others. The material consists of a PowerPoint lecture with interactive student components, a documentary film, and a group-guided facilitation activity regarding depression in youth. The BFFD curriculum includes a detailed facilitator's guide and supplementary materials. There is also a group discussion about stigma and other barriers against getting help, how the teens in the film negotiated and overcame these barriers, and what finally worked for them. Students are encouraged to seek help for themselves or their peers through a discreet and simple form that is given in each session.[42]

Other examples of depression awareness and suicide prevention curricula for high schools include More Than Sad: Teen Depression, More Than Sad: Preventing Teen Suicide (American Foundation for Suicide Prevention, 2010), and Linking Education and Awareness of Depression and Suicide (Suicide Awareness Voices of Education, 2008).

These interventions collectively highlight how clinicians can be helpful not only for diagnosing and treating depressive disorders in the school setting but also for serving as partners or implementers of best practice curricula to promote mental health, well-being, and education about the signs and symptoms of mood conditions to mitigate risk from developing serious depressive disorders. Prior research[42] has led to recommendations against 1-and-done presentations or assemblies that focus on depression or suicide prevention, because they may not be effective in changing knowledge over the long term or help-seeking behavior. Moreover, students (and school staff or parents) ought to have opportunities for questions, reflection, follow-up and support as needed. Thus, all of the curricula described in this section should be delivered over multiple sessions and monitored for effect.

An example of an evidence-supported program to enhance teacher self-efficacy in engaging with high-risk students is the Kognito: At Risk for Educators Program. It features interactive role-play simulations that build awareness, knowledge, and skills about mental health and suicide prevention, preparing educators in K12 settings to recognize and intervene with students in psychological distress, and, if needed, connect them with support services.[43] Because teachers are the most present adults directing the learning environment, it is important to engage with them early and often

Table 6
Examples of evidence-supported depression prevention and mental health awareness programs developed for schools

RAP-Kiwi[29]	Eleven-session manual-based program derived from cognitive-behavioral therapy, delivered by teachers; ages 13–15; depression scores were reduced significantly more by RAP-Kiwi than by placebo and were effective across cultural subgroups, at follow-up, postgroup, and 18 mo
MoodGYM[30]	Interactive, Web-based intervention designed to prevent and decrease depression symptoms; presented by classroom teacher for 1 h weekly over 5 wk, based on CBT; contains information, animated demonstrations, quizzes, and homework exercises; ages 13–17
Penn Resiliency Program[31]	Twelve-session group intervention for students aged 10–14; teaches CBT and problem-solving skills; widely researched and supported by 8 RCTs showing significantly positive results; among the most broadly researched depression prevention programs. Ten school-based trials for ages 10–14 y have been conducted since 2001. Significant effects found in 8 of the trials after follow-up. Delivery by teachers, mental health professionals, and graduate students[24]
Interpersonal Therapy, Adolescent Skills Training (IPT-AST)[32]	Based on IPT; goal is to prevent depression by teaching social and communication skills necessary to develop and maintain positive relationships; 2 individual and 8 group sessions for students 11–16 y old; significant positive results reported at 3- and 6-mo follow-ups in the areas of handling interpersonal role disputes, navigating role transitions, and addressing interpersonal deficits
Stress Inoculation Training[33]	Based on CBT; provides individual and group therapy for 15–18 y olds; 9–13 sessions delivered weekly with a 3-phase stress inoculation model: Conceptualization phase, skill acquisition phase, skill application phase; techniques taught include cognitive restructuring, problem solving, and relaxation. At least 2 universal school-based trials have found significant results
Brain Drivers Education[34,35] (https://www.massgeneral. org/psychiatry/assets/pdfs/ school-psych/Brain-Drivers-Education-Operators-Guide.pdf)	Based on CBT; developed by a child and adolescent psychiatrist at the Massachusetts General Hospital School Psychiatry Program at Harvard Program and an educator in the Boston schools; evidence-informed curriculum on emotional self-regulation; uses elements of CBT, DBT, and other widely accepted approaches for achieving well-being and healthy interpersonal relationships. Pilot study showed significant positive results regarding emotion regulation and conflict resolution; most students found the curriculum useful for their everyday lives
Positive Action[36]	An evidence-based educational program that promotes intrinsic learning and cooperation among peers; links positive actions to positive self-perception; adapted for various grade levels; shown to increase academic achievement and reduce problem behaviors. Intervention topics address mental health, physical health, behavior, family, academics, and substance use; designed for teachers to run in as little as 15 min per school day

Abbreviations: CBT, cognitive behavioral therapy; DBT, dialectical behavioral therapy; RCT, randomized controlled trials.

Modified from Calear AL. Depression in the classroom: considerations and strategies. Child Adolesc Psychiatr Clin N Am 2012;21(1):138; with permission.

in order to build a healthy and long-lasting supporting alliance. When children are younger, it may be quite easy for parents/guardians to engage with school staff through volunteering or chaperoning a school field trip, for example. It gets harder to stay engaged as a parent, as youth progress through middle and high school. Parent strategies for engaging with school staff can be found at https://community.understood.org/school-services/f/working-with-teachers.

THE SOCIOCULTURAL MILIEU OF TREATMENTS IN THE SCHOOL SETTING

In schools, culture influences important areas that are central to mental health, such as behavioral expectations and tolerance, language, emotion, attention, attachment, traumatic experiences, conduct, personality, motivation, limit setting, and other aspects of teaching in general. Cultural context plays an important role not only in structuring the school environment in which youth with emotional and behavioral disorders function but also in the way such children and teens are understood and treated.[44,45]

Teachers play a crucial role in promoting the overall health and academic engagement of their students, in addition to their social and emotional learning and development.

As McCullough and Quinlan[46] have highlighted:

Without a more direct focus on teacher well-being, the proposed strategies for promoting youth happiness may be futile, especially if the adults with whom they interact with most during the school day feel emotionally exhausted and overworked. Accordingly, Hills and Robinson[47] emphasized that "teachers need to be the first to put on their oxygen masks prior to supporting their students' social and emotional wellness" (p. 104).[6]

As parents engage with schools to advocate for accommodations for their children with mood conditions, it is important to know what their rights and resources are. In the United States, the main laws of relevance are the Individuals with Disabilities Education and Improvement IDEA, and section 504 of the Rehabilitation Act of 1973. A useful site that summarizes relevant information is https://www.understood.org/en/school-learning/special-services/504-plan/the-difference-between-ieps-and-504-plans.

FROM PREVENTION TO STATE POLICY AND A NEW LAW

In 2016, California became one of the first states to require that all public school districts serving students in grades 7 to 12 develop a suicide prevention board policy and administrative regulations. A model suicide prevention policy has been developed by the California Department of Education,[48] and a K12 Toolkit for Mental Health Promotion and Suicide Prevention[49] lists evidence-supported suicide prevention programs and social-emotional learning strategies that can begin even earlier than middle school, such as the Good Behavior Game (GBG), Promoting Alternative Thinking Strategies (PATHS),[50] and others that are especially suited for middle and older teens (Sources of Strength).[51] GBG is a classroom game where elementary school children are rewarded for displaying appropriate on-task behaviors during instructional times. It has shown long-term benefits in multiple social and emotional domains by strengthening inhibition, extending self-regulation, and improving social emotional scaffolding, in addition to being associated with significantly decreased suicide risk in later school years by those who participated in this game while in elementary school.[52] PATHS has shown effectiveness in enhancing the educational process and promoting social and emotional competencies in elementary school youth, while also reducing aggression and behavior problems.[4]

Sources of Strength is a universal suicide prevention program that builds protective influences and reduces the likelihood that vulnerable youth will become suicidal. It trains students as peer leaders and connects them with adult advisors at school and in the community. These trusted adults support the peer leaders in conducting well-defined messaging activities that aim to change peer group norms that influence coping practices and problem behaviors (eg, self-harm, drug use, unhealthy sexual practices). The program has benefits for both suicide prevention and well-being promotion. In an 18-school randomized controlled trial (RCT), Wyman and colleagues[51] demonstrated that the program led to changes in norms across the full population of high school students after 4 months of school-wide messaging.

SUMMARY

In this article, evidence-supported programs and approaches that to address depression in schools are highlighted. The process of school stakeholder buy-in and the cultivation of a supporting alliance among school staff, clinician, and parent are essential. A review of assessment tools, intervention strategies, and prevention programs is complemented by approaches that focus on well-being promotion. Virtual role-play software can assist teachers in implementing practical tools for responding to students in need, developing classroom management strategies for those in crisis, and referring them to resources. Programs such as the GBG in elementary schools and Sources of Strength in secondary schools can be used as school-wide positive behavior and suicide prevention programs and may also have important downstream prevention benefits in reducing adolescent risk-taking behaviors more broadly.[4] Finally, the importance of positive student-teacher relationships is emphasized in order to promote healthy school functioning and both student and teacher well-being.[46,47,49]

Box 1
Resources: useful school mental health web sites

1. Promising Practices Network on Children, Families, and Communities (http://www.promisingpractices.net/programs.asp); features summaries of programs and practices that have shown positive outcomes for children

2. Suicide Prevention Resource Center: Best Practices Registry for Suicide Prevention (http://www.sprc.org/featured_resources/bpr/index.asp)

3. National Center for School Mental Health (http://csmh.umaryland.edu): Up-to-date information about national school mental health training, practice, research, and policy

4. Center for Mental Health in Schools and Student/Learning Supports at University of California, Los Angeles (http://smhp.psych.ucla.edu): Clearinghouse of important mental health, school, and educational materials

5. Individuals With Disabilities Education Act (IDEA) Partnership (http://www.ideapartnership.org): Up-to-date information on changes in the IDEA parameters.

6. HEARD Alliance (Health Care Alliance for Response to Adolescent Depression; https://www.heardalliance.org): A collaborative Web site that features resources for suicide prevention and mental health promotion; features a best practice K-12 Toolkit for Mental Health Promotion and Suicide Prevention

7. National Child Traumatic Stress Network (http://www.nctsn.org): Contains very useful resources for educators to teach students with trauma, loss, and anxiety; also has useful tips for speaking with parents, children, and the media about the consequences of human-caused and natural disasters and resources for preventing burnout in educators

Data from Ref.[53]

REFERENCES

1. Results from the 2016 national survey on drug use and health (NSDUH). Available at: https://www.nimh.nih.gov/health/statistics/major-depression.shtml. Accessed February 11, 2019.
2. Suldo SM. Promoting student happiness: positive psychology interventions in schools. New York: Guilford Press; 2016.
3. Feinstein NF, Fielding K, Udvari-Solner A, et al. The supporting alliance in child and adolescent treatment: enhancing collaboration between therapists, parents and teachers. Am J Psychother 2009;63(4):319–44.
4. Joshi SV, Jassim N. School-based interventions for mood disorders. In: Singh MK, editor. A clinical handbook for the diagnosis and treatment of pediatric onset mood disorders. Washington, DC: Amer Psychiatric Press, Inc; 2019.
5. Centers for Disease Control and Prevention. Youth risk behavior survey 2017. Available at: https://www.cdc.gov/healthyyouth/data/yrbs/index.htm. Accessed February 11, 2019.
6. Rettew D, Satz I, Joshi SV. Teaching well-being: from kindergarten to child psychiatry training programs. Child Adolesc Psychiatr Clin N Am 2019;28(2):267–80.
7. Evans DW, Andrews LW. If your adolescent has depression or bipolar disorder- an essential resource for parents. New York: Oxford Univ Press; 2005. p. 198.
8. Fristad M, Goldberg Arnold JS. Raising a moody child: how to cope with depression and bipolar disorder. New York: Guilford Press; 2004. p. 260.
9. Calear AL. Depression in the classroom: considerations and strategies. Child Adolesc Psychiatr Clin N Am 2012;21:135–44.
10. Lewinsohn PM, Rohde P, Seeley JR. Treatment of adolescent depression: frequency of services and impact on functioning in young adulthood. Depress Anxiety 1998;7:47–52.
11. Williams SB, O'Connor EA, Eder M, et al. Screening for child and adolescent depression in primary care settings: a systematic evidence review for the US preventive services task force. Pediatrics 2009;123:e716–35.
12. Carnevale T. An integrative review of adolescent depression screening instruments: applicability for use by school nurses. J Child Adolesc Psychiatr Nurs 2011;24:51–7.
13. Allison VL, Nativio DG, Mitchell AM, et al. Identifying symptoms of depression and anxiety in students in the school setting. J Sch Nurs 2014;30(3):165–72.
14. Bernstein IH, Rush AJ, Trivedi MH, et al. Psychometric properties of the quick inventory of depressive symptomatology in adolescents. Int J Methods Psychiatr Res 2010;19(4):185–94.
15. Nandakumar AL, Vande Voort JL, Nakonezny PA, et al. Psychometric properties of the patient health questionnaire-9 modified for major depressive disorder in adolescents. J Child Adolesc Psychopharmacol 2019;29(1):34–40.
16. Richardson LP, Rockhill C, Russo JE, et al. Evaluation of the PHQ-2 as a brief screen for detecting major depression among adolescents. Pediatrics 2010;125:e1097–103.
17. Radloff LS. The use of the center for epidemiologic studies depression scale in adolescents and young adults. J Youth Adolesc 1991;20:149–66.
18. Siddawaya AP, Wood AM, Taylorb PJ. The Center for Epidemiologic Studies-Depression (CES-D) scale measures a continuum from well-being to depression:

testing two key predictions of positive clinical psychology. J Affect Disord 2017; 213:180–6.

19. D'Angelo EJ, Augenstein T. Developmentally informed evaluation of depression: evidence-based instruments. Child Adolesc Psychiatr Clin N Am 2012;21: 279–98.

20. Kessler RC, Andrews G, Colpe LJ, et al. Short screening scales to monitor population prevalences and trends in non-specific psychological distress. Psychol Med 2002;32:959–76.

21. Jensen-Doss A. Practice involves more than treatment: how can evidence-based assessment catch up to evidence-based treatment? Clin Psychol Sci Pract 2011; 18:173–7.

22. Craig SE. Reaching and teaching children who hurt. Baltimore (MD): Brookes; 2008.

23. Bostic JQ, Rauch PK. The 3 R's of school consultation. J Am Acad Child Adolesc Psychiatry 1999;38(3):339–41.

24. Waxman RP, Weist MD, Benson DM. Toward collaboration in the growing education–mental health interface. Clin Psychol Rev 1999;19(2): 239–53.

25. Chokroverty L. 100 questions and answers about your child's depression or bipolar disorder. Sudbury (MA): Jones and Bartlett; 2010. p. 203.

26. California Department of Education. Placer Co. Office of education and Minnesota association for children's health: a guide to student mental health and wellness in California. St. Paul (MN): Minnesota Association for Children's Health; 2014.

27. Calear AL, Christensen H. Systematic review of school-based prevention and early intervention programs for depression. J Adolesc 2010;33:429–38.

28. Mufson LH, Dorta KP, Olfson M, et al. Effectiveness research: transporting interpersonal psychotherapy for depressed adolescents (IPT-A) from the lab to school-based health clinics. Clin Child Fam Psychol Rev 2004;7(4): 251–61.

29. Merry S, McDowell H, Wild CJ, et al. A randomized placebo-controlled trial of a school-based depression prevention program. J Am Acad Child Adolesc Psychiatry 2004;43(5):538–47.

30. Twomey C, O'Reilly G. Effectiveness of a freely available computerized cognitive behavioural therapy programme (MoodGYM) for depression: meta-analysis. Aust N Z J Psychiatry 2016. Available at: https://moodgym.com.au/info/about. Accessed February 11, 2018.

31. Gillham JE, Reivich KJ, Freres DR, et al. School-based prevention of depressive symptoms: a randomized controlled study of the effectiveness and specificity of the Penn Resiliency Program. J Consult Clin Psychol 2007;75: 9–19.

32. Young JF, Mufson L, Davies M. Efficacy of interpersonal psychotherapy-adolescent skills training: an indicated preventive intervention for depression. J Child Psychol Psychiatry 2006;47(12):1254–62.

33. Hains AA, Ellmann SW. Stress inoculation training as a preventative intervention for high school youths. J Cogn Psychother 1994;8(3):219–28, 230–232.

34. Khan CK, Patterson AD, Joshi SV. Brain driver education: teaching kids emotion regulation skills through an innovative and integrative curriculum; presented at annual meeting of the Amer Acad of Child Adolesc Psychiatry. San Diego, October 20–25, 2014.

35. Blumenfeld K, Bostic JQ, Potter MP, et al. Massachusetts General Hospital. Brain Drivers Education. 2005. Available at: https://www.massgeneral.org/psychiatry/assets/pdfs/school-psych/Brain-Drivers-Education-Operators-Guide.pdf.   Accessed February 11, 2019.

36. Lewis KM, DuBois DL, Bavarian N, et al. Effects of positive action on the emotional health of urban youth: a cluster-randomized trial. J Adolesc Health 2013;53:706–11. Available at: https://www.positiveaction.net/research-outcomes. Accessed February 11, 2019.

37. Chi X, Bo A, Liu T, et al. Effects of mindfulness-based stress reduction on depression in adolescents and young adults: a systematic review and meta-analysis. Front Psychol 2018;9:1034.

38. Dray J, Bowman J, Wolfenden L, et al. Systematic review of universal resilience interventions targeting child and adolescent mental health in the school setting. Syst Rev 2015;4:186.

39. Zoogman S, Goldberg SB, Hoyt WT, et al. Mindfulness interventions with youth: a meta-analysis. Mindfulness (N Y) 2015;6:290–302.

40. Dunning DL, Griffiths K, Kuyken W, et al. The effects of mindfulness-based interventions on cognition and mental health in children and adolescents: a meta-analysis of randomised controlled trials. J Child Psychol Psychiatry 2019;60(3):244–58.

41. Boston Children's Hospital neighborhood partnerships program: break free from depression curriculum, revised. 2017. Available at: https://www.openpediatrics.org/course/break-free-depression. Accessed February 11, 2019.

42. Joshi SV, Hartley SN, Kessler M, et al. School-based suicide prevention: content, process, and the role of trusted adults and peers. Child Adolesc Psychiatr Clin N Am 2015;24(2):353–70.

43. Long MW, Albright G, McMillan J, et al. Enhancing educator engagement in school mental healthcare through digital simulation professional development. J Sch Health 2018;88:651–9.

44. Malik M, Lake J, Lawson W, et al. Culturally adapted pharmacotherapy and the integrative formulation. Child Adolesc Psychiatr Clin N Am 2010;19(4):791–814.

45. Lin K-M, Smith MW, Ortiz V. Culture and psychopharmacology. Psychiatr Clin North Am 2001;24(3):523–38.

46. McCullough M, Quinlan D. Universal strategies for promoting student happiness. In: Suldo SM, editor. Promoting student happiness: positive psychology interventions in schools. New York: Guilford Press; 2016. p. 103–21.

47. Hills KJ, Robinson A. Enhancing teacher well-being: put on your oxygen masks! Communique 2010;39:1–17.

48. California Department of Education. Model youth suicide prevention policy. 2017. Available at: https://www.cde.ca.gov/ls/cg/mh/suicideprevres.asp. Accessed September 22, 2018.

49. Joshi SV, Lenoir L, Ojakian M, et al. K-12 mental health promotion and suicide prevention Toolkit 2017. p. 300. Available at: http://www.heardalliance.org/help-toolkit/. Accessed February 11, 2019.

50. Promoting alternative thinking strategies (PATHS):information on classroom applications. Available at: http://www.pathstraining.com/main/curriculum/. Accessed July 2, 2018.

51. Wyman PA, Brown CH, LoMurray M, et al. An outcome evaluation of the Sources of Strength suicide prevention program delivered by adolescent peer leaders in high schools. Am J Public Health 2010;100(9):1653.

52. PAX Good Behavior Game: information on scientific basis. Available at: https://www.goodbehaviorgame.org/pax-science. Accessed July 2, 2018.
53. Bostic JQ, Hoover SA. School consultation. In: Martin A, Bloch MH, Volkmar F, editors. Lewis's child & adolescent psychiatry: a comprehensive textbook. 5th edition. Philadelphia: LWW; 2018. p. 956–74.

Transitional Age Youth and College Mental Health

Vivien Chan, MD[a,b,c,*], Jessica Moore, MD[d], Jennifer Derenne, MD[e],
D. Catherine Fuchs, MD[f]

KEYWORDS

- Depression • Major depressive disorder • Development • Adolescent • Psychiatry
- Transitional age youth • College • University

KEY POINTS

- A biopsychosocial formulation is key to treatment; improvements in identification and evidence-based treatment have allowed young adults with depression to succeed.
- Transitional age youth have unique developmental needs; neurobiologic development, including that of executive functioning, persists until age 25 years old.
- The transition to adulthood involves increasing independence, supported by coaching, in numerous domains, including self-management, health literacy, and advocacy.
- Transitional age youth are vulnerable to relapsing depression in the context of managing life stresses, including the process of separation and individuation, and identity formation.
- Substance use and sexual trauma are common; both increase risk for suicide, a tragic outcome that needs to be explicitly addressed with safety planning.

INTRODUCTION

The developmental epoch of late adolescence to early adulthood is a time of evolution. Young adults may change from a structured educational and home life to a more challenging environment, independent of adult oversight. Child and adolescent

Disclosure Statement: Dr V. Chan holds common stock in: Abbvie Inc, Abbot Labs, Bristol Myer Squibb, Eli Lilly, Johnson & Johnson, McKesson, and Omega Health Inc.
[a] Student Health Center, University of California Irvine, 501 East Peltason Drive, Irvine, CA 92697-5200, USA; [b] Department of Psychiatry and Human Behavior, UC Irvine Health, Orange, CA, USA; [c] Center for Resiliency, Wellness & Education, Children, Youth, Prevention and Intervention Behavioral Services, Orange County Healthcare Agency, Orange, CA, USA; [d] University of Texas Southwestern Medical Center, 5323 Harry Hines Boulevard, Dallas, TX 75390, USA; [e] Comprehensive Care Program, Division of Child and Adolescent Psychiatry, Lucille Packard Children's Hospital at Stanford, Stanford University, 401 Quarry Rd, Stanford, CA 94304, USA; [f] Division of Child and Adolescent Psychiatry, Vanderbilt University Medical Center, Vanderbilt Child and Adolescent Psychiatry, 1500 21st Avenue South, #2200, Nashville, TN 37212, USA
* Corresponding author. 501 East Peltason Drive, Irvine, CA 92697-5200.
E-mail address: vchan1@uci.edu

Child Adolesc Psychiatric Clin N Am 28 (2019) 363–375
https://doi.org/10.1016/j.chc.2019.02.008
1056-4993/19/© 2019 Elsevier Inc. All rights reserved.

psychiatrists can make a significant impact using developmental milestones to create care plans. Child and adolescent psychiatrists must consider strategies for prevention of depression occurrence or relapse while also identifying resources for treatment. We use an integrated case formulation model well-described by Henderson and Martin (**Tables 1** and **2**)[1] (ie, biopsychosocial and "Four Ps") to discuss the treatment of depression in this population. Most of this article focuses on major depressive disorder (MDD).

The diagnosis of MDD and its related conditions may seem straightforward, because many can memorize mnemonics that prompt the description of traditional neurovegetative symptoms that last for 14 serial days and cause functional impairments, with 2 months' duration of interceding recovery if possible. Clear differential diagnosis and comorbid anxiety should be considered through a longitudinal lens.[2]

Clinical diagnosis in this age group is complicated by individual developmental maturity, which is influenced by formative experiences, interpersonal connectedness, personal experience of autonomy, aptitude, impulse control and affective regulation, socioeconomic status, and a host of unique personal factors described by the "Four P's."[3] This age group is also vulnerable to the onset of MDD and suicidality (**Fig. 1**).[4–6] Clinicians are encouraged to incorporate these developmental factors into treatment planning.

YOUNG ADULTHOOD AS A DISTINCT DEVELOPMENTAL ENTITY: TRANSITIONAL AGE YOUTH

Singling out this population has its controversies, but child and adolescent psychiatrists are at the forefront of recognizing young adulthood as a unique stage.[7] Developmental assumptions about young adults are easily influenced by personal experience (eg, "I did that at that age") contributing to risk of implicit bias. Cultural factors may influence tolerance and permissiveness for social behaviors. Expectations are easily created regarding the subgroup of college students (eg, beliefs of higher functioning), contributing to missed opportunities for interventions. The term transitional age youth (TAY) originated from the Substance Abuse and Mental Health Services Administration (SAMHSA), because of early awareness of the lack of developmentally appropriate services and supports for youth exiting foster care by "aging out." Since 1995, SAMHSA grants have encouraged projects, drawing attention to services and

Table 1
Biopsychosocial model case formulation

Biologic	Psychological	Social
Family history	Emotional development	Family constellation
Genetics	Personality structure	Peer relationships
Physical development	Self-esteem	School
Constitution	Insight	Neighborhood
Intelligence	Defenses	Ethnic influences
Temperament	Patterns of behavior	Socioeconomic issues
Medical comorbidities	Patterns of cognition	Cultures
	Responses to stressors	Religions
	Coping strategies	

From Henderson SW, Martin A. Case formulation and integration of information in child and adolescent mental health. In: Rey JM, editor. IACAPAP e-Textbook of child and adolescent mental health. Geneva (Switzerland): International Association for Child and Adolescent Psychiatry and Allied Professions; 2014. p. 4; with permission.

Table 2
The "Four P's" and the biopsychosocial model intersection

The 'P' Characteristic and Trigger Question	Biologic	Psychological	Social
Predisposing *Why me?*	Genetic loading	Immature defensive structure	Poverty and adversity
Precipitating *Why now?*	Iatrogenic reaction	Recent loss	School stressors
Perpetuating *Why does it continue?*	Poor response to medication	No support at school	Unable to attend therapy sessions because of parents' work schedule
Protective *What can I rely on?*	Family history of treatment response	Insightful	Community and faith as sources of support

From Henderson SW, Martin A. Case Formulation and integration of information in child and adolescent mental health. In: Rey JM, editor. IACAPAP e-textbook of child and adolescent mental health. Geneva (Switzerland): International Association for Child and Adolescent Psychiatry and Allied Professions; 2014. p. 6; with permission.

systems of care, not just for foster care youth, but also to those aged 16 to 25 years old at risk of serious mental health conditions.[8] The term "emerging adult" was first published in 2000 by psychologist Arnett[9] to describe a discrete normal developmental phase for ages 18 to 25 years. The minimum age of maturity (18 vs 21 years) has been debated in the public health sector for use of potentially dependence-forming substances, such as alcohol, tobacco, and cannabis. Ethics writers have questioned adolescents' capacity "to appreciate the long-term consequences of their choices until the age of 21."[10] More recently, the upper age limit of adolescence itself has been

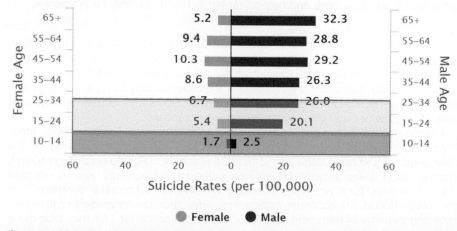

Suicide Rates for Males and Females by Age in the United States (2016)

Female Age	Female	Male	Male Age
65+	5.2	32.3	65+
55–64	9.4	28.8	55–64
45–54	10.3	29.2	45–54
35–44	8.6	26.3	35–44
25–34	6.7	26.0	25–34
15–24	5.4	20.1	15–24
10–14	1.7	2.5	10–14

Suicide Rates (per 100,000)

● Female   ● Male

Fig. 1. Suicide rates. (*Adapted from* the National Institute of Mental Health (NIMH). Mental Health Information. Available at: https://www.nimh.nih.gov/health/statistics/suicide.shtml. Accessed November 1, 2018; *Courtesy of* CDC.)

explored.[11,12] There is debate about current broad demographic divisions of 10 to 17 years and 18 to 65 years, and the quality of evidence (vs anecdote) to support the need for a separate developmental phase. Here, the authors use the terms TAY, emerging adult, late adolescence, and early adulthood as interchangeable and describe depression treatment considerations for the transition to adulthood.

Social Considerations

Culture, self, and identity

Predisposing dynamic relations among youth, family, and peers continue to evolve through adolescence. This leads to exploration about one's sense of self, with increasing awareness about having multiple identities and identifications. Peer relationships intensify and become more central, with the need to renegotiate familial relationships. Precipitating factors may include low preparation for the demands of independent living. Social scientists have expressed concern about college campus "coddling" from microaggressions and trigger warnings,[13] and developmental implications of social media on the "iGen[eration]."[14] Young adults who have depression may require more emotional, educational, and financial support from their families while striving for independence in these same areas.[15]

Studies of adverse childhood events (ACEs) indicate that ethnic and racial minority youth often have somatization, or anger as a presenting symptom of depression, instead of sadness.[16] Minority adolescents may also experience racism and prejudice that increase risk for MDD.[16] Risk factors of marginalization, discrimination, and isolation occur whenever diversity in minority and majority groups exist. Rodgers[17] validates that lesbian, gay, bisexual, transgender, and questioning late adolescents experience higher rates of bullying and victimization than heterosexual and cisgender peers, which directly relates to increased rates of depression and suicide; more than 40% seriously considered suicide overall and 29% considered suicide in the past 12 months. Issues of acculturation are significant when adolescents develop identities that diverge from their families of origin. Clinicians must explore their own personal biases and cultural beliefs whenever diversity of majority and minority issues arise. Rivas-Drake and Stein[18] remind us that identification with cultural assets, such as having a positive sense of ethnic-racial identity, and values, such as maintaining deference, bidirectional support, and respect for family members, may be protective.

Educational and vocational success

Pao[19] writes that the concept of a "successful" transition to adulthood is contextual, culturally dependent, but may have common themes. Pao[19] offers "because there is not one specific pathway to successful adulthood, and there will be tensions between personal, familial, and community ambitions, it is essential that TAY, parents or guardians, clinicians, educators, and policymakers recognize, clearly articulate and evaluate their vision together and clarify common goals of 'success.'"

A report in 1988 from the William T. Grant Foundation, "The Forgotten Half," identified clear divergences in economic, vocational, and marital success for the college-bound and noncollege bound 16 to 24 year olds.[20] For the noncollege bound, income was in "steep decline;" federal job training and support was used by less than 5% who qualified for it, and when offered, only lasted up to 4 months' duration.[20] For the college bound, the academic calendar provides structure for students with corresponding patterns of treatment utilization. Higher education for TAY may promote a sense of accomplishment but introduce perpetuating new stressors. Sood and Linker[21] describe that attending college full time may be somewhat protective toward suicidality (**Fig. 2**).

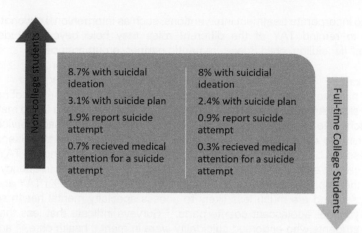

Fig. 2. Suicidality rates in noncollege students versus full-time college students in the last year. (*Data from* Sood AB, Linker J. Proximal influences on the trajectory of suicidal behaviors and suicide during the transition from adolescence to young adulthood. Child Adolesc Psychiatr Clin N Am 2017;26(2):235–51.)

A dramatic increase in college enrollment began in 1988.[22,23] However, many TAY complete baccalaureate credentials nearer to 6 years instead of the "expected" 4 years, extending time and financial consequences.[23] The updated reports posit that the new *Forgotten Half* are those who enroll in but do not complete college.[22] For this half, early adults who ultimately obtain technical/vocational certificates or associate's credentials have better outcomes financially than those who attain no credentials at all.[23] The "college for all" ideal, although well intentioned, contributes to the pressure for academic success. HalfofUs.com was founded on the premise that more than half of college students felt "so stressed" that they could not function.[24] A recent national college health survey (**Fig. 3**) shows the impact of depression in undergraduate students.[25] The distinctions between "stress," "depression," and duration of functional impairments should be clarified.

Students who have received Individual Education Plans or "504" accommodations in high school should be instructed to consider enrollment in the on-campus disability office and informed that accommodations in higher education require student-initiated requests.[25] Child and adolescent psychiatrists should discuss with students the absence of curricular modifications in higher education and the need to problem-solve options for support.[25] TAY in the workforce may need coaching on how to request needed workplace accommodations through the Americans with Disabilities Act.[26] Despite an early adult's focus on work or school success it is important for

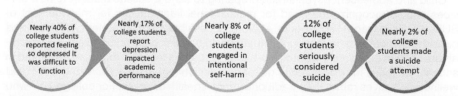

Fig. 3. American College Health Association-National College Health Association data. Fall 2017 reference group. (Data from Kisch J, Leino EV, Silverman MM. Aspects of suicidal behavior, depression, and treatment in college students: results from the Spring 2000 National College Health Assessment Survey. Suicide Life Threat Behav 2005;35(1):3–13.)[28]

clinicians to incorporate treatment interventions, such as interpersonal psychotherapy for MDD, to remind TAY of the different roles they hold beyond "student" or "employee," (ie, sibling, child, friend, romantic partner, group member).[27]

Accessing care

Many TAY have never independently managed their health care and may not have the necessary skills. An early adult who has no trouble calling or texting a friend may avoid calling to schedule an appointment; may not know how to use pharmacy services; and may not think to call to cancel, reschedule, or notify of running late. Skehan and Davis[15] describe best practices for meeting developmental needs, noting TAY terminate treatment at eight times the rate of mature adults. Despite the frequency of suicidality in the population, studies have shown that most (60%–80%) TAY are not in treatment,[28,29] and are much less likely to access specialty mental health services than their younger adolescent counterparts.[15] Surveys indicate that less than 20% of college students who endorsed suicidality were in mental health care,[28] and 86% of college students who completed suicide had not sought local campus counseling center assistance.[30] This low mental health service utilization is only partially correlated with change in insurance status.[31] In the past 10 years, stigma reduction has contributed to increased numbers of college students seeking treatment from 19% to 33%.[32] TAY in foster care or the juvenile justice system are particularly vulnerable, with eligibility-related abrupt discontinuation of services, and need additional considerations for finances, housing, transportation, and access to care.[33] Lee and Morgan[34] offer that subgroups of foster youth from the Midwest Study describe themselves as "accelerated adults" by virtue of "growing up fast."

Examining transition age youth substance use disorders: parallels with major depressive disorder and access to college mental health care

Substance use and substance use disorders (SUDs) are highest in the TAY age group; 63% of young adults have tried an illicit drug, and 37% have tried an illicit drug other than cannabis.[35]

Campuses receiving federal funds are required to be drug free, regardless of state laws on recreational use. Colleges and universities typically define residential halls as areas of sobriety, yet enforcement is challenging. Routine screening for SUDs is rare on college campuses; however, there are many programs providing education and support services for students. The assumption is that students will make informed decisions as adults. Screening, when done, is often by online anonymous survey (eg, e-CHUG, or e-TOKE),[36,37] or BASICS, a brief strengths-based, motivational-type interview.[38] Impacted campuses may develop more recovery supports, such as on-campus 12-step groups, peer programs, or alcohol and other drug counseling with capitated session numbers. Medical or psychiatric evaluations are less common.

Child and adolescent psychiatrists preparing to send a college student to new services should recognize the need for multifactorial interventions for management of SUD. Clinicians and TAY should explore accessible SUD treatment services and consider dedicated recovery living situations. In parallel, child and adolescent psychiatrists need to be aware that campus-based resources for MDD may also be limited in scope. The focus may be screenings for depression (eg, PHQ-9, CCAPS-34)[39,40] and wellness initiatives rather than traditional mental health services. For college TAY who do screen at risk for MDD, they are often first referred to counseling instead of psychotherapy or psychiatric services. Colleges and universities vary significantly in the number of sessions that they are able to provide, and some facilities refer to off-campus resources for ongoing psychotherapies, or specialty psychiatric care. The availability of high-quality, convenient, accessible, affordable mental health professionals is also variable. Child and adolescent psychiatrists should provide additional guidance regarding an unfamiliar system of care, including location-specific nuances of insurance, and the changes in parental access to information and privacy rights.

TAY continuing treatment may also find it difficult to shift from the developmental approach of a child and adolescent psychiatrist to an approach that emphasizes autonomy as an adult. The focus on autonomy is important, yet vulnerable young adults with MDD may need a developmental approach to individuation, including consent for parental and other third-party communications to protect from deterioration under stress in an unsupervised environment.

Psychological Considerations

Insight
Age and experience influence self-awareness and interpretation of symptoms. An emerging adult may not realize how much narrative shaping and collateral history provided by parents and family has occurred in the past until it is absent. Subjective expectations of "normal" may be misunderstood, interfering with proactive use of wellness initiatives for college-attending TAY, thereby limiting opportunities for support. Nascent self-care and efforts at self-management may affect treatment adherence. It may be difficult to incorporate daily structure, such as medication compliance, or symptom monitoring, into regular habits.

Trauma
ACEs are correlated with dose-response poorer health outcomes later in life.[41] A study of low-income young adults in an urban setting suggests that childhood adversities, were associated with more depressive symptoms with onset in early adulthood.[41] Several factors put TAY with prior diagnoses of post-traumatic stress disorder at greater risk for destabilization when in a college or university setting, Including substance use and sexual assaults on campus. One in five women and 6% of men experience attempted or completed sexual assault during the college years, with higher rates of sexual violence for racial/ethnic minorities.[42] There are also federal campus regulations that require "timely warning" to the campus community, usually via email or text, when a crime has occurred on campus, including sexual assault.[43] These alerts may trigger and exacerbate distress for those who have experienced previous assaults. Students who experience an assault during this epoch may have new onset of post-traumatic stress disorder and acute stress disorder, potentially generating new mood symptoms or exacerbating current mood symptoms.

Emotional development and regulation
It is critical for clinicians to carefully consider risk and protective factors when assessing mood and anxiety symptoms. In addition, the context of behaviors must be considered in light of typical development in TAY. Inability to cope with transitions may be easily misinterpreted as pathology. Child and adolescent psychiatrists should explore symptoms through the biopsychosocial lens to avoid overpathologizing behavior. For example, psychiatrists may diverge on bipolar disorder diagnostic criteria, with some clinicians following the "three soft sign spectrum" conceptualizations[44]; some counting irritability without elation[45]; and others requiring the combination of elation, grandiosity, flight of ideas, decreased need for sleep, and hypersexuality as pathognomonic.[46] Cues, such as spendthrift money management, brief decreased need for sleep with ensuing next-day functionality, and simultaneous pursuit of several dating interests should be clarified against the backdrop of perceived peer and social normative behaviors.

Depression may negatively impact the individual's sense of self, contributing to increased sensitivity to interpersonal slights. This age group may also interpret time-transient symptoms as perpetual and enduring. Several descriptive behaviors of different personality disorders may present in transient ways during the transition to adulthood. Personality disorders are often considered immutable and chronic; however, longitudinal studies indicate variability in diagnostic stability, pathologic severity, and psychosocial functioning.[47,48] Clinicians should encourage psychotherapy to process and challenge maladaptive character traits and related behaviors.

Biologic Considerations

Brain development

Chung and Hudziak[49] describe several changes in the maturation of the "transitional age brain." They emphasize the interplay between mature subcortical areas and immature regulatory areas, with more fully developed areas governing risk-taking overriding still-maturing executive functioning areas.[49] Other studies of brain development highlight early brain plasticity with observed patterning based on enrichment from experience or thinning when deprived states, such as ACEs and trauma, exist.[49] Gray and white matter cortical pruning occurs from 0 to 3 years with a second critical period occurring from age 13 to 25 years.[49] Continuation of white matter maturation occurs through age 30 years in the tracts implicated in executive functioning.[49] Note that different white and gray matter areas develop at different times.[49] The authors propose a "mismatch hypothesis" among three main structures to explain TAY behavior.[49] The nucleus accumbens, site for motivation and pleasure, and the amygdala, which integrates positive and unpleasant emotional reactions, may develop ahead of the prefrontal areas that manage attention control and mood regulation.[49] Emotional regulation is continually modified through life experience.[49] This plasticity leads Chung and Hudziak[49] to suggest positive shaping of brain structures and intervention through treatment and therapies including during the TAY stage.

Neurovegetative symptoms

A chronologic and detailed history is a foundation of clinical practice. TAY often find it challenging to engage in regular self-care as they shift to a more independent lifestyle; this may obscure recognition of a clinical MDD by TAY, parent, and peer perspectives on "normal." Clinicians and patients must clarify colloquial use of the term "depressed," and identify expectations of positive and negative emotions. Many emerging adults have unrealistic expectations for happiness as they individuate from caregivers. The clinician can initiate discussions about "well-being" and the differences among happiness, joy, pleasure, and optimism, aided by the modified Differential Emotions Scale.[50] Queries about anhedonia should explore longitudinal patterns of interests from middle school and high school activities. Appetite and weight changes need to be captured in the context of scheduled meals and their nutritional balances. References to MyPlate guides, snacking, and timing of meals may assist, as may widely available calculators of basal energy expenditure and body mass index.[51] Accessibility to convenience processed foods, body image expectations and peer comparisons, and impressions about nutritional supplement and diet trends should be explored. College-age youth may be tempted to restrict eating to avoid gaining the "freshman 15," or may overeat in the context of unlimited buffet-style cafeterias.

Similarly, sleep habits, hygiene, and waking experience should be explicitly reviewed. When still living with parents, teenagers often have enforced bedtimes and curfews supporting healthy behaviors. Often, independent waking and bedtime are skewed as a natural extension of adolescent sleep patterns, such as sleep latency and waking delay.[52] Inadequate sleep preparation and sleep hygiene may impact sleep latency and the perception of excessive nighttime cognitions interfering with sleep. Expectations for minimum adequate sleep may be ignored, impacting concentration. Patients often require education that *minimum* sufficient sleep for TAY is 6 to 11 hours, with a new age division of 18 to 25 years from the National Sleep Foundation.[53] The National Sleep Foundation also raises caution that more than half of fall-asleep crashes involve drivers younger than 25 years old. Psychomotor changes may also be missed in the absence of collateral sources who know the premorbid baseline. Physical activity at 150 to 300 minutes per week should be recommended.[54] Organized sports and physical education classes are less common in this patient population, contributing to a risk of individuals becoming sedentary, or alternatively, using exercise in an unhelpful way to manage stress and anxiety. Fatigue can be monitored using a 2-week sleep diary, or electronic apps, provided healthy screen use.[55,56] Energy and concentration, peer comparisons, identity transitions, pressure about daily productivity, and occupational goals can affect self-image and worthlessness. Concentration, particularly for the student, should be reviewed as task- and interest-dependent, because of many popular press articles touting only seconds-to-minutes' worth of normal attention span, and a dearth of academic literature describing healthy attention.[57]

Suicide is critical to address, because it remains one of the leading causes of death in this population.[58] Sood and Linker[21] note that prior experiences of suicidality may lead to habituated suicidal behaviors in a subset of TAY. A 2009 study surveyed college students about suicidal ideation, identifying more than half with lifetime suicidal ideation (**Fig. 4**). The survey appropriately separated undergraduates from graduate/professional students as a developmental group.[59] This study indicates that clinicians overemphasize verbalizations of suicidality and underrecognize suicidal risk factors. Child and adolescent psychiatrists should guide safety plans, including review of crisis hotlines with any patient and include parents and support networks in the discussion when allowed. They should routinely ask about suicide at any clinical contact. Following SAMHSA's direction to provide comprehensive

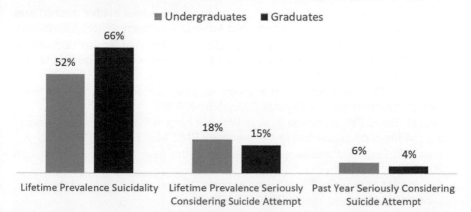

Fig. 4. College student survey of suicidality data. (*Adapted from* Drum DJ, Brownson C, Denmark AB, et al. New data on the nature of suicidal crises in college students: shifting the paradigm. Prof Psychol Res Pract 2009;40(3):213–22; with permission.)

systems of care, child and adolescent psychiatrists working with depressed and suicidal early adults should incorporate available community resources in treatment planning.[60,61]

SUMMARY

The developmental transition from adolescence to early adulthood is a mutilayered, dynamic process. Child and adolescent psychiatrists and clinicians working with this population should promote comprehensive treatment by using their developmental training in a biopsychosocial model. As *The Forgotten Half* stated in 1988, "Although rich in material resources, our society seems unable to ensure that *all* our youth will mature into young men and women able to face their futures with a sense of confidence and security." TAY who have MDD may have additional setbacks and challenges. Child and adolescent psychiatrists may provide true impact in their patient's life trajectories by providing anticipatory guidance, treatment, resources, and life skills through a developmental lens.

REFERENCES

1. Henderson SW, Martin A. Case formulation and integration of information in child and adolescent mental health. In: Rey JM, editor. IACAPAP e-textbook of child and adolescent mental health. Geneva (Switzerland): International Association for Child and Adolescent Psychiatry and Allied Professions; 2014. p. 1–20.

2. American Psychiatric Association. Diagnostic and statistical manual of mental disorders. 5th edition. Arlington (VA): American Psychiatric Association; 2013.

3. Partridge BC. Adolescent psychological development, parenting styles, and pediatric decision making. J Med Philos 2010;35:518–25.

4. Zisook S, Lesser I, Stewart W, et al. Effect of age at onset on the course of major depressive disorder. Am J Psychiatry 2007;164(10):1539–46.

5. Burke K, Burke JD, Reiger DA, et al. Age at onset of selected mental disorders in five community populations. Arch Gen Psychiatry 1990;47:511–8.

6. Mental health information > statistics > suicide. National Institute of Mental Health. Available at: https://www.nimh.nih.gov/health/statistics/suicide.shtml. Accessed November 1, 2018.

7. Wilens TE, Rosenbaum JF. Transitional aged youth: a new frontier in child and adolescent psychiatry. J Am Acad Child Adolesc Psychiatry 2013;52(9):887–90.

8. Now Is the Time Technical Assistance Center. Substance Abuse and Mental Health Services Administration. Available at: https://www.samhsa.gov/nitt-ta. Accessed September 2, 2018.

9. Arnett JJ. Emerging adulthood a theory of development from the late teens through the twenties. Am Psychol 2000;55(5):469–80.

10. Hein M, Troost PW, Broersma A, et al. Why is it hard to make progress in assessing children's decision-making competence? BMC Med Ethics 2015;16(1):1–6.

11. Stetka B. Extended adolescence: when 25 is the new 18. Scientific American 2017.

12. Sawyer SM, Azzopardi PS, Wickremarathne D, et al. The age of adolescence. Lancet Child Adolesc Health 2018;2(3):223–8.

13. Lukianoff G, Haidt J. The coddling of the American mind: how good intentions and bad ideas are setting up a generation for failure. New York: Penguin Press; 2018.

14. Twenge JM. iGen: why today's super-connected kids are growing up less rebellious, more tolerant, less happy – and completely unprepared for adulthood and what that means for the rest of us. 2nd edition. New York: Atria Books; 2017.

15. Skehan B, Davis M. Aligning mental health treatments with the developmental stage and needs of late adolescents and young adults. Child Adolesc Psychiatr Clin N Am 2017;26(2):177–90.

16. Pumariega A. Practice parameter for cultural competence in child and adolescent psychiatric practice. J Am Acad Child Adolesc Psychiatry 2013;1101–15.

17. Rodgers SM. Transitional age lesbian, gay, bisexual, transgender and questioning youth: issues of diversity, integrated identities and mental health. In: Martel AM FDTH, ed. Child and adolescent psychiatric clinics of North America. vol. 26 (2). Transitional Age Youth and Mental Illness: Influences on Young Adult Outcomes ed: Elsevier; 2017.

18. Rivas-Drake D, Stein GL. Multicultural Developmental Experiences Implications for Resilience in Transitional Age Youth. In: Martel AM, Fuchs DC, Trivedi H, eds. Child and Adolescent Psychiatric Clinics of North America. Vol 26(2). Transitional Age Youth and Mental Illness: Influences on Young Adult Outcomes ed: Elsevier; 2017.

19. Pao M. Conceptualization of success in young adulthood. Child Adolesc Psychiatr Clin N Am 2017;26(2):191–8.

20. Resources. American youth policy Forum. Available at: http://www.aypf.org/resources/the-forgotten-half-pathways-to-success-for-americas-youth-and-young-families-1988/. Accessed September 16, 2018.

21. Sood AB, Linker J. Proximal influences on the trajectory of suicidal behaviors and suicide during the transition from adolescence to young adulthood. Child Adolesc Psychiatr Clin N Am 2017;26(2):235–51.

22. 1998 American Youth Policy Forum, Inc, editor. The forgotten half revisited: American youth and young families, 1988-2008. Washington, DC: Samual Halperin; 2010. ISBN 1-887031-63-4.

23. Rosenbaum J, Rosenbaum J, Ahearn C, et al. The new forgotten half and research directions to support them: The William T. Grant Foundation Inequality Paper 2015. Available at: https://wtgrantfoundation.org/library/uploads/2015/09/The-New-Forgotten-Half-and-Research-Directions-to-Support-Them.pdf. Accessed September 16, 2018.

24. MTVU and The Jed Foundation. Feeling stressed. Half of us. Available at: http://www.halfofus.com/feeling/stress/. Accessed September 03, 2018.

25. Chan V. Special needs: scholastic disability accommodations from k-12 and transitions to higher education. Curr Psychiatry Rep 2016;18(2):21.

26. United States Code. Americans with Disabilities Act of 1990, As Amended. Available at: https://www.ada.gov/pubs/ada.htm. Accessed November 1, 2018.

27. Markowitz JC, Weissman MM. Interpersonal psychotherapy: principles and applications. World Psychiatry 2004;3(3):136–9.

28. Kisch J, Leino EV, Silverman MM. Aspects of suicidal behavior, depression, and treatment in college students: results from the spring 2000 National College Health Assessment Survey. Suicide Life Threat Behav 2005;35(1):3–13.

29. Substance Abuse and Mental Health Services Administration. Major depressive episode among full-time college student and other young adults, age 18 - 22: National Survey and Drug Use and Health Report 2012. Available at: https://www.samhsa.gov/data/sites/default/files/NSDUH060/NSDUH060/SR060CollegeStudentsMDE2012.pdf. Accessed September 22, 2018.

30. Pistorello J, Coyle TN, Locey NS, et al. Treating suicidality in college counseling centers: a response to polychronis. J College Stud Psychother 2017;31(1):30–42.
31. Copeland WE, Shanahan L, Davis M, et al. Increase in untreated cases of psychiatric disorders during the transition to adulthood. Psychiatr Serv 2015;66: 397–403.
32. Lipson SK, Lattie EG, Eisenberg D. Increased rates of mental health service utilization by U.S. college students: 10-year population-level trends (2007-2017). Psychiatr Serv 2018. https://doi.org/10.1176/appi.ps.201800332.
33. Osgood DW, Foster EM, Courtney ME. Vulnerable populations and the transition to adulthood. Future Child 2010;20:209–29.
34. Lee T, Morgan W. Transitioning to adulthood from foster care. In: Martel AM FDTH, ed. Child and Adolescent Clinics of North America. Vol. 2 (26): Elsevier; 2017.
35. Bukstein OG. Challenges and gaps in understanding substance use problems in transitional age youth. Child Adolesc Psychiatr Clin N Am 2017;26(2):253–69.
36. Hustad JT, Barnett NP, Borsari B, et al. Web-based alcohol prevention for incoming college students: a randomized controlled trail. Addict Behav 2010; 35:183–98.
37. Elliot JC, Carey KB, Vanable PA. A preliminary evaluation of a web-based intervention for college marijuana use. Psychol Addict Behav 2014;28:288–93.
38. Borsari B, Carey KB. Effects of a brief motivational intervention with college student drinkers. J Consult Clin Psychol 2000;68:728–33.
39. Kroenke K, Spitzer RL, Williams JBW. The PHQ-9 validity of a brief depression severity measure. J Gen Intern Med 2001;16:606–13.
40. Locke BD, McAleavey AA, Zhao Y, et al. Development and initial validation of the counseling center assessment of psychological symptoms - 34. Meas Eval Couns Dev 2012;45(3):1–19.
41. Topitzes J, Reynolds AJ. Impacts of adverse childhood experiences on health, mental health, and substance use in early adulthood: a cohort study of an urban, minority sample in the U.S. Child Abuse Negl 2013;37:917–25.
42. Preventing sexual violence on college and university campuses: a summary of CDC activities. Centers for Disease Control and Prevention; 2016. Available at: https://www.cdc.gov/violenceprevention/pdf/campusvsummary.pdf.   Accessed November 1, 2018.
43. Federal Register. Jeanne Clery Disclosure of Campus Security Policy and Campus Crime Statistics Act of 1990, as Amended. Available at: https://www. govinfo.gov/content/pkg/FR-2014-10-20/pdf/2014-24284.pdf#page=33. Accessed November 1, 2018.
44. Aiken C. Modern medicine network. Psychiatric Times 2017. Available at: http:// www.psychiatrictimes.com/bipolar-disorder/secret-life-bipolar-disorder.   Accessed September 16, 2018.
45. Hunt J, Birmaher B, Leonard H, et al. Irritability without elation in a large bipolar youth sample: frequency and clinical description. J Am Acad Child Adolesc Psychiatry 2009;40(7):730–9.
46. Geller B, Zimmerman B, Williams EA. DSM-IV mania symptoms in a and early adolescent bipolar disorder phenotype compared to attention-deficit hyperactive and normal controls. J Child Adolesc Psychopharmacol 2002;12(1):11–25.
47. Wright AGC, Hopwood CJ, Skodol AE, et al. Longitudinal validation of general and specific structural features of personality pathology. J Abnorm Psychol 2016;125(8):1120–34.
48. Reich D, Zanarini MC. Developmental aspects of borderline personality disorder. Harv Rev Psychiatry 2001;9(6):294–301.

49. Chung WW, Hudziak JJ. The transitional age brain: "the best of times and the worst of times". Child Adolesc Psychiatr Clin N Am 2017;26(2):157–75.
50. Fredrikson B. Chapter one - positive emotions broaden and build. Adv Exp Soc Psychol 2013;47:1–53.
51. United States Department of Agriculture. Available at: ChooseMyPlate.Gov https://www.choosemyplate.gov/. Accessed September 3, 2018.
52. The National Sleep Foundation. Adolescent sleep needs and patterns research report and resource guide. Washington, DC: National Sleep Foundation; 2000. Available at: https://www.sleepfoundation.org/sites/default/files/2019-02/sleep_and_teens_report1.pdf. Accessed November 1, 2018.
53. Hirshkowitz M, Whiton K, Albert M, et al. National Sleep Foundation's sleep duration recommendations: methodology and results summary. Sleep Health 2015;1: 40–3.
54. Cancer Prevention and Control Physical Activity Guidelines. Center for Disease Control and Prevention CDC 24/7 Saving Lives, Protecting People. 2008. Available at: https://www.cdc.gov/cancer/dcpc/prevention/policies_practices/physical_activity/guidelines.htm. Accessed September 03, 2018.
55. Sleep Diary. National Sleep Foundation. Available at: https://sleepfoundation.org/sites/default/files/SleepDiaryv6.pdf. Accessed September 03, 2018.
56. PTSD: National Center for PTSD. Mobile App: CBT-i Coach. U.S. Department of Veterans Affairs. Available at: https://www.ptsd.va.gov/professional/materials/apps/cbticoach_app_pro.asp. Accessed September 03, 2018.
57. Bradbury NA. Attention span during lectures: 8 seconds, 10 minutes, or more? Adv Physiol Educ 2016;40:509–13.
58. National Institute of Mental Health. Statistics Suicide. Mental Health Information. Available at: https://www.nimh.nih.gov/health/statistics/suicide.shtml. Accessed August 19, 2018.
59. Drum DJ, Brownson C, Denmark AB, et al. New data on the nature of suicidal crises in college students: shifting the paradigm. Prof Psychol Res Pract 2009;40(3): 213–22.
60. Chan V, Rasminsky S, Viesselman JO. A Primer for working in campus mental health: a system of care. Acad Psychiatry 2015;39(5):533–40.
61. Rasminsky SR, Chan V. Managing the suicidal college student: advice for community providers. Psychiatric Times 2015;32(11).

Telepsychiatry
A New Treatment Venue for Pediatric Depression

David E. Roth, MD[a],*, Ujjwal Ramtekkar, MD, MPE, MBA[b],
Sofija Zeković-Roth, LAc, DOM[a]

KEYWORDS

- Telepsychiatry • Telehealth • Telemedicine • Depression • Child psychiatry
- Adolescent psychiatry

KEY POINTS

- Telepsychiatry is being deployed to treat pediatric depression in several different models of care. The benefits of using it to provide direct care in homes, schools, primary care offices, juvenile correction centers, and residential facilities are well established.
- Telepsychiatry has the potential to improve prevention, early identification, and treatment of pediatric depression. Telepsychiatry removes the geographic barrier between patients and providers, which lowers the cost of providing treatment and decreases the time, effort, and lost income usually associated with transporting either patients/families or providers to rural and underserved communities.
- Telepsychiatry outcomes and patient satisfaction ratings are sometimes superior to sessions held in traditional face-to-face venues.
- Engaging, building relationships, and communicating with telepsychiatry patients are significantly different from traditional medical settings.
- Effective use of telepsychiatry requires Webside manners and the intentional shaping of both an authentic treatment experience and provider-patient relationships. When telepsychiatry staging and nonverbal and verbal communication skills are properly used, telepsychiatry sessions feel authentic to both patients and providers, and treatment outcomes meet or exceed traditional face-to-face venues.

 Video content accompanies this article at www.childpsych.theclinics.com.

Disclosure Statement: None of the authors has any relationship with a commercial company that has a direct financial interest in subject matter or materials discussed in article or with a company making a competing product.
[a] Mind & Body Works, Inc., 3340 Wauke Street, Honolulu, HI 96815-4452, USA; [b] Partners for Kids, Nationwide Children's Hospital, 700 Children's Way, Columbus, OH 43215, USA
* Corresponding author.
E-mail address: drroth@mind-bodyworks.com

Child Adolesc Psychiatric Clin N Am 28 (2019) 377–395
https://doi.org/10.1016/j.chc.2019.02.007
1056-4993/19/© 2019 Elsevier Inc. All rights reserved.

childpsych.theclinics.com

INTRODUCTION

Contemporary children and adolescents are immersed in interactive media, including social media, online videos, video chat, and video games. It is estimated that more than 70% of teenagers are interacting on 1 or more social media sites on the Internet and approximately 25% of teenagers are constantly connected to Internet.[1] Although caution has been advised against such excessive media use, it reflects the exposure and comfort level youth have with technology. Because they are already using video technology to socialize and play, telepsychiatry is a good fit and appropriate treatment venue with most youth.

TELEPSYCHIATRY
Definition

The Centers for Medicaid & Medicare Services defines telehealth as the use of telecommunications and information technology to provide access to health assessment, diagnosis, intervention, consultation, supervision, and information across distance that seeks to seeks to improve a patient's health by permitting 2-way, real-time, interactive communication between a patient and a physician or practitioner at a distant site. This electronic communication means the use of interactive telecommunications equipment that includes, at minimum, audio and video equipment.[2] The term, *telepsychiatry*, refers to behavioral and mental health services that are provided via synchronous telecommunications technologies, including discipline-specific applications, such as telepsychiatry and telepsychology. Telepsychiatry refers to the use of secure, Health Insurance Portability and Accountability Act (HIPAA)–compliant videoconferencing to connect the psychiatric provider at the destination site with youth and/or their families at the origination site. If the videoconference is live, it is called synchronous telepsychiatry or simply telepsychiatry. If the interaction involves the exchanging of information at different times over a period of time, it is considered asynchronous telepsychiatry.

Laws

The prescription of medications by a telepsychiatrist is impacted by clinical and legal requirements. The clinical monitoring responsibility can be shared with a physician extender or clinician at the origination site or the youth's primary care provider. Standard tools, however, such as the Abnormal Involuntary Movement Scale and other neuropsychiatric assessments, can be used reliably over videoconferencing[3] to monitor for neurologic side effects. When depressed youth have comorbid conditions, such as attention-deficit/hyperactivity disorder or anxiety, the telepsychiatrist has to comply with federal regulations when prescribing Schedule II controlled substances, including stimulant medications and benzodiazepines. These federal regulations began in 2008 with the Ryan Haight Online Pharmacy Consumer Protection Act and were updated in late 2018. The current regulations include specific situations that require special registration with the Drug Enforcement Administration and a requirement that at least 1 in-person visit occurs before prescription of the controlled substances.[2] The federal government update to this act in 2018 provides a special registration for telepsychiatry. This allows a provider to prescribe controlled substances without an in-person visit in 7 categories of clinical practice. These include public health emergencies, working with the Indian Health Service, collaboration with another practitioner at the patient site, and during medical emergencies. A good summary of this special registration is available online from the Congressional Research Service. Telepsychiatrists must maintain active medical licenses for the state(s) in which the patient and provider are located at the time of treatment. Similar restrictions often apply to hospital credentialing and malpractice insurance. Several states have additional requirements and regulations, so the authors recommend telepsychiatrists regularly consult with agencies that track these changes. These include the Center for Connected Health Policy (www.cchpca.org), the American Telemedicine Association (www.americantelemed.org), and the Center for Telehealth and e-Health Law (www.ctel.org).

USING TELEPSYCHIATY TO TREAT DEPRESSION
Proved Efficacy

Landmark studies of the efficacy, feasibility, and acceptability of telepsychiatry service for children living in nonmetropolitan communities found high satisfaction rates in pediatric providers as well as youth. The service was shown to be feasible with good utilization rates in primary care settings.[4,5] Treating youth via telepsychiatry is well accepted by families and they report high satisfaction with the care delivered.[6] Telepsychiatry actually has several advantages over traditional face-to-face sessions. Youth treated with telepsychiatry feel a greater sense of safety and control when dealing with an unfamiliar adults (psychiatrists and other mental health professionals) and greater sense of personal space. They miss less school for sessions, and coordination of care with their other providers and teachers is improved.

Child and adolescent mental health studies of diagnostic accuracy and effectiveness of telepsychiatry treatment demonstrated positive outcomes for children in different settings.[7,8] The growing body of pediatric telepsychiatry literature also includes clinical guidelines for practicing telepsychiatry. The American Academy of Child and Adolescent Psychiatry has published clinical guidelines based on the systematic review and recommendations of the telepsychiatry committee.[2] The American Telemedicine Association published "Practice Guidelines for Telemental Health With Children and Adolescents" in 2017.[9]

Decrease Barriers to Care

Pediatric depression is associated with significant morbidity, including suicide. Despite the potential safety risks of this condition, only a small proportion of youth with depression receive adequate treatment in a timely manner due to barriers (discussed previously). The gap between the high need for care and limited access to care can be mitigated by telepsychiatry. Telepsychiatry has the potential to improve prevention, early identification, and treatment of pediatric depression. Telepsychiatry removes the geographic barrier between patients and providers, which lowers the cost of providing treatment and decreases the time, effort, and lost income usually associated with transporting either patients or providers to rural and underserved communities.[10–12]

Better Collaboration

Telepsychiatry potentially facilitates collaboration between child and adolescent mental health providers and other professionals. Schools and primary care providers can obtain consultations and collaborate with these providers through telehealth with a frequency and intensity usually unobtainable because of logistical barriers.[13] This makes telepsychiatry less expensive and more cost effective than other medical specialties that require additional technological devices necessary for physical examinations and testing. Cost savings have been demonstrated most clearly with newer programs that do not rely on expensive equipment and use the recently available array of secure technology.[14]

Cost Benefits

Mental health disorders affect approximately 15 million children and adolescents in the United States and are a national public health concern. Pediatric depression not only clinically impairs children but also disrupts family systems, often reducing children's adult functioning when it persists into adulthood. Pediatric depression is a clinical burden to the patients and their families, and it is also a financial burden to our society. Although the cost of pediatric depression alone has not been definitively determined, because the total annual cost of adult depression is estimated to be more than $83 billion, pediatric depression is likely a substantial portion of the total annual cost of all pediatric mental health disorders, which is at least $247 billion.[15,16] The overall impact and cost of this mental health burden are expected to rise due to several barriers in providing timely and adequate treatment. These include a critical shortage of child and adolescent psychiatrists, inadequate access to mental health providers with specialized training in treating children, significant geographic distances to reach rural communities, and socioeconomic/resource disparities in rural areas where primary medical care facilities are less concentrated and specialty care access is often suboptimal.[17] These access issues pose overall disadvantages with regard to social determinants of health, such as financial burden to afford transportation, lost wages from attending sessions, specialist copays, affordability of medications, lack of health insurance, poverty, unstable housing, and decreasing income due to worsening economies in those areas.[18] The social determinants related to finances and access often result in the delay of early identification and intervention for childhood mental illness, nonadherence to treatment, inadequate frequency of therapeutic interventions, and overall poor long-term functional outcomes.

MODELS OF TELEPSYCHIATRIC CARE
Direct Care and Collaborative Care/Consultation

Telepsychiatry is being deployed to treat pediatric depression in several different models of care. The benefits of using it to provide direct care in homes, schools, primary care offices, emergency departments, juvenile correction centers, and residential facilities are well established.[19–21] Rapid adoption is being facilitated by the falling cost of telemedicine hardware and the ubiquity of Internet-connected personal devices capable of running telemedicine apps. Recently, collaborative care telepsychiatry consultation models have been adopted because Medicare is reimbursing these consultations. In this model of care, the treatment plan is devised collaboratively with the consulting psychiatrist, but the primary care provider is responsible for implementation of the treatment plan, including medication management, care coordination, monitoring, and follow-up. This collaborative relationship supports the primary care provider and improves patient access to quality care.[22]

Project Extension for Community Healthcare Outcomes

Another model of telepsychiatry consultation is Project Extension for Community Healthcare Outcomes (ECHO). This hub-and-spoke model aims to improve primary care providers' abilities to confidently screen and provide care for children with mild to moderate psychiatric disorders. Project ECHO model outcomes indicate that it is an effective and potentially cost-saving model that increases participant knowledge and patient access to health care in remote locations.[23]

ENGAGING PATIENTS, BUILDING RAPPORT, AND DEVELOPING GOOD WEBSIDE MANNERS

Engaging, building relationships, and communicating with patients in the telepsychiatry venue are significantly different from traditional medical settings. Cameras, microphones, and speakers alter voices, change how participants are seen, and flatten emotional expressions. In order to appear as genuine, trustworthy, and empathic as they normally do in traditional clinical settings, telepsychiatrists need to adjust their communication patterns. Many of these adjustments are techniques used by newscasters, actors, and television studios to engage viewers and ensure clear and emotionally congruent communication with the audience.

Like an actor stepping onto the stage, telepsychiatrists must immediately engage a patient's attention and convince the patient that they are trustworthy, competent, empathic, and responsive to their needs.[24] Providers who seem naturally empathic and create good rapport are instinctually communicating well both verbally and nonverbally with their patients.[25] Adolescent depression treatment outcomes are better when the alliance is strong.[26]

The importance of using and observing congruent nonverbal communication cannot be overstated. More than two-thirds of communicated meaning comes from nonverbal messages, not the actual words spoken.[27] If a provider's nonverbal communication does not reinforce and support the verbal communication, the provider seems odd or insincere.[28] Insufficient, unobserved, or incongruent nonverbal communication weakens the provider-patient relationship.[29] It is often not what is said, but how it is said, that matters most to patients.[25,30]

A provider's bedside manner is the unique mixture of verbal and nonverbal communication used when communicating In a professional role with different patients in different settings.[31] During medical training, providers learned how to modify their bedside manner (consciously or unconsciously) to fit the clinical setting (hospital, emergency department, clinic, nursing home, or nursery). These modifications promote good communication that are appropriately nuanced to engage patients of different ages, genders, maturity, and cultures. It is the authors' opinion that telepsychiatry is not a technology but rather a new clinical setting in which providers must adjust how they communicate to engage patients and maintain therapeutic relationships. Telepsychiatrists must adapt their bedside manners to this venue, a communication style often called Webside manners.

This unspoken need to operate differently In a new clinical venue may be a contributing factor to the pervasive but gradually decreasing resistance to telepsychiatry among established providers. A better understanding of nonverbal communication and mastery of the conscious adjustments providers can make, however, give novice telepsychiatrists more confidence and help them overcome the limitations of this technology. This article reviews the categories of nonverbal communication and how telepsychiatrists can intentionally use and monitor nonverbal communication to successfully engage, diagnose, and treat children and adolescents suffering from depression. This article also reviews the nonverbal impact of the physical setting, including room selection, participant arrangement, and camera framing, on engagement and rapport.

ADOPTING GOOD WEBSIDE MANNERS

A provider's physical appearance, grooming, uniform/dress, and interactions become a more significant part of how patients make a first impression and how they judge a provider as trustworthy, competent, and empathic.[25,32] The provider's physical appearance is restricted by the camera frame, which limits patients' ability to see the provider and surroundings. Patients have less visual information about the provider and where the provider is working to inform and influence their perception and acceptance of the provider (**Box 1**).

Erect and open body posture (**Fig. 1**) communicates to patients that a provider is a confident, nonjudgmental, and trustworthy authority figure who is paying attention to their needs.[33,34] Moving toward or away from the camera approximates the effect of interpersonal space during in-person sessions. For example, moving slightly closer to the camera communicates more interest or attention. If a depressed patient seems defensive, moving slightly away from the camera conveys the perception of giving the patient more space. The picture-in-picture function on the monitor helps providers to monitor how their image is projected and stay within the frame.

Because patients can see only the facial expressions, gestures, movements, and activities that fall within the camera frame, providers must replace large gestures with smaller ones that are seen more easily.[35] Common gestures, like outstretched arms, can be replaced with hand gestures or emotionally congruent facial expressions.[36] Hand gestures, like waving and the thumbs-up sign, also can replace engaging physical contacts like handshakes and fist bumps. Children especially seem to enjoy these hand gestures (**Fig. 2**).

A provider's tone of voice affects the relationship.[37] The provider must sound honest, compassionate, and intelligent while speaking slowly, loudly, and clearly enough to be easily heard and understood through the microphone but without sounding robotic. Many novice providers speak robotically due to performance anxiety or distractions by the electronics, for example, a medical record that is simultaneously projected onto a monitor during the session. Smiling while speaking makes a provider sound warm and approachable. Placing a smiley face sticker next to the camera is a good reminder for those who often look or sound too serious.

There is a transmission delay during synchronous telepsychiatry sessions that, although brief, affects communication. Therefore, pauses and turn-taking are more important for providers to manage. Giving the patient an extra moment to reply in conversation may seem like a long pause but replicates a normal pause during in-person conversation. If there is a significant lag between 1 or more parties in a multicenter session, the provider may need to allow for even longer pauses. When patients feel they are encouraged to speak, they are more likely to feel their needs were fulfilled.[38]

Box 1
Limitations of telepsychiatry technology on the provider

- See the patient
- Be seen by the patient
- Be heard and understood
- Make gestures
- Maintain eye contact
- Touch
- Smell
- Demonstrate usual good bedside manner

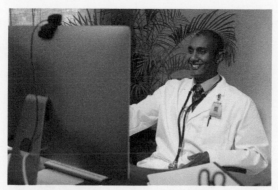

Fig. 1. Good posture suggests to others that you are healthy, confident, and deserving of their respect. (*Courtesy of* D. Roth, MD, FAAP, FAPA, Honolulu, HI.)

Due to the slight audio transmission delay, verbal encouragers, like "yes," "tell me more," and "go on," are harder to use during telepsychiatry. If participants have already resumed speaking, they stop speaking to listen to the encourager, thereby interfering with communication. Therefore, experienced providers frequently use gestures, such as the thumbs-up gesture, to facilitate the reciprocal exchange of information while maintaining engagement and without interrupting the speaker (**Fig. 3**). The other approach is to nod and smile. After thousands of telepsychiatry sessions, the authors suggest the most important nonverbal rapport-building strategy is to periodically nod and smile while a patient is talking. Nodding and smiling reassure patients that a provider is listening and encourages them to continue.[25] Consider placing a sticky note that says "Nod and Smile!" on the monitor until these become natural.

OPTIMIZING THE AUTHENTICITY OF THE EXPERIENCE
Room Selection

Optimizing the telepsychiatry experience begins with appropriate room selection (**Box 2**). In telepsychiatry, the camera is turned on and—boom!—the provider is suddenly meeting with the patient. There are no grand hospital architecture, professional decor, and staff interactions to mentally prepare a patient for the clinical encounter. To

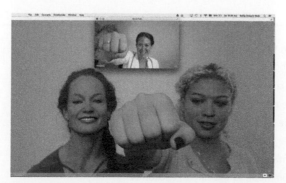

Fig. 2. A fist bump or hand waving gesture can help open and close a session. This gesture replaces the physical contact like handshakes normally used as part of greeting patients. (*Courtesy of* D. Roth, MD, FAAP, FAPA, Honolulu, HI.)

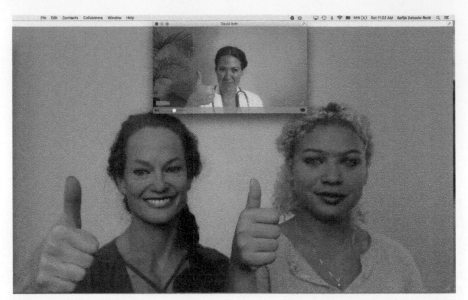

Fig. 3. Using the thumbs-up and other meaningful gestures can signal agreement or other thoughts without interrupting the speaker. Audio transmission delays make it difficult to rapidly state an affirmative verbally without talking over the other speaker. These gestures also are helpful when many participants want to signal agreement or vote on an idea at the same time. (*Courtesy of* D. Roth, MD, FAAP, FAPA, Honolulu, HI.)

make matters worse, a patient's site may be a home, school, or another provider's office—all settings the provider cannot control. It is entirely up to the provider to make it feel like an authentic medical experience.

Good room selection begins with thoughtful selection, arrangement, and appearance of the rooms at both patient and provider sites. Telepsychiatrists often have to work with a wide range of rooms, but with the right setup, sessions can be conducted successfully in classrooms, conference rooms, treatment rooms, offices, living rooms, and bedrooms. After the room at the patient's site is selected, it should be tailored to support videoconferences, accommodate the routine number of participants, and maximize participants' focus during the session. If a child's motor skills, play,

---

Box 2
Room selection in telepsychiatry

Room selection should ensure that

- Everyone feels comfortable

- Distractions are minimized

- Everyone is able to see each other

- Everyone is able to hear each other

- The room maintains visual and auditory privacy

- Room size accommodates the clinical encounter

- Décor minimizes camera distortions

exploration, and movements are being assessed, the room should be large enough for these activities to fit within the camera frame (**Fig. 4**).

Power and Network

One of the most important considerations in room selection for sites using consumer-based equipment or cloud videoconferencing is proximity to the Wi-Fi router to maintain a strong Internet connection. If connecting through a computer, it should be plugged into the router with an ethernet cable to provide the strongest and most stable video and auditory signals. Plugging the router, modem, computer, and monitor(s) into a combination surge protector and battery backup ensures that the connection does not drop if there is a momentary electrical surge or loss of power.

Privacy

Commercial telepsychiatry vendors advertise whether they meet HIPAA standards, including software encryption, and if they would sign a HIPAA Business Associate Agreement. Many popular video chat programs like FaceTime and Viber are not HIPAA-compliant.

Both sites must ensure that they can restrict access to the session. Family sessions may be best accommodated in a kitchen or family room, but these are high-traffic areas. Individual sessions, and some parent-child sessions, may be conducted away from other family in a bedroom, office, or porch. Many depressed teenagers prefer the privacy of a bedroom. If the telepsychiatrist routinely wants a parent's input during the session, it should be set up to occur at the beginning and/or end of the session. This helps with consent for treatment changes and getting parental input about home and school functioning. It gives the telepsychiatrist a chance to assess the parent's feelings about the youth and treatment efficacy while preserving the youth's

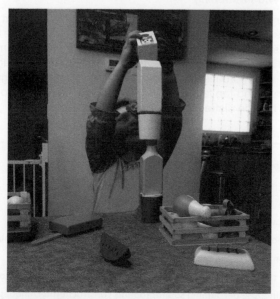

Fig. 4. When working with children, it is necessary to widen the camera's field of view to appreciate the task given to the child or to observe the child's behavior. (*Courtesy of* D. Roth, MD, FAAP, FAPA, Honolulu, HI.)

privacy, as appropriate. It may be helpful to tell the parent when to join the session. This decreases parent and youth anxiety about who should be in the room and who has input into the session, and the provider can avoid being carried around the home as the youth looks for the parent.

Audio privacy may be the largest obstacle to privacy (**Box 3**). The privacy of the patient site is held to the same HIPAA standards as a traditional clinic, nursing home, school, or hospital. Like any other clinical setting, the provider's voice and the patient's voice should be difficult or impossible to hear outside of the videoconferencing room.

Another privacy concern is whether to include a clinical staff member as a coordinator/presenter at the patient site during the session. Coordinators can provide valuable assistance with the telepsychiatry technology, emotionally support the patient, and provide immediate help in a clinical crisis. Additionally, they can provide educational material to patients' families, assist with follow-through on recommendations, and help ensure continuity of care. The presence of a coordinator in the session, however, may negatively affect the therapeutic relationship with a depressed patient. An uncomfortable patient may withhold disclosing critical information to a provider, and shy patients may not ask the coordinator to leave the room. Technical, confidentiality, and ethics trainings for the coordinator are highly encouraged.

Room Setup

Selecting a room with a camera-friendly color scheme makes it easier a the camera to focus on the participant instead of the background. The camera should be focused on a wall that is painted a soft neutral shade to help the participant's image stand out from the wall. Decorations in the provider's room should be minimal and professional, reflecting the services delivered.

Camera Framing and Positioning

The telepsychiatry provider has to overcome the visual field deficit created by the camera. Cameras have a limited field of view, whereas the human eye has both central and peripheral vision. How the provider positions and zooms the camera determines what the participants see and can have a profound impact on engagement with the participant. It is a compromise between being too close, which greatly limits the viewing of gestures, and too far, which makes the provider harder to see and harder to hear and may include distracting background objects.

Box 3
Audio privacy in telepsychiatry

Ways to improve audio privacy

- Close windows
- Block gaps below doors
- Place a white noise machine outside and beside the door to the telepsychiatry room.
- Put carpet or an area rug on the floor.
- Add pillows to couches, curtains on windows, and/or tapestries on walls to absorb sound
- When remodeling, use decoupling soundproofing construction techniques.
- Consider using a headset microphone

The telepsychiatry provider should sit approximately 2 ft to 4 ft directly back from the camera. This usually put the image in the middle of the frame. Providers should check this self-monitoring image at the beginning of each session to ensure their image is large, centered, and in focus. Telepsychiatry providers can then adjust their chair height or camera until the eyes are approximately one-third down from the top of the self-monitor image (**Fig. 5**). This creates the natural-looking framing commonly used to make television newscasters appear attentive and engaging. Encourage the patient to similarly adjust positioning and camera framing at the beginning of the session.

Thoughtful camera placement improves the mental status examination. A participant's camera should be positioned at a sufficient distance to allow visualization of a child's motor abilities and play as well as dysmorphic facial features, facial expressions, hygiene, clothing, tics, and gestures.

Provider eye contact is significantly related patients' perceptions of a provider's connectedness and empathy.[39] The camera may not be located above the monitor, however, causing participants to make eye contact in the wrong direction. Therefore, the provider's camera should be directly in front of the provider, positioned at eye level, and immediately above or below the participant's image (**Fig. 6**). If a separate Web camera is available, place it on top of the computer or on a shelf so that it is positioned directly over the patient's image on the screen.

When using a portable device for a telepsychiatry session, place it on a desk or table so it does not move around. Handheld devices should be propped up at shoulder height and at arm's length from the user's body to make the eye contact feel more natural. This also prevents excessive camera movement, which causes the camera to lose focus, degrades image quality, and can make the other participants feel seasick (Video 1). If a single participant is using a phone or tablet, it should be positioned in vertical/portrait orientation. This improves the eye contact between participants because the other participant's eyes are closer to the camera. If the device needs to capture 2 or more people in the frame, turning the device to the horizontal/landscape position often creates a larger frame that encompasses more of the room, but eye contact may be misaligned.

If an electronic medical record (EMR) is used during the session and can be projected onto the screen, place it in a window below the participants' images. This causes the provider to constantly nod up and down in a positive and affirmative

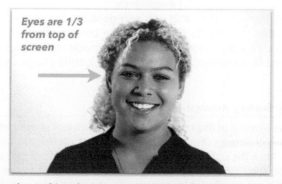

Fig. 5. Follow this rule used in television studios: when framing a person for a videoconference, have the person's eyes approximately one-third below the top of the frame and in the center of the frame. (*Courtesy of* D. Roth, MD, FAAP, FAPA, Honolulu, HI.)

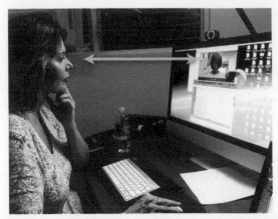

Fig. 6. Virtual eye contact is created when you appear to be looking at the person because you have juxtaposed the participant's image and your camera. When juxtaposed, you are looking at the camera when you are looking at the participant's image on your screen. This is much easier than trying to look at a camera lens. (*Courtesy of* D. Roth, MD, FAAP, FAPA, Honolulu, HI.)

manner when glancing at the EMR (**Fig. 7**). By contrast, if the EMR window is placed lateral to the participant images, the provider is constantly making negative, head-shaking gestures during the session. Medical providers spend 30% of the visit length gazing at the EMR.[39] Telepsychiatrists should minimize the time spent looking at the EMR to maintain eye contact and rapport with the patient, even if this means charting very little during the session.

Staying Within the Camera Frame

Drifting out of the camera frame is a common problem, because people move around in their chairs and often slouch (**Fig. 8**). Most software displays the provider's picture as a smaller self-monitor image on the screen. Even if providers are uncomfortable watching themselves on camera, they need to monitor their image. If they do not, they run the danger of disappearing from the other participants' screens, diminishing their ability to perceive the provider and distracting them. When the provider moves out of the frame the participants are reminded they are not face-to-face and this detracts from the authenticity of the experience.

Providers should ensure their hand and arm gestures are visible within the frame. Exclude moving objects like fans from the frame because they are distracting and degrade the picture. Digitally rendering these movements uses up valuable bandwidth and computer processing power, causing the participant's image and voice clarity to degrade.

Youth and Family Seating Arrangement

If there is only 1 participant at the remote site, the participant should sit 2 ft to 4 ft away from the camera and screen (**Fig. 9**). Each additional participant should be moved another 2 ft back from the camera (**Fig. 10**). If 2 people to 3 people want to sit within 3 ft of the camera, they have to sit shoulder to shoulder to fit in the frame (**Fig. 11**). Although armchairs are comfortable, chairs with straight backs and without armrests accommodate 2 people to 3 people closer to the camera. This often is necessary when the microphone or speakers are marginally adequate to the task.

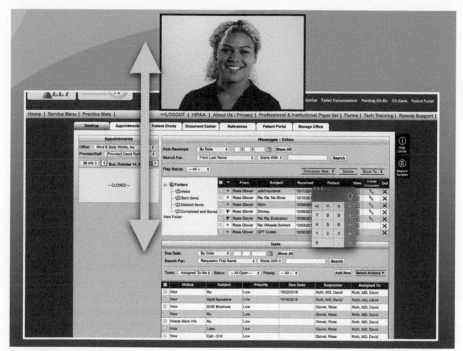

Fig. 7. By stacking a patient's image above or below the EMR, your head is moving up and down in a "yes" movement every time you reference the EMR. When arranged side-by-side, your head repeatedly makes a "no" movement. (*Courtesy of* D. Roth, MD, FAAP, FAPA, Honolulu, HI.)

When working with families, have them position the camera far enough away to see most of the room and keep all the participants within the frame so they do not have to adjust it during the session. Many seating arrangements can work for children. Children can sit next to a parent, between parents, on a parent's lap, or in front of parents

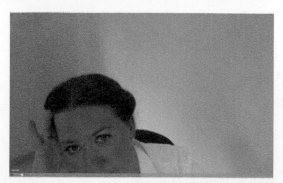

Fig. 8. Drifting out of the frame reminds the patient that you are on a screen and takes away from immersion in the experience. This often happens when telehealth providers turn off or hide their self-monitoring image. The way self-consciousness novice providers feel when seeing themselves on camera commonly fades with practice. (*Courtesy of* D. Roth, MD, FAAP, FAPA, Honolulu, HI.)

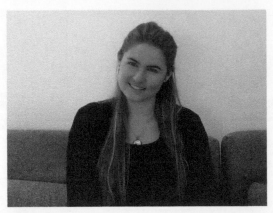

Fig. 9. If there is only 1 participant at the remote site, the participant should sit 2 ft to 4 ft feet away from the camera and screen. (*Courtesy of* D. Roth, MD, FAAP, FAPA, Honolulu, HI.)

in either their own chair or on the floor (**Fig. 12**). When focusing on a single youth who can remain in a chair, have the youth sit close to the camera. The chairs should be stationary to keep children from rolling them out of the frame and light enough for the parent to reposition them. Sometimes a hyperactive or agitated youth cannot remain in the camera frame. Consider keeping the parent(s) in the frame and call the child back to the camera when needed to answer a question (Video 2). Occasionally anxious, depressed, and defiant youth refuse to sit within the camera frame. If behavior management strategies fail to move the youth, then prior to the next session instruct the parent or session facilitator to turn off the self-monitor image and sit the youth farther away from the camera. This makes it more likely that the youth is at least partially within the camera frame.

Lighting

Lighting affects quality of the videoconferencing session.[35] Cameras need more light than human eyes to produce a clear image with accurate colors. An insufficiently illuminated room prevents participants from seeing each other clearly, detecting

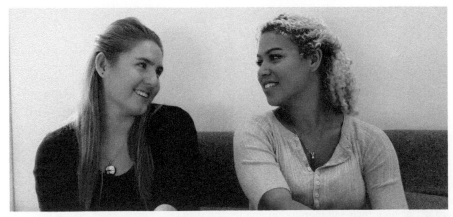

Fig. 10. Move each additional participant 2 ft or more back from the camera. (*Courtesy of* D. Roth, MD, FAAP, FAPA, Honolulu, HI.)

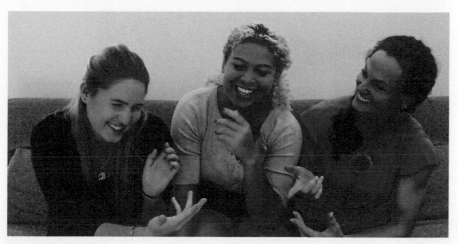

Fig. 11. If 2 people or 3 people want to sit within 3 ft of the camera, they have to sit shoulder-to-shoulder to fit in the frame. (*Courtesy of* D. Roth, MD, FAAP, FAPA, Honolulu, HI.)

nonverbal communication, and identifying physical signs and symptoms and detracts from the authenticity of the experience.[32] Backlighting should be avoided. This occurs when a bright light comes from behind the person, such as when participants are seated with their backs to a window or bright light (**Fig. 13**).

Room lighting should be considered early in room selection and when the position of the camera is determined. Copious indirect lighting, such as floor lamps that bounce light off the ceiling, is key to a good lighting plan (**Fig. 14**). It looks natural and softer and does not cause glare or shadows. Removing or covering reflective surfaces that cause glare also helps optimize the video image.

Audio Quality

Rooms should be selected to minimize common interfering sounds, including printers, air conditioners, fans, intercoms, animals, lawn equipment, and outside traffic. Most

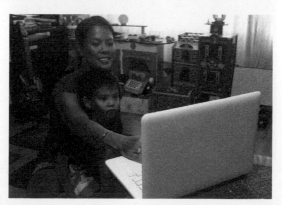

Fig. 12. When working with small children, having children sit on a parent's lap is a good way to keep them within the camera frame and engaged in the session. (*Courtesy of* D. Roth, MD, FAAP, FAPA, Honolulu, HI.)

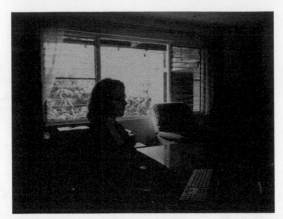

Fig. 13. Backlighting is a common problem in telehealth sessions. Cameras need more light in front of the subject rather than behind or to the side. When the light is misplaced, the camera is unable to properly render colors and light balance and keep the people brighter than the background. (*Courtesy of* D. Roth, MD, FAAP, FAPA, Honolulu, HI.)

rooms are not perfectly quiet, however, and the provider should work with staff at the patient site to implement strategies to decrease background noise. If the provider is the only person in the room, the provider could use a headset microphone that eliminates most background sounds, minimizes keyboard clicks, and also ensures that participants' voices are not overheard.

Telepsychiatry providers must have a backup plan in case the audio connection fails. Usually, a conference speakerphone or smartphone can provide an adequate duplex connection, allowing the session to continue with suboptimal but sufficient video.

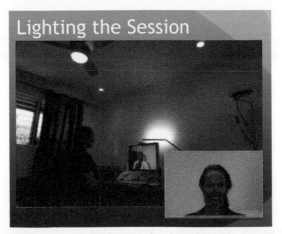

Fig. 14. Telehealth sessions need to be lit more brightly than other rooms to appear as they normally do to the human eye. Cameras need more light to correctly render the image details including color, contrast, and depth of field. A simple rule to follow is have 1 additional light in front of the subject or indirectly (and off camera) lighting the whole room to make the room seem as bright on camera as it does in face-to-face sessions. (*Courtesy of* D. Roth, MD, FAAP, FAPA, Honolulu, HI.)

SUMMARY

Telepsychiatry is rapidly becoming an established medical venue for treating depressed children and adolescents. Effective use of telepsychiatry requires Web-side manners and the intentional shaping of both an authentic treatment experience and provider-patient relationships. When these staging and nonverbal and verbal communication skills are properly used, telepsychiatry sessions feel authentic to both patients and providers, and treatment outcomes meet or exceed traditional face-to-face venues and improve access to care. With sufficient practice, providers can become as effective and comfortable treating depressed pediatric patients via telepsychiatry as they are in other clinical venues. Additional resources for optimizing the telepsychiatry session are available at www.telepsychiatryguide.org, www.telepsychiatryresourcecenter.org, and www.americantelemed.org.

SUPPLEMENTARY DATA

Supplementary data to this article can be found online at https://doi.org/10.1016/j.chc.2019.02.007.

REFERENCES

1. Council on Communications and Media. Media use in school-aged children and adolescents. Pediatrics 2016. https://doi.org/10.1542/peds.2016-2592.
2. American Academy of Child and Adolescent Psychiatry (AACAP) Committee on Telepsychiatry and AACAP Committee on Quality Issues. Clinical update: telepsychiatry with children and adolescents. J Am Acad Child Adolesc Psychiatry 2017. https://doi.org/10.1016/j.jaac.2017.07.008.
3. Amarendran V, George A, Gersappe V, et al. The reliability of telepsychiatry for a neuropsychiatric assessment. Telemed J E Health 2011. https://doi.org/10.1089/tmj.2010.0144.
4. Myers KM, Valentine JM, Melzer SM. Feasibility, acceptability, and sustainability of telepsychiatry for children and adolescents. Psychiatr Serv 2007. https://doi.org/10.1176/ps.2007.58.11.1493.
5. Myers KM, Valentine JM, Melzer SM. Child and adolescent telepsychiatry: utilization and satisfaction. Telemed J E Health 2008. https://doi.org/10.1089/tmj.2007.0035.
6. Gloff NE, Lenoue SR, Novins DK, et al. Telemental health for children and adolescents. Int Rev Psychiatry 2015. https://doi.org/10.3109/09540261.2015.1086322.
7. Elford R, White H, Bowering R, et al. A randomized, controlled trial of child psychiatric assessments conducted using videoconferencing. J Telemed Telecare 2000. https://doi.org/10.1258/1357633001935086.
8. Nelson E-L, Barnard M, Cain S. Treating childhood depression over videoconferencing. Telemed J E Health 2003. https://doi.org/10.1089/153056203763317648.
9. Myers K, Nelson E-L, Rabinowitz T, et al. American telemedicine association practice guidelines for telemental health with children and adolescents. Telemed J E Health 2017;23(10):779–804.
10. Yilmaz SK, Horn BP, Fore C, et al. An economic cost analysis of an expanding, multi-state behavioural telehealth intervention. J Telemed Telecare 2018. https://doi.org/10.1177/1357633X18774181.
11. Russo JE, McCool RR, Davies L. VA telemedicine: an analysis of cost and time savings. Telemed J E Health 2016;22(3):209–15.

12. Bashshur RL, Shannon GW, Bashshur N, et al. The empirical evidence for tele-medicine interventions in mental disorders. Telemed J E Health 2016;22(2): 87–113.
13. Scott Kruse C, Karem P, Shifflett K, et al. Evaluating barriers to adopting telemed-icine worldwide: a systematic review. J Telemed Telecare 2018;24(1):4–12.
14. Behere PB, Mansharamani HD, Kumar K. Telepsychiatry: reaching the un-reached. Indian J Med Res 2017;146(2):150–2.
15. Nelson EL, Cain S, Sharp S. Considerations for conducting telemental health with children and adolescents. Child Adolesc Psychiatr Clin N Am 2017;26(1):77–91.
16. Greenberg PE, Kessler RC, Birnbaum HG, et al. The economic burden of depres-sion in the United States: how did it change between 1990 and 2000? J Clin Psy-chiatry 2003. https://doi.org/10.4088/JCP.v64n1211.
17. Merikangas KR, He JP, Burstein M, et al. Service utilization for lifetime mental dis-orders in U.S. adolescents: results of the national comorbidity surveyAdolescent supplement (NCS-A). J Am Acad Child Adolesc Psychiatry 2011. https://doi.org/10.1016/j.jaac.2010.10.006.
18. Allen J, Balfour R, Bell R, et al. Social determinants of mental health. Int Rev Psy-chiatry 2014. https://doi.org/10.3109/09540261.2014.928270.
19. Butterfield A. Telepsychiatric evaluation and consultation in emergency care set-tings. Child Adolesc Psychiatr Clin N Am 2018;27(3):467–78.
20. Nelson E-L, Barnard M, Cain S. Feasibility of telemedicine intervention for child-hood depression. Couns Psychother Res 2006. https://doi.org/10.1080/14733140600862303.
21. Thomas JF, Novins DK, Hosokawa PW, et al. The use of telepsychiatry to provide cost-efficient care during pediatric mental health emergencies. Psychiatr Serv 2018;69(2):161–8.
22. Martínez V, Rojas G, Martínez P, et al. Remote collaborative depression care pro-gram for adolescents in araucanía region, Chile: randomized controlled trial. J Med Internet Res 2018;20(1):e38.
23. Zhou C, Crawford A, Serhal E, et al. The impact of project ECHO on participant and patient outcomes: a systematic review. Acad Med 2016. https://doi.org/10.1097/ACM.0000000000001328.
24. Feldman RS. Applications of nonverbal behavioral theories and Research 1992. Available at: https://www.taylorfrancis.com/books/9781317782667. Accessed September 15, 2018.
25. Riess H, Kraft-Todd G. E. M. P. A. T. H. Y.: A tool to enhance nonverbal commu-nication between clinicians and their patients. Acad Med 2014;89(8):8–10.
26. Shirk SR, Gudmundsen G, Kaplinski HC, et al. Alliance and outcome in cognitive-behavioral therapy for adolescent depression. J Clin Child Adolesc Psychol 2008; 37(3):631–9.
27. Leathers D. Successful nonverbal communication: principles and applications. 3rd edition 1997. Available at: https://www.taylorfrancis.com/books/9781315542317. Accessed September 15, 2018.
28. Knapp ML, Hall JA, Horgan TG. Nonverbal communication in human interaction, eighth edition, international edition 2007. Available at: https://books.google.com/books?hl=en&lr=&id=rWoWAAAAQBAJ&oi=fnd&pg=PP1&dq=6.%09Knapp+M,+Hall+J,+Horgan+T:+Nonverbal+Communication+in+Human+Interaction,+8th+Ed.+Wadsworth,+Boston,+2014.&ots=4RqBTSsXcC&sig=Bq_1D2B9mKHi7N Nemn5HfNS6abs. Accessed September 15, 2018.
29. Henry SG, Fuhrel-forbis A, Rogers MAM, et al. Patient Education and Counseling Association between nonverbal communication during clinical interactions and

outcomes : a systematic review and meta-analysis86. Elsevier; 2012. p. 297–315. https://doi.org/10.1016/j.pec.2011.07.006.

30. Burgoon J, Guerrero L, Floyd K. Nonverbal communication, vol. 201, 2015. p. 1–6. Available at: https://content.taylorfrancis.com/books/download?dac= C2015-0-61479-2&isbn=9781317346074&format=googlePreviewPdf. Accessed September 15, 2018.

31. Patel RA, Hartzler A, Pratt W, et al. Visual feedback on nonverbal communication : a design exploration with healthcare professionals. Pervasive Heal 2013. https:// doi.org/10.4108/icst.pervasivehealth.2013.252024.

32. Glueck D. Establishing therapeutic rapport in telemental health. In: Myers K, Turvey C, editors. Telemental health. Waltham (MA): Elsevier; 2013. p. 29–46. https://doi.org/10.1016/B978-0-12-416048-4.00003-8.

33. Brugel S, Postma-nilsenová M, Tates K. The link between perception of clinical empathy and nonverbal behavior : the effect of a doctor' s gaze and body orientation. Patient Educ Couns 2015;98(10):1260–5.

34. Ebner N, Thompson J. @ Face value? Nonverbal communication & trust development in online video-based mediation. Int J Online Disput Resolut 2016;1–7. https://doi.org/10.1089/105072502761016494.

35. Onor ML, Misan S. The clinical interview and the doctor–patient relationship in telemedicine. Telemed J E Health 2005;11(1):102–5.

36. Savin D, Glueck DA, Chardavoyne J, et al. Bridging cultures: child psychiatry via videoconferencing. Child Adolesc Psychiatr Clin N Am 2011;20(1):125–34.

37. McHenry M, Parker PA, Baile WF, et al. Voice analysis during bad news discussion in oncology: reduced pitch, decreased speaking rate, and nonverbal communication of empathy. Support Care Cancer 2012;20(5):1073–8.

38. Dijkstra H, Albada A, Klöckner Cronauer C, et al. Nonverbal communication and conversational contribution in breast cancer genetic counseling. Patient Educ Couns 2013;93(2):216–23.

39. Montague E, Asan O. Dynamic modeling of patient and physician eye gaze to understand the effects of electronic health records on doctor – patient communication and attention. Int J Med Inform 2013;83(3):225–34.

Depression in Youth with Autism Spectrum Disorder

Florencia Pezzimenti, MEd[a], Gloria T. Han, MA[b], Roma A. Vasa, MD[c], Katherine Gotham, PhD[d],*

KEYWORDS

- Depression • Mood • Dysthymia • Autism • ASD • Psychiatric comorbidity
- Assessment • Treatment

KEY POINTS

- Depression is a commonly cooccurring disorder in individuals with autism spectrum disorder (ASD), with lifetime rates approximately 4 times greater than the general population when pooled across age ranges (7.7% in child ASD samples; 40.2% in adults with ASD).
- Depression in ASD compromises adaptive functioning and quality of life and is associated with increased risk of medication and service use, suicidality, other forms of self-injury, and caregiver burden.
- Assessment and diagnosis of depression in young people with ASD are challenging because of symptom overlap between the disorders and lack of validated psychometric instruments for assessing depressive symptoms in ASD.
- Evidence for effective treatment of depression in youth with ASD is limited, but adapted psychotherapies show some promise.

INTRODUCTION

For several decades, the focus on understanding autism spectrum disorder (ASD) seemed to leave little room for research on cooccurring affective disorders. In addition, diagnostic overshadowing, or the tendency for clinicians to overlook or dismiss depressive symptoms or behaviors as attributes of ASD, largely obscured clinical awareness of depression in youth with ASD. Pioneering work[1,2] raised awareness of

Disclosure Statement: Sources of support included the National Institute of Mental Health R01-MH113576, K01-MH103500, T32-MH18921. Content is solely the responsibility of the authors and does not necessarily represent the official views of the NIH. No funding body or source of support had a role in the study design, data collection, analysis, or interpretation, or writing of this manuscript.
[a] Department of Psychiatry and Behavioral Sciences, Vanderbilt University Medical Center, 1500 21st Avenue South, Village at Vanderbilt, Room 2246, Nashville, TN 37212, USA; [b] Department of Psychology, Vanderbilt University, 111 21st Avenue South, Wilson Hall, Room 205, Nashville, TN 37240, USA; [c] Department of Psychiatry and Behavioral Sciences, Johns Hopkins University School of Medicine, Kennedy Krieger Institute, 3901 Greenspring Avenue, Baltimore, MD 21211, USA; [d] Department of Psychiatry and Behavioral Sciences, Vanderbilt University Medical Center, 1500 21st Avenue South, Village at Vanderbilt, Room 2252, Nashville, TN 37212, USA
* Corresponding author.
E-mail address: katherine.gotham@vanderbilt.edu

Child Adolesc Psychiatric Clin N Am 28 (2019) 397–409
https://doi.org/10.1016/j.chc.2019.02.009
1056-4993/19/© 2019 Elsevier Inc. All rights reserved.

childpsych.theclinics.com

the syndrome of depression in ASD, and over the past decade, there has been a sharp increase in the number of research publications on this topic. The number of youth presenting with cooccurring ASD and depression often exceeds the clinical capacity to intervene in many (possibly most) regions throughout North America as well as globally. Stakeholders and funding agencies are swiftly coming to realize the importance and urgency of research on depression in ASD. Here, the authors provide an overview of the prevalence, impact, presentation, and risk factors associated with cooccurring depression in children and adolescents with ASD. Clinical guidelines for the assessment and treatment of depression in the ASD population are also provided, with the caveat that these are emerging fields in which research is ongoing.

PREVALENCE AND IMPACT OF DEPRESSION IN AUTISM SPECTRUM DISORDER

Establishing accurate and reliable prevalence rates of depression in ASD is challenging due to method variance (eg, population-based vs convenience sample estimates; self-report vs caregiver report of depressive symptoms). However, the literature suggests that depression commonly cooccurs with ASD, with prevalence estimates that exceed estimates from the general population and comparable subpopulations, such as those with intellectual disability.[3] In samples of children and adolescents with ASD, current rates of depression generally fall in the range of 1% to 10% as diagnosed by parent report; these same studies tend to report elevated subsyndromal depression rates for an additional 10% to 15% of their samples.[4,5] In a convenience sample of 1272 youth with ASD enrolled in the Autism Speaks Autism Treatment Network, parents reported depression diagnoses for 20.2% of adolescents aged 13 to 17.[6] By approximate comparison, 8.4% of typically developing early adolescents (13–14 year olds) had major depressive disorder or dysthymia in a large US representative study.[7]

A recent meta-analysis[8] found that individuals with ASD are approximately 4 times more likely to experience depression compared with the general population when age ranges are pooled. Significantly elevated lifetime depression rates in ASD are associated with the following:

- Increasing age (40.2% in adult samples vs 7.7% in samples <18 years old)
- Average to above average IQ (52.8% vs 12.2% when mean IQ is below average)
- Structured interviews to assess depression (28.5% vs 6.7% for other assessment instruments)
- Self-report (48.6% vs 14.4% via caregiver report)

Cooccurring depression has significant emotional, social, and behavioral consequences for individuals with ASD, including the following:

- Exacerbated impairments associated with ASD (eg, diminished social motivation and adaptive functioning)[1,9,10]
- Diminished quality of life, and increased caregiver burden, medication, and service use[11,12]
- Heightened physical (eg, gastrointestinal problems, seizures), emotional (eg, anxiety), and behavioral (eg, aggression, inattention) comorbidities[6,13]
- Increased suicidality in a population with elevated rates of suicidal ideation and attempts compared with the general population[14,15,16]

PHENOMENOLOGY OF DEPRESSION IN AUTISM SPECTRUM DISORDER

Individuals with ASD exhibit traditional *Diagnostic and Statistical Manual of Mental Disorders* (Fifth Edition)[17] depressive symptoms (eg, sadness, decreased pleasure in most activities, cognitive and somatic symptoms, and suicidality). As shown in **Table 1**, they may also exhibit more atypical presentations of depression[10,18,19] that focus on changes in engagement of special interests or other repetitive behaviors and decreases in adaptive behavior skills and self-care. Within the heterogeneous autism spectrum, depression presentation likely depends on a variety of factors, several covered below in the section on vulnerability factors. Although lacking prototypical benchmarks, the authors offer hypothetical "snapshots" of cases here:

- Cognitively able and socially motivated youth with ASD may experience sadness, increased irritability, anhedonia, sleep disturbance, diminished appetite, self-deprecatory thoughts, coupled with an exacerbation of their ASD symptoms (eg, more intense circumscribed interests and increased rigidity).
- Youth with ASD and intellectual disability may present with increased crying, self-injury, aggression, perseveration, weight gain or loss, and toileting accidents.

ASD and depression have overlapping features in several key areas (**Fig. 1**), most notably more constricted or flat affect and social withdrawal. Historically, this has led to diagnostic overshadowing, which has hindered awareness, characterization, and diagnostic precision of depression in ASD samples.

Little is known about the course of depression in children and adolescents with ASD, although preliminary data indicate that depression may persist longitudinally. Specifically, girls may show a steeper increase in depressive symptoms throughout adolescence, on par with typically developing girls, whereas boys with ASD may have elevated symptoms in school-aged years (compared with typically developing children and with girls with ASD) that persist into adulthood.[20] Depressive symptoms may also be more likely to persist in children who are experiencing bullying or greater social communication difficulties.[21]

RISK FACTORS

Researchers have posited several potential vulnerability factors for depression in ASD. Most of these come from independent studies of ASD and of typically developing depressed samples, with no direct comparison of the 2 clinical populations. Very few studies have used longitudinal designs to capture the interplay between

Table 1	
Symptom presentation of depression in autism spectrum disorder	
Prototypical Depression Symptoms that Commonly Mark Depression in ASD	**Depression Symptoms that May be More Specific to ASD**

• Depressed and/or irritable mood
• Loss of pleasure in previously enjoyed activities
• Hopelessness and tearfulness
• Negative beliefs about oneself
• Feelings of failure or worthlessness
• Constricted affect
• (Increased) Social withdrawal
• Change in appetite (increased or decreased)
• (Increased) Sleep problems
• Poor concentration abilities
• Lack of motivation
• Thoughts about death or suicidal ideation
	• Increased irritability
	• Changes in circumscribed interests (CI):
	  ○ Decreased pleasure in CI
	  ○ Increased intensity
	  ○ Change to darker/morbid content
	• Increased repetitive behaviors
	• Increased anxiety or insistence on sameness
	• Increase in aggression or self-injury
	• Regressive behavior
	• Decline in self-care

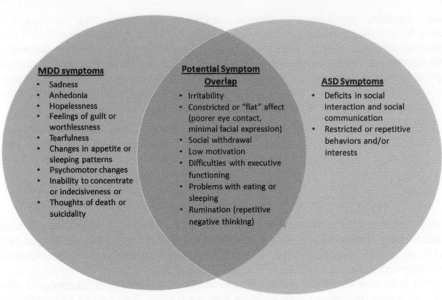

Fig. 1. Potential symptom overlap in major depressive disorder (MDD) and ASD.

depressed mood and ASD symptoms over time. A summary of data is presented on potential candidate vulnerability factors associated with ASD and/or depression that may further the understanding of their cooccurrence.

Genetic/Neurobiological

- Higher familial rates of affective disorders have been reported in family members of individuals with autism, even before having a child with a developmental disability.[22]
- ASD, major depressive disorder, and other mental health conditions have been found to share common genetic variance.[23] Serotonin and dopamine gene variants have been linked to more severe depressive symptoms in children with ASD.[13]
- Atypical neural processes related to serotonin,[24] microglia (indicating inflammatory processes),[25] amygdala anatomy and function,[26] and other functional or connectivity disruptions[27] have been associated with both depression and ASD in independent samples.

Demographic and Individual Characteristics

- Age: Evidence suggests that the risk for depression in ASD increases in adolescence,[8,20,21] similar to patterns observed in the general population.[7] Adult ASD depression rates are significantly higher still than child rates in ASD[8] (several studies report lifetime depression rates ranging from 50% to 77% in adults with ASD[28,29]), which provides context for the importance of recognizing and treating this issue at younger ages.
- Sex/gender: It is still unclear whether girls with ASD are at a greater risk for depression than are boys, in line with general population findings.[30] Studies suggest that girls with ASD are at equal, greater, or less risk of developing depression than boys with ASD.[13,27] With emerging data on more frequent nonbinary

interpretations of gender in youth with ASD, it will also be important to study how gender identity influences mood in this special population.[31]

- Intellectual and verbal ability: Individuals with lower ASD severity and average to above average IQ are at greater risk for depressive symptoms and suicidality.[8] This finding suggests that greater insight into their social difficulties might confer risk for depression, and/or depressive symptoms are more easily overlooked in individuals with lower verbal ability and intellectual disability.[27]
- Poor emotion regulation, and maladaptive coping strategies and/or thought patterns:
  - Children, adolescents, and transition-age youth with ASD have been reported to exhibit higher rates of negative self-perceptions (eg, guilt, shame, feelings of worthlessness), maladaptive coping strategies (eg, repetitive negative thinking), and perceived stress and inability to cope, all of which are associated with depression in the general population.[27]
  - Children with ASD who use adaptive coping strategies (ie, problem-solving, seeking social support) compared with those who engage in rumination and other maladaptive coping strategies appear to be at lower risk of depression.[32]
- Other psychiatric comorbidities: Depression is associated with the presence of additional psychiatric comorbidities, such as anxiety, in children and adolescents with ASD.[33]
- Social motivation: A desire to make meaningful connections paired with social communication impairments and negative social feedback in ASD could increase risk for depression.[34,35] In adults with ASD as a proxy, greater social interest was associated with loneliness,[36] and loneliness in turn has been associated with higher rates of depression and suicidality in individuals with ASD.[36–38]

External Variables that May Function as Vulnerability Factors for Depression in Autism Spectrum Disorder

- Socioeconomic status (SES): The limited research on SES and depression risk in ASD is inconclusive, with findings of no relationship or a significant positive relationship.[39–41]
- Social support: Adults with ASD who perceived greater social support and acceptance reported lower depressive symptoms,[42] whereas lower perceived social support and social satisfaction have been associated with elevated depressive symptoms.[38] The equivalent data in children are not known, but this suggested pathway may reasonably apply across the lifespan.
- Life stress/trauma: People with ASD tend to have higher rates of stressful life experiences, including stigma, bullying, and poor prospects for independence, employment, and romantic fulfillment.[43] Bullying and other stressful life experiences that were considered traumatic have been associated with depression in transition age youth and young adults with ASD in independent studies.[21,44]

DIAGNOSTIC EVALUATION OF DEPRESSION
Multimethod Multi-Informant Approach

Because diagnostic instruments for assessing depression in ASD have not yet been psychometrically validated, and given the diagnostic complexity due to symptom overlap, a multimethod, multi-informant approach is strongly recommended to assess symptoms across multiple contexts. This approach includes gathering information from the individual with ASD, parents, teachers, and other professionals. The psychiatric evaluation includes but it is not limited to assessing the following domains:

- Current and past psychiatric history, onset and phenotype of depressive symptoms, typical and atypical presentations, teasing apart overlapping symptoms between depression and ASD, presence of other cooccurring conditions
- Family history of affective disorders and other psychopathology
- Developmental history and current level of functioning
- Educational placement and supports
- Psychosocial history, which includes family functioning, trauma, and current stressful life events (eg, recent traumatic experiences, bullying, changes in the home environment, social support)
- Psychological and interpersonal functioning (eg, social interests, friendships, self-awareness of disability, isolation, recreational activities, ego strengths, self-attitude)
- Assessment of baseline behavior to determine recent behavioral changes and impact on functioning
- Medical history to rule out other conditions that may be contributing to depression (eg, anemia, hypothyroidism)
- Suicidal risk assessment
- Mental status examination

Special Diagnostic Considerations in Autism Spectrum Disorder

While conducting these assessments, clinicians are encouraged to keep in mind several factors that are unique to the diagnostic assessment in the ASD population. These factors include the following:

- Assessing symptom overlap between mood problems and autism (eg, irritability, sleep and eating problems, inconsistent eye contact, constricted affect, and social isolation) (see **Fig. 1**). Some symptoms may be part of the ASD, depression, or both. It is therefore important to carefully assess whether symptoms are new or are an exacerbation of baseline symptoms.
- Determining the validity of self-report: Social-communication deficits and inability to recognize and label emotions (ie, alexithymia)[45] may prevent individuals on the spectrum from identifying and expressing emotional states, causing depressive symptoms to be overlooked by family and clinicians.
- Using depression measures with caution: At this time, there is not enough evidence to determine if instruments designed for the general population may be valid to assess depressed mood in ASD.[46]
- Assessing for atypical presentations of depression in ASD (see **Table 1**).
- Evaluate for other comorbidities, particularly anxiety, gastrointestinal problems, seizures, and others known to cooccur with depression in ASD.[13]
- Screening for suicidality at every visit: Individuals with ASD are at high risk for suicidal thoughts and behaviors.[47] In addition to well-established suicidality assessment practices, it is important to gauge impulsivity and the repetitive nature of thinking about death or self-harm in patients with ASD.

TREATMENT OF DEPRESSION IN AUTISM SPECTRUM DISORDER

Development of evidence-based practices for treating depression in ASD is an ongoing and emerging area of research. Preliminary evidence indicates the effectiveness of adapted psychotherapeutic interventions from the general population to the ASD population. Medications for depression in typically developing youth can be also considered, although data are lacking for their use in ASD.

Clinicians are encouraged to consider the following when making treatment decisions:

- Use a multimodal approach that tailors the intervention to the patient's needs and interests (the authors refer readers to these detailed case studies[27])
- Use a multidisciplinary care team with coordination of services across relevant systems (ie, home, social, educational, and vocational environments)
- Coordinate treatment modality with patient's level of cognitive functioning and social-emotional insight

Fig. 2 presents therapeutic options with consideration of the patient's cognitive and verbal abilities and social-emotional insight. As noted in the bottom band of **Fig. 2**, all patients may benefit from healthy living behaviors that have been shown to ameliorate and prevent depressive symptoms for the general population. Approaches that rely less on meta-cognitive skills (eg, behavioral activation [BA]) may be better initial choices for minimally verbal or intellectually disabled patients with depression. Finally, cognitive behavioral and interpersonal therapies may be more appropriate for individuals with requisite cognitive, social, and emotional insight. Importantly, these treatment options are not equivalently evidenced-based and must be considered of potential utility on a case-by-case basis.

Psychotherapeutic Treatments

Recent evidence suggests that *cognitive behavioral therapy* (CBT) can be effective in treating children and adolescents with comorbid ASD and depression.[48,49] CBT approaches focus on helping clients identify and change common unhelpful thoughts and behaviors to encourage improvement in mood and overall functioning.[50] Modifications to CBT protocols for ASD populations (see Kerns and colleagues[51]) include incorporating or considering the following:

- Psychoeducation to increase the individual's understanding of the depression diagnosis as a descriptor for maladaptive emotional symptoms (eg, prolonged sadness), physical symptoms (eg, fatigue, aberrant sleep patterns), and social consequences (eg, social withdrawal and isolation), which helps to identify core skills for symptom improvement
- Hands-on interactive activities (eg, role-playing, games)
- Visual analogue scales (eg, fear thermometer)
- Technology (eg, using telephone applications to monitor daily mood)
- Parent and family involvement
- Group therapy to foster a community of social support and accountability and to help the adolescent transition from family-centered support to peer support

The well-validated depression treatment protocol known as *behavioral activation or BA*[52] also may benefit youth on the spectrum. People with depression tend to isolate themselves and withdraw from pleasant activities. Using BA, individuals work on modifying behavior to increase opportunities for rewarding and positive experiences, thus improving mood over time. With less emphasis on insight and cognitive work, BA might be considered a first-line treatment for patients with cooccurring intellectual disability and depression. In addition, BA may be particularly effective in the following circumstances:

- During transition periods (eg, moving, changing schools, transitioning into adulthood), because it provides structured activities to promote goal setting, to attain goals, and to mitigate tendencies for social withdrawal and isolation.[51]

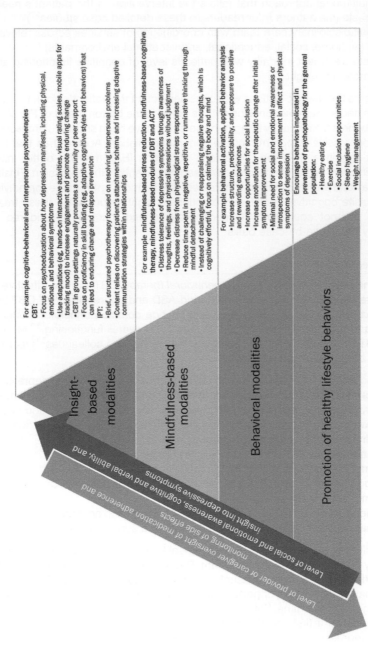

Fig. 2. Considerations in potential treatments for depression in ASD. These treatment modalities are neither equivalently nor thoroughly evidenced based at this point in time, particularly with regard to *youth* with ASD, and must be considered of potential utility on a case-by-case basis. ACT, acceptance and commitment therapy; DBT, dialectical behavioral therapy; IPT, interpersonal therapy.

- Patients with high levels of negative affect and minimal motivation for change. Increasing patient's access to rewarding experiences facilitates initial improvement in affect to provide hope and readiness to engage in other psychosocial interventions (eg, CBT).

Finally, some studies have provided support for *mindfulness-based interventions* in decreasing depressive symptoms in adults with ASD,[53,54] so results of child research on this modality are awaited. This approach is defined as being aware of thoughts, feelings, physical sensations, and experiences in the present moment, without judgment.[55] Through meditation exercises (eg, breathing, guided imagery, relaxation methods), patients learn to accept their feelings as a temporary state of mind, without overanalyzing the causes of their thoughts and emotions. Mindfulness interventions reduce maladaptive coping strategies, such as rumination, which is seen in ASD and in depressed individuals in the general population.[56,57] Although research is limited, mindfulness remains a promising treatment for reducing depression in ASD.

Psychopharmacological Treatments

Despite pharmacologic evidence supporting the use of selective serotonin reuptake inhibitors (SSRIs) for depression in typically developing youth,[58] evidence for their efficacy in children and adolescents with ASD is lacking. In fact, to date, there are no randomized controlled trials of antidepressant medications for the treatment of depression in children and adolescents with ASD. However, SSRIs are one of the most commonly prescribed classes of medications in individuals on the spectrum.[59] Existing studies examining the efficacy of SSRIs for other conditions (eg, repetitive behaviors) in youth ASD indicate high rates of BA (eg, impulsivity, aggression, disinhibition[60]; note that this is different from BA mentioned above as a therapeutic modality). Therefore, these medications should be prescribed cautiously for depression in youth with ASD with careful analysis of the risk/benefit ratio and close monitoring. Particular considerations when prescribing SSRIs include the following:

- Obtaining consent from the parent and from the individual with ASD if possible
- Eliciting a family history of bipolar disorder
- Starting with low doses and titrating slowly
- Routine monitoring of side effects, making every effort to elicit information from both the caregiver and individual with ASD
- Psychoeducation about medication side effects, with particular attention to providing parents with a clear plan about how to address BA and risk of mania should this occur
- Identifying objective treatment targets that can be tracked over time
- Establishing a timeline for assessing treatment efficacy, with a plan to taper and discontinue the medication if there is no benefit

SUMMARY AND FUTURE DIRECTIONS

Depression is common in youth with ASD, particularly for adolescents and those individuals with average or greater cognitive ability. Depression is associated with several negative outcomes, including functional impairments beyond those associated with autism itself and significant burden on the family system. Accurate screening and assessment of depression in people with ASD are complicated by uncertain validity of self-report, alexithymia and poor insight common to ASD, and overlapping symptoms between ASD and depression. Research is needed to elucidate the presentation of depression in people with ASD across age, gender, and ability ranges, in order to refine assessment practices for this commonly cooccurring disorder. In addition, identifying specific pathways to mood problems in this population will be important to understanding risk factors and contributing mechanisms, potentially informing targets for more precise and effective intervention.

REFERENCES

1. Ghaziuddin M, Ghaziuddin N, Greden J. Depression in persons with autism: implications for research and clinical care. J Autism Dev Disord 2002;32(4): 299–306.
2. Lainhart JE, Folstein SE. Affective disorders in people with autism: a review of published cases. J Autism Dev Disord 1994;24(5):587–601.
3. Mayes SD, Calhoun SL, Murray MJ, et al. Anxiety, depression, and irritability in children with autism relative to other neuropsychiatric disorders and typical development. Res Autism Spectr Disord 2011;5(1):474–85.
4. Simonoff E, Pickles A, Charman T, et al. Psychiatric disorders in children with autism spectrum disorders: prevalence, comorbidity, and associated factors in a population-derived sample. J Am Acad Child Adolesc Psychiatry 2008;47(8): 921–9.
5. Leyfer OT, Folstein SE, Bacalman S, et al. Comorbid psychiatric disorders in children with autism: interview development and rates of disorders. J Autism Dev Disord 2006;36(7):849–61.
6. Greenlee JL, Mosley AS, Shui AM, et al. Medical and behavioral correlates of depression history in children and adolescents with autism spectrum disorder. Pediatrics 2016;137(Suppl):S105–14.
7. Merikangas KR, He J, Burstein M, et al. Lifetime prevalence of mental disorders in U.S. adolescents: results from the National Comorbidity Survey Replication–Adolescent Supplement (NCS-A). J Am Acad Child Adolesc Psychiatry 2010; 49(10):980–9.
8. Hudson CC, Hall L, Harkness KL. Prevalence of depressive disorders in individuals with autism spectrum disorder: a meta-analysis. J Abnorm Child Psychol 2018. https://doi.org/10.1007/s10802-018-0402-1.
9. Magnuson KM, Constantino JN. Characterization of depression in children with autism spectrum disorders. J Dev Behav Pediatr 2011;32(4):332–40.
10. Stewart ME, Barnard L, Pearson J, et al. Presentation of depression in autism and Asperger syndrome: a review. Autism 2006;10(1):103–16.
11. Cadman T, Eklund H, Howley D, et al. Caregiver burden as people with autism spectrum disorder and attention-deficit/hyperactivity disorder transition into adolescence and adulthood in the United Kingdom. J Am Acad Child Adolesc Psychiatry 2012;51(9):879–88.
12. Joshi G, Wozniak J, Petty C, et al. Psychiatric comorbidity and functioning in a clinically referred population of adults with autism spectrum disorders: a comparative study. J Autism Dev Disord 2013;43(6):1314–25.
13. Menezes M, Robinson L, Sanchez MJ, et al. Depression in youth with autism spectrum disorders: a systematic review of studies published between 2012 and 2016. Rev J Autism Dev Disord 2018. https://doi.org/10.1007/s40489-018-0146-4.
14. Cassidy S, Bradley P, Robinson J, et al. Suicidal ideation and suicide plans or attempts in adults with Asperger's syndrome attending a specialist diagnostic clinic: a clinical cohort study. Lancet Psychiatry 2014;1(2):142–7.

15. Cassidy S, Rodgers J. Understanding and prevention of suicide in autism. Lancet Psychiatry 2017;4(6):e11.
16. Storch EA, Lewin AB, Collier AB, et al. A randomized controlled trial of cognitive-behavioral therapy versus treatment as usual for adolescents with autism spectrum disorders and comorbid anxiety: CBT for Adolescents with ASD and Anxiety. Depress Anxiety 2015;32(3):174–81.
17. American Psychiatric Association. Diagnostic and statistical manual of mental disorders: DSM-5. 5th edition. Arlington (VA): American Psychiatric Association; 2013. p. 2013.
18. Charlot L, Deutsch CK, Albert A, et al. Mood and anxiety symptoms in psychiatric inpatients with autism spectrum disorder and depression. J Ment Health Res Intellect Disabil 2008;1(4):238–53.
19. Chandrasekhar T, Sikich L. Challenges in the diagnosis and treatment of depression in autism spectrum disorders across the lifespan. Dialogues Clin Neurosci 2015;17(2):219–27.
20. Gotham K, Brunwasser SM, Lord C. Depressive and anxiety symptom trajectories from school age through young adulthood in samples with autism spectrum disorder and developmental delay. J Am Acad Child Adolesc Psychiatry 2015;54(5): 369–76.e3.
21. Rai D, Culpin I, Heuvelman H, et al. Association of autistic traits with depression from childhood to age 18 years. JAMA Psychiatry 2018;75(8):835–43.
22. Bolton PF, Pickles A, Murphy M, et al. Autism, affective and other psychiatric disorders: patterns of familial aggregation. Psychol Med 1998;28(2):385–95.
23. Cross-Disorder Group of the Psychiatric Genomics Consortium. Identification of risk loci with shared effects on five major psychiatric disorders: a genome-wide analysis. Lancet 2013;381(9875):1371–9.
24. Muller CL, Anacker AMJ, Veenstra-VanderWeele J. The serotonin system in autism spectrum disorder: from biomarker to animal models. Neuroscience 2016;321:24–41.
25. Frick LR, Williams K, Pittenger C. Microglial dysregulation in psychiatric disease. Clin Dev Immunol 2013;2013:1–10.
26. Dichter GS, Damiano CA, Allen JA. Reward circuitry dysfunction in psychiatric and neurodevelopmental disorders and genetic syndromes: animal models and clinical findings. J Neurodev Disord 2012;4(1). https://doi.org/10.1186/1866-1955-4-19.
27. Gotham K, Pezzimenti F, Eydt-Beebe M, et al. Co-occurring mood problems in autism spectrum disorder. In: White S, Mazefsky C, Maddox B, editors. The Oxford Handbook of Psychiatric Comorbidity in Autism. Oxford, UK: Oxford University Press; In press.
28. Lugnegård T, Hallerbäck MU, Gillberg C. Psychiatric comorbidity in young adults with a clinical diagnosis of Asperger syndrome. Res Dev Disabil 2011;32(5): 1910–7.
29. Gotham K, Siegle G, Han G, et al. Pupil response to social-emotional materials is associated with rumination and depressive symptoms in adults with autism spectrum disorder. PLoS One 2018;13(8):e0200340.
30. Hankin BL, Abramson LY, Moffitt TE, et al. Development of depression from pre-adolescence to young adulthood: emerging gender differences in a 10-year longitudinal study. J Abnorm Psychol 1998;107(1):128–40.
31. van Schalkwyk GI, Klingensmith K, Volkmar FR. Gender identity and autism spectrum disorders. Yale J Biol Med 2015;88(1):81–3.

32. Rieffe C, De Bruine M, De Rooij M, et al. Approach and avoidant emotion regulation prevent depressive symptoms in children with an Autism Spectrum Disorder. Int J Dev Neurosci 2014;39:37–43.
33. Vasa RA, Kalb L, Mazurek M, et al. Age-related differences in the prevalence and correlates of anxiety in youth with autism spectrum disorders. Res Autism Spectr Disord 2013;7(11):1358–69.
34. Meyer JA, Mundy PC, Van Hecke AV, et al. Social attribution processes and co-morbid psychiatric symptoms in children with Asperger syndrome. Autism 2006; 10(4):383–402.
35. Sterling L, Dawson G, Estes A, et al. Characteristics associated with presence of depressive symptoms in adults with autism spectrum disorder. J Autism Dev Disord 2008;38(6):1011–8.
36. Han GT, Tomarken AJ, Gotham KO. Social and non-social reward moderate the relation between autism symptoms and loneliness in adults with ASD, depression, and controls. Autism Res 2019. [Epub ahead of print].
37. Mazurek MO. Loneliness, friendship, and well-being in adults with autism spectrum disorders. Autism 2014;18(3):223–32.
38. Hedley D, Uljarević M, Foley K-R, et al. Risk and protective factors underlying depression and suicidal ideation in Autism Spectrum Disorder. Depress Anxiety 2018;35(7):648–57.
39. Gray K, Keating C, Taffe J, et al. Trajectory of behavior and emotional problems in autism. Am J Intellect Dev Disabil 2012;117(2):121–33.
40. Midouhas E, Yogaratnam A, Flouri E, et al. Psychopathology trajectories of children with autism spectrum disorder: the role of family poverty and parenting. J Am Acad Child Adolesc Psychiatry 2013;52(10):1057–65.e1.
41. Taylor JL, Seltzer MM. Changes in the autism behavioral phenotype during the transition to adulthood. J Autism Dev Disord 2010;40(12):1431–46.
42. Cage E, Di Monaco J, Newell V. Experiences of autism acceptance and mental health in autistic adults. J Autism Dev Disord 2018;48(2):473–84.
43. Henninger NA, Taylor JL. Outcomes in adults with autism spectrum disorders: a historical perspective. Autism 2013;17(1):103–16.
44. Taylor JL, Gotham KO. Cumulative life events, traumatic experiences, and psychiatric symptomatology in transition-aged youth with autism spectrum disorder. J Neurodev Disord 2016;8(1). https://doi.org/10.1186/s11689-016-9160-y.
45. Bird G, Cook R. Mixed emotions: the contribution of alexithymia to the emotional symptoms of autism. Transl Psychiatry 2013;3(7):e285.
46. Cassidy SA, Bradley L, Bowen E, et al. Measurement properties of tools used to assess depression in adults with and without autism spectrum conditions: a systematic review. Autism Res 2018;11(5):738–54.
47. Horowitz LM, Thurm A, Farmer C, et al. Talking about death or suicide: prevalence and clinical correlates in youth with autism spectrum disorder in the psychiatric inpatient setting. J Autism Dev Disord 2018;48(11):3702–10.
48. Keefer A, White SW, Vasa RA, et al. Psychosocial interventions for internalizing disorders in youth and adults with ASD. Int Rev Psychiatry 2018;30(1):62–77.
49. Santomauro D, Sheffield J, Sofronoff K. Depression in adolescents with ASD: a pilot RCT of a group intervention. J Autism Dev Disord 2016;46(2):572–88.
50. Beck AT, Rush AJ, editors. Cognitive therapy of depression. New York: Guilford Press; 1979. 13. Print.
51. Kerns CM, Roux AM, Connell JE, et al. Adapting cognitive behavioral techniques to address anxiety and depression in cognitively able emerging adults on the autism spectrum. Cogn Behav Pract 2016;23(3):329–40.

52. Jacobson NS, Martell CR, Dimidjian S. Behavioral activation treatment for depression: returning to contextual roots. Clin Psychol Sci Pract 2006;8(3):255–70.
53. Spek AA, van Ham NC, Nyklíček I. Mindfulness-based therapy in adults with an autism spectrum disorder: a randomized controlled trial. Res Dev Disabil 2013; 34(1):246–53.
54. Sizoo BB, Kuiper E. Cognitive behavioural therapy and mindfulness based stress reduction may be equally effective in reducing anxiety and depression in adults with autism spectrum disorders. Res Dev Disabil 2017;64:47–55.
55. Kabat-Zinn J. Mindfulness-based interventions in context: past, present, and future. Clin Psychol Sci Pract 2003;10:144–56.
56. Hayes SC. Acceptance and commitment therapy, relational frame theory, and the third wave of behavioral and cognitive therapies. Behav Ther 2004;35(4):639–65.
57. Jain S, Shapiro SL, Swanick S, et al. A randomized controlled trial of mindfulness meditation versus relaxation training: effects on distress, positive states of mind, rumination, and distraction. Ann Behav Med 2007;33(1):11–21.
58. March J, Silva S, Petrycki S, et al. Fluoxetine, cognitive-behavioral therapy, and their combination for adolescents with depression: treatment for adolescents with depression study (TADS) randomized controlled trial. JAMA 2004;292(7): 807–20.
59. Houghton R, Ong RC, Bolognani F. Psychiatric comorbidities and use of psychotropic medications in people with autism spectrum disorder in the United States. Autism Res 2017;10(12):2037–47.
60. King BH, Hollander E, Sikich L, et al. Lack of efficacy of citalopram in children with autism spectrum disorders and high levels of repetitive behavior: citalopram ineffective in children with autism. Arch Gen Psychiatry 2009;66(6):583–90.

Depression in Deaf and Hard of Hearing Youth

Jana Dreyzehner, MD[a],*, Karen A. Goldberg, MD[b]

KEYWORDS

- Deafness • Hard of hearing • Depression • Mental health • Children

KEY POINTS

- Factors important to consider in deafness that may increase risk of depression include language and communicative functioning, individual and familial stresses, and adverse experiences.
- A primary goal for clinicians in the evaluation and management of deaf children is to minimize language barriers during the assessment and treatment process.
- Interventions building psychosocial skills, including communication and emotion regulation skills, are needed to decrease the risk of depression in deaf and hard of hearing individuals.

INTRODUCTION

The prevalence of depression in deaf and hard of hearing (DHH) youth has been difficult to ascertain with certainty. Screening measures used for hearing youth may underrepresent or overrepresent rates of depression in DHH because of differences in language acquisition and expression among deaf youth. Most measures to assess depression in DHH youth have been normed among hearing youth, further complicating the ability to accurately determine prevalence of depression in DHH youth.[1] Despite the challenges, prior studies have used routine screening measures and have found that DHH youth are more at risk for depression than their hearing counterparts.[1–5] Van Eldik and colleagues[4] found that DHH youth were 2 to 4 times more likely to show internalizing problems on the Child Behavior Checklist, including depressive symptoms. Fellinger and colleagues[5] used the structured diagnostic interview measure (Kinder-DIPS) and found that 26% of the DHH youth met criteria for clinical depression. This increase in vulnerability to mental distress likely stems from communicative barriers in a hearing world and adverse experiences related to stigma and discrimination.[5,6] According to the National Association for the Deaf (NAD) position

Disclosures: None.
[a] Life Connect Health, Tennessee School for the Deaf, Knoxville, TN, USA; [b] Behavioral Health Services, eQHealth Solutions, 5802 Benjamin Center Drive, Suite 105, Tampa, FL 33634, USA
* Corresponding author. 415 Church Street #2802, Nashville, TN 37219.
E-mail address: DrD@LifeConnectHealth.com

Child Adolesc Psychiatric Clin N Am 28 (2019) 411–419
https://doi.org/10.1016/j.chc.2019.02.011
1056-4993/19/© 2019 Elsevier Inc. All rights reserved.

statement on mental health services for deaf children (2008), DHH youth are subject to increased risks and barriers to mental health because of language barriers and overall inadequacy of the mental health system to address the unique needs of deaf children.[7] The position statement asserts that "mental health services should be made culturally affirmative and linguistically accessible to deaf children...regardless of mode of communication."[7]

There are a variety of factors specific to or important to consider in deafness that may contribute to the increased risk of depression and must be considered in the assessment and treatment of DHH youth. Rates of emotional and behavioral problems in DHH youth are about 2 times higher than in their hearing peers.[3,5] Language and developmental deficits contribute to behavioral and psychosocial difficulties. When language level, signed or spoken, is high, psychosocial difficulties are no more frequent for DHH than for hearing individuals.[8] Fellinger and colleagues,[5] relating this to the language and communication environment of the family, found that deaf children who could not make themselves understood in the family were 4 times more likely to be affected by mental health disorders than those from families who successfully communicate. In contrast, DHH youth from families in which early communication is good are likely to develop rich psychological resources and perceived quality of life, generally decreasing the risk of depression.[9]

In addition to language and communicative functioning as factors affecting risk of depression, adverse childhood experiences must also be considered. Childhood adverse experiences increasing risk of depression include maternal depression and other forms of or reactions to parental stress, including sexual or physical abuse, and feeling ostracized from the family if unable to communicate needs or be understood.[10,11] Because greater than 90% of DHH children are born to hearing parents without previous experience of deafness, many families experience considerable emotional distress with a new diagnosis of deafness in a child. This distress includes feelings of grief, guilt, anger, depression, and feeling overwhelmed and unprepared to care for a deaf child.[12] Only about 25% of hearing parents of a deaf child whose preferred communication is sign language regard their competence in sign language as good.[13] DHH children whose parents do not obtain competency in sign language may experience isolation and impoverished communication and language development and the relationship with their parents may suffer, all potentially increasing the risk of depression.[12,14]

In addition, studies by Bess and colleagues[15] showed DHH children's increased stress levels as indicated by increased cortisol levels at awakening. This pattern is consistent with adults experiencing burnout, a condition characterized by fatigue, loss of energy, and poor coping skills. This condition may suggest a physiologic need to mobilize energy promptly, in preparation for the new day, increasing risk of fatigue and concentration problems.[15] The intuitive assumption that DHH children are at increased risk for hearing-related fatigue and associated effects on concentration, energy, and potentially mood and social interactions has long been supported by anecdotal reports from parents and teachers, and self-reports from persons with hearing loss.[16–18]

ASSESSMENT

The evaluation and management of deaf children is intimately related to the child's communication, and a primary goal for clinicians is to minimize the language barriers during the assessment and treatment process.[19,20]

Special considerations in interacting with deaf patients:

- Using the general techniques of child psychiatry interviewing, clinicians should be prepared to function within the child's preferred mode of communication. This approach requires learning the child's preferred communicative approach before the assessment. A multi-informant approach including input from parents, teachers, and others with significant data on background history and communication mode preference may be essential. If visual or additional challenges are present, any augmentative communication devices used in classroom or daily life should also be made available during the assessment.[2,10,20]
- Plan for extra time for the assessment, knowing that good communication with deaf patients requires more time than with hearing patients because of large communication and education needs.[10]
- Deaf children rely on visual communication in addition to the use of any residual or augmented hearing, so attention to the lighting and ambient sounds is important. Having clinicians well lit without a bright light or window behind them avoids creating shadows or eyestrain. Avoidance of competing background noises, such as other voices, air conditioners, or echoing or reverberating sound in larger rooms without carpeting, is important in facilitating communication and attention.
- If sign language is preferred, a qualified professional sign language interpreter must be engaged rather than using a parent or family member to communicate for the child to allow the child to communicate confidentially and, if needed, to be reverse voice interpreted accurately without coming through a parent filter. An interpreter with experience in children's mental health is preferable, and ideally an interpreter who both knows and is known to the child, because deaf patients report fear, mistrust, and frustration in health-care settings and do appreciate efforts from providers to improve communication.[10]
- Even if an interpreter is being used, it is important for the clinician to engage the patient warmly and directly, making eye contact with and speaking directly to the child rather than to the interpreter. Speaking to and making eye contact with the interpreter directly may alienate the child. Side conversations with the interpreter are also signed to the deaf individual because professional interpreters do not step out of the interpreting role to make personal commentary. Thus, attempted side conversations generally add to confusion and mistrust that the hearing clinician is talking behind the deaf persons back.
- Making eye contact as often and for as long as possible is helpful because deaf culture tends to place a great deal of emphasis on eye contact. Glickman[21] (1996) found that clients who are deaf generally held eye contact for a full 5 seconds compared with 1 second for hearing clients.
- Positioning the interpreter beside the clinician provides an unobstructed view of both clinician and interpreter for the deaf person and facilitates the direct eye contact between the clinician and patient.
- Attention to one's own nonverbal behavior is important.[22] Making it clear to the deaf patient when eye contact and focus need to shift away during the assessment, such as to write or to look at a computer, adds to understanding and trust because the deaf person is better able to anticipate what is coming. It is helpful to be aware that it is difficult for deaf people to attend to simultaneous speech and action while moving about, such as talking while examining a patient or preparing materials. Communicating first, then acting, promotes comprehension and avoids unnecessary anxiety.[10]

- Gaining the child's attention before speaking or eliciting joint attention is helpful. The recommended strategies are also those commonly used by deaf mothers, which studies show are most successful in promoting communication and language development in deaf children. These strategies include gaining the child's attention using the child's preference of visual (moving or waving hands) or tactile signals (touching physically) and waiting to obtain the child's visual attention before signing or communicating.[23]
- Awareness of the limitations of lip reading is also important. Even good speech readers understand only a limited percentage of the mouth and lip formations without additional cues. Lip reading accuracy has ranged in studies from 12.4% to 30%,[24,25] and requires constant concentration and some guessing on the part of the speech reader. To help with the limited effectiveness and fatigue involved with lip reading, clinicians may add clear visual elements to the discourse, such as writing notes, using gestures, and the use of drawings and visual aids. Using simple language and short sentences but speaking at a natural volume and speed is most helpful. Speaking at louder than a natural volume or too slowly can distort the sound and lip and mouth movements, making speech reading more difficult.[2,10]
- Meaningful communication requires comprehension. Assessing for comprehension with a deaf person is best accomplished by requesting that the person summarize some essential points. Asking whether the person understands is not effective because a head nod might not mean comprehension.[10]
- Be aware that language problems and associated developmental deficits and behavior problems may make individuals appear more ill than they really are.[8] Because language and cognitive functioning are greatly affected by prelingual hearing loss, mental status examination of deaf patients requires understanding of communicative behavior differences such as occur in healthy deaf people and differentiation between the effects of any restricted language proficiency and various mental or neurologic disorders.[10]

Some dimensions of the mental status examination affected by deafness and use of visual language during assessment include appearance, affect, thought, and cognition.[10] A person using animated gestures and facial expressions may give a misleading appearance of being agitated to a clinician unfamiliar with sign language and how facial expressions serve specific linguistic functions. Language deficits may be mistaken as thought disorder. Aspects in the domain of cognition that may show differences in individuals who are deaf include attention, alertness, and visuospatial functioning.[26,27] There are neurodevelopmental differences that must be considered during assessment of the deaf child so as not to apply the same expectations for attention and vigilance as the clinician may to a hearing child. There are differences specifically in the neural systems important in the perception of visual motion and in visual attention. Bavelier and colleagues[27] found an enhancement of peripheral processing of motion stimuli in deaf signers that is not present in hearing native signers, indicating that deafness, rather than signing, is the source of the effect. Deaf signers are faster than hearing controls at reorienting their attention to new incoming information, supporting the finding that, in the absence of using hearing to monitor extrapersonal space, deaf individuals devote greater processing resources to monitoring of the peripheral visual field. Abrupt motion onsets in that periphery efficiently recruit orienting mechanisms to quickly reorient attention.[27]

Consideration of these neurologic system differences during evaluation of the deaf child provides important context, especially in assessing the ability to focus, sustain, and appropriately shift attention. It prepares the clinician to look at the environmental context and interactions. Learning more about the child's perceptions and functioning, rather than simply applying the typical criteria for symptom assessment, such as being off task for the symptom of inattention, is important. Without this context, these developmental differences and resulting behaviors are at risk to be misinterpreted and incorporated into potentially inappropriate diagnoses such as attention-deficit/hyperactivity disorder, psychosis, autism spectrum, posttraumatic stress disorder, and other mood disorders. For example, the enhancement of peripheral attention may be misinterpreted as inattention to a centrally located stimulus, such as eyes wandering rather than focusing on the task in front of the child, or defiance, the child choosing to not focus on the task when it appears the child is capable of sustained attention in some settings. The rapid shift of focus to a motion in the periphery could mimic repetitive visual fixations such as looking out of corner of the eye or stereotypy or visual self-stimulatory behavior. It can also be perceived as hypervigilance or hyperarousal, assuming an exaggerated state of awareness, or as paranoia, especially if the peripheral motion is created by another person. Sign language is a visual language that incorporates use of eye contact and direction of gaze and attention to indicate subject content. It is important to consider that deaf persons who communicate with visual language, who see a person in their periphery glance toward the deaf individual, may interpret that look as having been included in that person's thoughts or conversation. This point is in addition to the frequently held belief, often true, within the deaf culture that hearing people talk about them without signing so it is effectively behind their backs.

TREATMENT

A biopsychosocial wraparound approach is important in the treatment of depression in deaf and hard of hearing youth to properly assess and monitor needs and strengths and to support the youth with specific needs related to deafness in the school, home, and community environments. Psychotherapeutic approaches are important primary interventions and support any psychopharmacologic interventions. The use of psychotropic medications in combination with psychotherapy for the treatment of depression is similar to that in hearing youth for deaf or hard of hearing individuals who have meaningful language and communication ability, but with the addition of specific cultural awareness and necessary adaptations for the clinician to operate in the individual's preferred mode of communication. However, for deaf youth with significant language deprivation and deficiencies in behavioral, social, and emotional adjustment, additional focus on the deficits is necessary.[8,20] Glickman[8] reports a greater tendency to use a medical model and treat symptoms of depression in this population with only medication, especially when various therapy modalities are not readily accessible. However, in "Lessons Learned from 23 Years of a Deaf Psychiatric Inpatient Unit," Glickman[8] cautions that medications are easily overused without efficacy. He notes that the pressures on clinicians toward treating these problems as if they resulted primarily from brain disorders, rather than from a lack of language and skills development, ignores what he conceptualizes as a language deprivation disorder.[8]

Effective treatment and management includes family therapy and supportive measures to empower and increase the confidence of the parents. It is important to identify and assist parents with resolution of their grief and/or anger. Unresolved grief and anger may manifest as maternal depression, which has been shown to negatively affect deaf children's future mood states and outcomes. Depressed mothers have been found to be less sensitive to their children's needs and less effective with nurturing language and psychosocial development in their children.[28] A strength-based approach in treatment is important in both providing hope for the parents as well as countering the historically disorder-based approach, which frames deafness as a defect contributing to lower self-esteem and self-concept than for hearing individuals.[21] An important consideration in being effective in treating children who are deaf and dependent on visual communication includes both the clinician and parents having an understanding and appreciation for the deaf culture because there are some members of the deaf community and their advocates who argue that their deafness is not a disability but rather their identity, and should be celebrated rather than fixed or grieved.[22,29] Multiple studies have found that the level of depressive symptoms in a child is unrelated to the degree of hearing loss.[1] Turning to state this in the positive, nurturing children who are happy and well adjusted does not depend on having a certain level of hearing.[13]

Many investigators have pointed to the importance of focusing on the development of psychosocial skills, including communication and emotion regulation skills, in the prevention and treatment of depression in deaf and hard of hearing individuals.[1,13,26,30,31] Important in the family treatment is facilitation of communication and the relationship between the parent and child. Research has shown that difficulties in understanding basic communication with parents increases the likelihood of development of depression. When holding all other variables constant, depression was 8 times more likely to be reported in persons who retrospectively indicated they could understand little to none of what the same-sex parent said. Thus promoting healthy communication, especially between deaf and hard of hearing girls and their mothers and deaf or hard of hearing boys and their fathers, may reduce the later emergence of depressive symptoms.[14] Communication between deaf children and hearing parents tends to have shorter and less complex interactions, fewer questions, and less use of abstract concepts having the effect of impoverishing communication.[32] For many deaf and hard of hearing children, this impoverished communication may contribute to difficulty labeling and articulating experiences and emotional state, which has been identified as one of the factors leading to gaps in social-emotional development.[33] Communication is enhanced by intentionally including the child in the day-to-day occurrences of the family, which includes labeling not only things but also feelings and emotions. It takes extra time to stop the flow of conversation and explain to deaf youth what just occurred and to include them in the resulting emotional reactions, but this type of parental involvement, emotional availability, and effective communicative interaction has been found to be a powerful predictor of language development.[34,35]

In addition, focusing on development of adequate coping strategies is important because proficiency with these strategies seems to have a direct relationship with the level of depression reported in deaf and hard of hearing youth.[1] Fellinger and colleagues[13] emphasized the need for supporting deaf children in educational settings with earlier identification and therapy for those at risk for mental disorders. Several psychotherapy models have adaptations described for deaf and hard of hearing persons, including cognitive-behavior therapy, dialectical behavioral therapy (DBT), and solution-focused brief and constructionist therapies.[10,36–38] An adaptation of the DBT Skills System for deaf persons with comorbid intellectual and developmental disability is underway using the DBT informed approach.[39] However, clinicians experienced in these adaptations are not accessible to many deaf individuals in need. Use of telehealth and telepsychiatry can improve accessibility for some and is generally well accepted when done in a culturally and linguistically competent manner.[10] Additional attention, research, and resources are needed to support children and their families early on to reduce the impact associated with deafness and to improve prevention and treatment of depression in this vulnerable population.

REFERENCES

1. Bozzay M, O'Leary K, De Nadia A, et al. Adolescent depression: differential symptom presentations in deaf and hard-of-hearing youth using the patient health questionnaire-9. J Deaf Stud Deaf Educ 2017;22(2):195–203.
2. Theunissen S, Rieffe C, Kouwenberg M, et al. Depression in hearing-impaired children. Int J Pediatr Otorhinolaryngol 2011;75:1313–7.
3. Van gent T, Goedhart A, Hindley P, et al. Prevalence and correlates of psychopathology in a sample of deaf adolescents. J Child Psychol Psychiatry 2007;48: 950–8.
4. Van Eldik T, Treffers P, Veerman J, et al. Mental health problems of deaf Dutch children as indicated by parents' responses to the child behavior checklist. Am Ann Deaf 2004;148:390–5.
5. Fellinger J, Holzinger D, Sattel H, et al. Correlates of mental health disorders among children with hearing impairments. Dev Med Child Neurol 2009;51: 635–41.
6. Kvam M, Loeb M, Tambs K. Mental health in deaf adults: symptoms of anxiety and depression among hearing and deaf individuals. J Deaf Stud Deaf Educ 2007;12:1.
7. National Association of the Deaf position statement on mental health services for deaf children. 2008. Available at: https://www.nad.org/about-us/position-statements/position-statement-on-mental-health-services-for-deaf-children/. Accessed January 14, 2019.
8. Glickman N. Lessons learned from 23 years of a deaf psychiatric inpatient unit: part 1. J Am Deaf Rehab 2010;44:225–42.
9. Hintermair M. Self-esteem and satisfaction with life of deaf and hard-of-hearing people- a resource-oriented approach to identity work. J Deaf Stud Deaf Educ 2008;13:278–300.
10. Fellinger J, Holzinger D, Pollard R. Mental health of deaf people. Lancet 2012; 379:17–23.
11. Felitti V, Anda R, Nordenberg D, et al. Relationship of childhood abuse and household dysfunction to many of the leading causes of death in adults. Am J Prev Med 1998;14:245–58.
12. Aranda B, Sleeboom-Van Raaij I. Mental health services for deaf people: treatment advances, opportunities and challenges. Washington, DC: Gallaudet University Press; 2015.
13. Fellinger J, Hozinger D, Sattel H, et al. Mental health and quality of life in deaf pupils. Eur Child Adolesc Psychiatry 2008;17(7):414–23.
14. Kushalnagar P, Bruce S, Sutton T, et al. Retrospective basic parent-child communication difficulties and risk of depression deaf adults. J Dev Phys Disabil 2017; 29(1):25–34.
15. Bess F, Gustafson S, Corbett B, et al. Salivary cortisol profiles of children with hearing loss. Ear Hear 2015;37(3):334–44.
16. Bess F, Hornsby B. Commentary: listening can be exhausting-fatigue in children and adults with hearing loss. Ear Hear 2014;35:592–9.

17. Bess F, Dodd-Murphy J, Parker R. Children with minimal sensorineural hearing loss: prevalence, educational performance, and functional status. Ear Hear 1998;19:339–54.

18. Griswold M. Take five! the importance of listening breaks for students with hearing loss. Mainstream News 2015;34:1–3.

19. Mathos K, Broussard E. Outlining the concerns of children who have hearing loss and their families. J Am Acad Child Adolesc Psychiatry 2005;44(1):96–100.

20. Goldberg K, Dreyzehner J. Psychiatric care of the deaf, blind or deaf-blind child. In: Martin A, Volkmar F, Bloch M, editors. Lewis' child and adolescent psychiatry: a comprehensive textbook. 5th edition. Philadelphia: Wolters Kluwer; 2017. p. 123–37.

21. Glickman N. What is culturally affirmative psychotherapy?. In: Glickman N, Harvey M, editors. Culturally affirmative psychotherapy with deaf persons. New York: Routledge; 1996. p. 1–55.

22. Peters S. Cultural awareness: enhancing counselor understanding, sensitivity, and effectiveness with clients who are deaf. J Multi Coun Dev 2007;35(3):182–90.

23. Loots G, Devise I. The use of visual-tactile communication strategies by deaf and hearing fathers and mothers of deaf infants. J Deaf Stud Deaf Educ 2003;8: 31–42.

24. Altieri N, Pisoni D, Townsend J. Some normative data on lip-reading skills. J Acoust Soc Am 2011;130(1):1–4.

25. Conrad R. The deaf schoolchild. London: Harper & Row Ltd; 1979.

26. Barker D, Quittner A, Fink N, et al, CDaCI Investigative Team. Predicting behavior problems in deaf and hearing children: the influences of language, attention, and parent-child communication. Dev Psychopathol 2009;21(2):373–92.

27. Bavelier D, Brozinsky C, Tomann A, et al. Impact of early deafness and early exposure to sign language on the cerebral organization for motion processing. J Neurosci 2001;21(22):8931–42.

28. Chaudhury S. Anxiety and depression in mothers of deaf children: awareness needed. Med J D.Y. Patel University 2014;7:720–1.

29. Andrews J, Leigh I, Weiner M. Deaf people: evolving perspectives from psychology, education and sociology. Boston: Pearson; 2003.

30. Grinker R, Vernon M, Mindel E, et al. Psychiatric diagnosis, therapy and research on the psychotic deaf. No. Research Grant number RD-2407-S. Washington, DC: US Department of Health, Education and Welfare; 1969.

31. Southam-Gerow M, Kendall P. Emotion regulation and understanding: implications for child psychopathology and therapy. Clin Psychol Rev 2002;22(2): 189–222.

32. Marschark M, editor. Raising and educating a deaf child. 2nd edition. New York: Oxford University Press; 2007.

33. Calderon R, Greenberg M. Social and emotional development of deaf children: family, school and program effects. In: Marschark M, Spencer P, editors. Oxford handbook of deaf studies, language, and education. New York: Oxford University Press; 2003. p. 177–89.

34. Moeller M. Early intervention and language development in children who are deaf and hard of hearing. Pediatrics 2000;106:1–9.

35. Yoshinaga-Itano C. From screening to early identification: discovering predictors to successful outcomes for children with significant hearing loss. J Deaf Stud Deaf Educ 2003;8:11–30.

36. O'Hearn A, Pollard R. Modifying dialectical behavior therapy for deaf individuals. Cogn Behav Pract 2008;15(4):400–14.

37. Estrada B, Beyebach M. Solution-focused therapy with depressed deaf persons. J Fam Psychol 2007;18(3):45–63.
38. Munro L, Knox M, Lowe R. Exploring the potential of constructionist therapy: deaf clients, hearing therapists and a reflecting team. J Deaf Stud Deaf Educ 2008; 13(3):307–23.
39. Brown J, editor. The emotion regulation skills system for cognitively challenged clients: a DBT-informed approach. New York: Guilford Press; 2015.

Depression in Medically Ill Children and Adolescents

Nasuh Malas, MD, MPH[a,b,]*, Sigita Plioplys, MD[c], Maryland Pao, MD[d]

KEYWORDS

- Depression • Pediatrics • Child • Adolescent • Physically ill • Medically ill

KEY POINTS

- Clinicians should have early awareness of depression in medically ill youth.
- Developmental, psychological, biological, and familial risk factors contribute to the unique presentation of depression in medically ill youth.
- Depression in this population can result from a primary depressive disorder, poor adjustment to medical illness, and/or directly from the medical illness.
- Multidisciplinary collaboration across all care settings, with awareness of potential bidirectional interactions between physical and mental health, is important in the care of depression in medically ill youth.
- Depression treatment in medically ill youth requires understanding of other unique medical and psychiatric needs of a given patient and being flexible to adapt care based on an evolving medical course, adjustments in medical treatment, and response to psychotherapeutic and pharmacologic interventions.

INTRODUCTION

Pediatric medical illness is increasing in developed countries and affects more than 25% of youth in the United States.[1] The increase is multifactorial and influenced by environmental toxin exposure, changes in lifestyle, dietary practices, psychosocial stressors, and advances in medical technologies.[1–3] Although most medically ill youth are resilient and function well, illness effects can worsen daily functioning, self-esteem, mood, and quality of life, with systemic impacts on family and schooling.[3–5]

[a] Department of Psychiatry, University of Michigan Medical School, Ann Arbor, MI, USA; [b] Department of Pediatrics and Communicable Diseases, University of Michigan Medical School, Ann Arbor, MI, USA; [c] Department of Child and Adolescent Psychiatry, Ann and Robert H. Lurie Children's Hospital of Chicago, Feinberg School of Medicine, Northwestern University, 225 East Chicago Avenue Box# 10, Chicago, IL 60611, USA; [d] Intramural Research Program, National Institutes of Health, National Institute of Mental Health, Clinical Research Center, NIH Building 10, CRC East 6-5340, MSC 1276, Bethesda, MD 20892-1276, USA
* Corresponding author. C.S. Mott Children's Hospital, University of Michigan Health System, 1500 East Medical Center Drive, UH South, F6315, Ann Arbor, MI 48109.
E-mail address: nmalas@med.umich.edu

Child Adolesc Psychiatric Clin N Am 28 (2019) 421–445
https://doi.org/10.1016/j.chc.2019.02.005
1056-4993/19/© 2019 Elsevier Inc. All rights reserved.

The relationship between medical illness and depression is bidirectional, with medical illness being a risk factor for depression.[4,5] Depression may increase treatment non-adherence, worsen physical disease, and lead to poor functioning, greater health care use, and increased school absenteeism.[3,6,7]

This article focuses on early identification, assessment, diagnosis, and management of medically ill youth with comorbid depression. It highlights specific considerations related to unique medical disease contributors to the presentation and management of depression with examples from common pediatric medical disorders in which depression is prevalent. The article highlights the importance of collaborative and integrative care while understanding the unique biopsychosocial factors influencing each child's presentation.

SPECIFIC RISKS FOR DEPRESSION IN MEDICALLY ILL YOUTH

Developmental Factors

The experience of medical illness and expression of depression is affected by the child's developmental stage (**Fig. 1**). Caution should be taken to not overidentify depressive symptoms in emotionally healthy youth with normative negative reactions to medical illness. However, vegetative symptoms accompanied by hopelessness, guilt, and low self-esteem need to be thoroughly evaluated for possible subsyndromal depression or major depressive disorder.

Preschool Age:
- Limited understanding of illness, care, and environment
- Often misperceive physical disease as punishment
- Respond to medical treatment with behavioral changes, increased irritability, tantrums, and defiance that may be short-lived
  - Prolonged symptoms with associated changes in child's mood, may suggest emergence of depression

School Age:
- Understand physical factors result in generation of disease
- May worry about bodily harm, loss of control of either their body or their environment
- Chronic worry can result in feeling overwhelmed and may progress to depression

Adolescents:
- More abstract and nuanced understanding of physical disease and relationship between physical and emotional health
- Experience uncertainty around emerging physical symptoms while undergoing diagnostic assessment
  - Can result in hypervigilance, somatization and psychological distress
  - Can be devastated by initial delivery of diagnosis with mixed emotions including disbelief, anger, sadness, anxiety and detachment

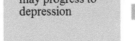

Fig. 1. Development factors influencing depression in medically ill youth.

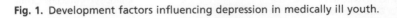

Biological Factors

Most medical illnesses have clinical manifestations that can mimic, overlap, or exacerbate depressive illnesses. Medications, particularly immunomodulators, anticonvulsants, antibiotics, anticholinergics, opioids, and benzodiazepines, can all directly affect the presentation of depression and should be carefully reviewed. Depressive symptoms can be a harbinger of emerging medical illnesses such as hypothyroidism, autoimmune encephalitis, anemia, catatonia, or delirium. The severity of medical illnesses is directly correlated with depression risk.[8,9] Depression can also affect medical illness course through direct neuroendocrine and inflammatory pathways.[8,10,11]

Psychosocial Factors

Medically ill youth with preexisting maladaptive coping, anxious temperament, poor self-esteem, poor premorbid functioning, history of trauma, and limited social supports have increased risk of depression.[8] Missed school and illness-related social isolation can generate a sense of loss, loneliness, and feelings of guilt or hopelessness. Medical illness can result in youth perceiving themselves as different or deficient. This perception can lead to avoidant behavior that diminishes further risk of anticipated emotional, psychological, or physical harm, which may result in rejection and a poor self-concept. Medically ill youth are also more likely to be bullied because of their physical appearance, functional limitations, or psychological vulnerabilities, which can perpetuate further physical and emotional insult.[12]

Family Factors

Medical illness can have dramatic effects on family functioning and result in disruptions in family life, loss of relational and financial stability, and impaired parenting. Primary caregivers can be particularly vulnerable to the distress of observing their child impaired or in discomfort.[5] The child's helplessness and worry can engender a variety of responses from the primary caregiver, ranging from avoidance to hypervigilance and overprotection. However, parents may underestimate the impact of physical disease on the child, and underreport the presence of depression. Similarly, parents often overfocus on the medical illness management and do not recognize changes in the child's mood. These strong emotions, coupled with physical exhaustion and difficulty juggling multiple competing roles, can result in caregiver burnout and increased risk of parental depression or anxiety.[13] Parents of medically ill youth have a higher prevalence of depression that further affects their parenting and emotional availability.[5] Furthermore, sibling well-being can be neglected while focusing of the care of medically ill youth, leading to increased family and sibling conflict.[14]

IDENTIFICATION AND ASSESSMENT

Astute clinicians have a high index of suspicion for depressive symptoms early and often in medically ill youth.

- Detailed understanding of medical disease course, medication use, and past medical experiences should be thoroughly explored.
- Prudent assessment involves obtaining information from multiple sources longitudinally, and strategic use of screening instruments.
- Important to engage child's primary care provider (PCP) and other subspecialists to understand direct and indirect influences of medical illness on child's mood.

Parents of medically ill children can have strong biases and misattribute emerging mood symptoms to medical illness or its treatment. Medically ill youth with depression may show greater somatization, poor insight, maladaptive coping, and habituation to responding to emotional distress through physical symptoms.[3,6] Therefore, the child's general clinical presentation and diagnostic conceptualization should be regularly reviewed and revised while incorporating new, relevant medical information.

Screening

Medically ill youth may be naive to discussions of their emotional and behavioral health in the medical setting. Routine depression screening can normalize conversations regarding depressive symptoms. Screening can aid in monitoring depressive symptom evolution and response to intervention over time. Several professional pediatric organizations recommend routine screening for depression in medically ill youth, particularly adolescents, including the American Academy of Pediatrics, American Academy of Child and Adolescent Psychiatry, International Committee on Mental Health in Cystic Fibrosis, American Diabetes Association, American College of Gastroenterology, US Preventive Services Task Force, American Diabetes Association, and the Child Neurology Society.[15–21] Several depression screening instruments are available that are well suited for use with medically ill youth (**Table 1**).

Differential Diagnosis

Depressive symptoms in medically ill youth can originate from 3 causes, either in isolation or more commonly in combination:

- Poor adjustment to medical illness
- Primary depressive disorder
- Medical illness, and/or treatment, directly inducing depressive symptoms

Establishing the relative contribution of these 3 sources to a child's mood presentation is important to diagnosis and management. Maladjustment and depression stemming from persistent difficulty coping with medical illness can lead to behavioral regression characterized by separation anxiety, treatment nonadherence, frequent deference to family, withdrawal from normal activities and routines, social avoidance, and dramatic displays of emotion and behavior.[3,15] Grief and traumatic loss in the setting of lost functioning or terminal illness can compound depression in medically ill youth.[26]

It is important to recognize difficulty with illness-related adjustment early to prevent progression to a major depressive disorder. Differentiation between adjustment disorder and primary depression can be challenging, requiring an exploration of past psychiatric history and the timing of mood symptom development. Poor self-esteem, hopelessness, anhedonia, guilt, suicidal ideation/behavior, and the pervasiveness of mood symptoms over time are more typical of primary depression, particularly if they precede a medical illness.[27] Negative emotions and behavioral changes specific to a medical illness burden also distinguish adjustment disorder from depression. Youth experiencing difficulties adjusting generally do not have underlying issues with self-esteem.[26] Poor adjustment and potential progression to depression is influenced by disease burden, cognitive effects related to disease, psychosocial supports, bullying and psychological trauma, as well as the ability of the child and family to balance the competing and parallel processes of grief and survival in chronic illness.[26] Family history of depression may also suggest current primary depression.[3]

Depressive symptoms can also arise from the direct pathophysiologic effects of medical illness and/or its treatment.[9,10] In these cases, depression onset is temporally associated with the medical illness development or its treatment.

Table 1
Depression screening instruments

Name	Description	Content (%)	Cost
Patient Health Questionnaire-9	Most commonly used screening tool in the pediatric medical setting because of easy completion and scoring	Sensitivity: 89.5 Specificity: 77.5	Free
Patient Health Questionnaire-2	Very brief, 2-question screen with greater sensitivity and less specificity for busy practice	—	Free
Children's Depression Rating Scale Revised	Focuses on specific symptoms of depression, helps in distinguishing primary depressive disorder from depression related to medical illness	—	$2.50 per scale, $76.00 for manual
Children's Depression Inventory	Anhedonia subscale can be useful in early identification of depression, and subclinical manifestations in medical settings	Sensitivity: 83 Specificity: 83	$3–4 dollars per scale, $92.00 for manual
Abbreviated Children's Depression Inventory	10-item version	Sensitivity: 93 Specificity: 70	—
Hospital Anxiety and Depression Screen	14-item self-administered instrument designed to minimize the symptoms that might be ascribed to somatic disorders such as dizziness, insomnia, and fatigue	—	Not free

Data from Refs.[22–25]

SPECIFIC MEDICAL ILLNESS CONSIDERATIONS

Summarized in **Table 2** are epidemiologic and risk factors, disease-specific evaluation considerations, and evidence-based depression management strategies for youth with common pediatric medical illnesses.

TREATMENT

Non-pharmacologic Interventions

Education of the child, family, and within interdisciplinary teams is critical early and often in managing depression in medically ill youth (**Box 1**). Building off routine education and communication, psychotherapy is fundamental to the management of depression in medically ill youth. It is particularly important given the value of adaptive coping and the potential intolerance to psychiatric medications in this population.

Providing psychotherapies in medically ill youth can be challenging. Mental health clinicians must be able to tolerate frequent disruptions to psychotherapeutic interventions caused by fluctuations in medical illness course, particularly medical hospitalizations, which can be chaotic and potentially traumatic.[101] This ability requires strong

Table 2
Specific considerations in the evaluation and management of depression in common pediatric medical illnesses

Disease	Prevalence of Depression (%)	Risk Factors	Evaluation and Management
Asthma	27–45[28,29]	• Need for regular asthma maintenance treatment, white race, tobacco smoke, poor family functioning, increased psychosocial stress associated with increased depression risk[29,33,34]	• SSRIs can alleviate depression and directly target asthma potentially through immunosuppression and anticholinergic regulation[35,36] • Asthma-related cholinergic dysregulation directly affects depression pathophysiology through downstream effects on neuronal nicotinic acetylcholine receptors[30,31] • Asthma and depression each independently associated with proinflammatory states with bidirectional impact[32]

Cystic fibrosis	8–29[13,37]	• 2–3 times greater depression risk than community with greatest risk in women, those with hemoptysis or pneumothorax in past 6 mo, comorbid anxiety, and parents with mental illness[13]
		• Depression associated with decreased lung function, lower body mass index, poor treatment adherence, worse quality of life, frequent hospitalizations, longer length of hospital stay, increased mortality following lung transplant, and increased health care costs[7,13,18]
			• Consensus statements for screening and treatment of depression published by The International Committee on Mental Health in Cystic Fibrosis, the Cystic Fibrosis Foundation, and European Cystic Fibrosis Society[18,38]
			  ○ Antidepressant medication, namely SSRIs, should be prescribed jointly with psychological interventions for moderate to severe depression
			  ○ To reduce drug-drug interactions, prescribers should be informed of all daily, cycled, or as-needed medications, including linezolid, an antibiotic that acts as a mild monoamine oxidase inhibitor and that should be used cautiously with SSRIs

Congenital heart disease	9–33[39,40]	• Depression risk increased with female gender, older age, poor social support, disease severity, lower IQ, low education level, presence of more than 1 cardiac defect, cyanotic disease, moderate to severe residual lesions, coexisting CNS abnormalities, and a history of more than 1 cardiac catheterization[39–42]	• Although there are no specific psychological interventions for this population, general psychotherapeutic intervention and SSRI use is safe and preferably provided in specialized, multidisciplinary service settings[43,44]

Epilepsy	22–35[45–47]	• Presence of depression results in more complicated epilepsy course[45–47] • Female gender, academic impairment, poor socialization, younger age at seizure onset and longer duration of epilepsy, unpredictability and high frequency of seizures, antiepileptic medications, and direct seizure effects on brain function[45,46] • Depressed youth with epilepsy have increased suicide risk compared with depressed physically healthy peers[45]	• SSRIs and SNRIs are safe and effective medications for treatment of depression[48] • Immediate-release bupropion has a higher risk for seizures (0.4%) than extended-release bupropion (0.1%) at total daily doses of 300–450 mg and should be avoided in this patient population[49]
DM	30[50]	• Adolescents with type 2 DM may be at higher risk for depression compared with type 1 DM[51] • Increased depression risk with disease chronicity, dietary restrictions, stigma, DM management regimen, and need for close family involvement increases risk of psychosocial distress and depression[50,52] • Depression can lead to worse glycemic control, treatment nonadherence, increased frequency and duration of hospitalization, and higher rates of diabetic ketoacidosis[53]	• Clinical course of early DM can overlap with depression, including fatigue, irritability, poor concentration, and psychomotor agitation • Early depressive symptoms may be attributed to DM symptoms, so youth with DM should be screened and monitored for depression early and regularly, particularly because youth with DM are at increased risk of suicidal ideation and self-injurious behavior compared with physically healthy peers with depression[52,54] • Depression treatment positively affects mood, glycemic control, and DM course[55] • Psychosocial interventions, namely CBT and supportive therapy, are effective in improving depression and hemoglobin A1c levels in youth with diabetes compared with treatment as usual or psychoeducation alone[55,56] • Fluoxetine and sertraline show improvements in glycemic control and depression[57] • Bupropion is promising in addressing both depression and glycemic control[55] • Cost-effective stepped care and multimodal collaborative interventions, such as the Pathways Intervention and IMPACT are available for youth with diabetes[55]

(continued on next page)

Table 2
(continued)

Disease	Prevalence of Depression (%)	Risk Factors	Evaluation and Management
Obesity	>35[58,59]	• Sleep disturbance, fatigue, apathy, and sedentary behavior have synergistic and compounding effects on the progression of obesity and depression[60] • Risk factors for depression are female gender, extent of body fat, HPA axis activation, increased cortisol level, and chronic stress[58,61,62] • Both depression and obesity promote relative systemic proinflammatory state with release of interleukin-6 and effects on HPA[60] • Obesity can result in lower quality of life, social difficulties and stigma, poor self-perception, suicidal thoughts and attempts, bullying, comorbid mental disorder, and depression in adulthood[61] • Emotional eating to cope with negative emotions and depression affects development of obesity[63]	• No current formal recommendations for evaluation and treatment of depression in obese youth[64] • National Institute of Mental Health 2009 report emphasizes need for increased study of associations and treatments in care of obese youth with depression[65] • Most recent expert guidelines for pediatric obesity published in 1998 are directed at PCPs and recommend use of Primary Care Evaluation of Mental Disorders questionnaire and Children's Depression Inventory for screening[64] ○ Recommends screening for depression and psychological intervention if identified. Recommendations affirmed in 2011 Expert Panel on Integrated Guidelines for Cardiovascular Disease in Children and Adolescents[66] • SSRIs can be effective in depression treatment but may increase abdominal obesity (OR = 1.4) and hypercholesterolemia (OR = 1.36) [67]
CA	Up to 33[68,69]	• Uncertainty in CA disease course and outcomes with lingering prospect of future morbidity and mortality increases risk for depression[70,71] • Depression leads to greater health care use, longer hospital stays, greater recidivism, and increased morbidity[11]	• Both CA and depression can present with poor appetite, weight loss, fatigue, low energy, amotivation, irritability, and insomnia[68] • CA pathophysiology and treatments can have direct impact on depression development[68,69] • Regular screening for early depression symptoms is recommended with well-validated approaches, including the Distress Thermometer and the PAT [72]

- Pediatric Preventive Psychosocial Health Model uses public health framework and uses PAT, which stratifies patients based on risk with matched treatment strategies[73]
  - Most families have temporary distress and minimal risk with sufficient resources to cope and adapt to disease
  - Smaller group of families are high risk and require multimodal, intensive, evidence-based treatments
- Psychosocial, psychotherapeutic, and pharmacologic interventions are efficacious in depression treatment in patients with cancer[74]
- Psychotherapy may be only therapeutic intervention needed for milder forms of depression
  - Psychoeducation, CBT, relaxation strategies, and problem solving are efficacious[75]
  - Supportive-expressive psychotherapy may aid in processing grief and loss in terminal illness[76]
  - Other beneficial evidence-based therapies include meaning-centered group therapy, dignity therapy, mindfulness-based meditation[77–79]
- SSRIs are effective in moderate to severe depression, or for those who do not respond to psychotherapy alone[74]
  - Depression treatment must be guided by limiting side effects and targeting comorbid somatic complaints such as poor appetite, disturbed sleep, fatigue, pain, and hot flashes
  - Sertraline, escitalopram, and citalopram have fewest drug-drug interactions and a low potential side effect burden[80]
- Second-generation neuroleptics, such as quetiapine or olanzapine, may be used for symptom palliation; eg, sleep and nausea respectively, mitigating delirium risk, and adjunctive depression management[81]
  - Requires caution because of potential adverse and long-term metabolic effects

(continued on next page)

Table 2
(continued)

Disease	Prevalence of Depression (%)	Risk Factors	Evaluation and Management
			• Mirtazapine can promote sleep regulation, reduce nausea, and improve appetite[81] • Stimulants can be used in palliative setting, or in youth without enteral access but who can tolerate transdermal medication transmission, to address depressive symptoms given their rapid onset of action[74] • Even after illness remission, depression risk is increased because of disruptions in daily life, family dysfunction, poor self-perception, disfigurement or disability, and worries about CA recurrence[71]
IBD	10–25[8,82–85]	• Illness-related effects, such as lifelong IBD course with frequent relapses, colonic resection and diverting ostomies, abdominal pain, physical discomfort, worsening inflammation, and sleep disturbances are risk factors for depression[8,82–86] • Depression risk most significant after IBD onset, with 5-fold increase in first year of disease onset compared with general population[85,86] • Little differentiation in depression risk between ulcerative colitis, Crohn, or mixed disease[86] • Loss of control and poor self-perception can lead to stigma and increased risk for depression[85,86] • Youth with hopelessness, tearfulness, and suicidal ideation have longer IBD duration, more ostomies, and greater pain[83] • Depression, maladaptive coping and heightened somatization worsen visceral hypersensitivity, abdominal pain, IBD disease activity, and are more predictive of physical symptom development than many medical variables[82,87]	• High risk of suicidal ideation and behavior with as many as 22% of subjects in 1 cohort endorsing lethality[82,83] • Treatment with steroids and immunosuppressants can worsen mood, increase fatigue, and disturb sleep, but can also improve depression through improvement in underlying medical illness[83,84] • Supportive therapy and CBT show significant reductions in depression and in IBD disease activity, leading to decreased hospital stay and use of intensive medical services and testing, with improved quality of life and adaptive coping, school attendance, and parental response to the child's physical symptoms[82,84] • SSRIs are safe in the treatment of depression[82]

Chronic pain and pain-related disorders	24[88,89]	• Particularly high risk in illnesses with prominent pain component (eg, SCD), in which prevalence of depression can be as high as 46%.[88,89] 　o Youth with SCD and depression have more acute vasoocclusive pain crises, acute chest syndrome–related visits, end-organ complications, greater health care use with higher SCD-related costs[89] • Pain causes considerable social and physical dysfunction, disruption to family interactions, and psychological distress leading to increased health use, disability, depression, and anxiety[90] • Pain-related impairment is associated with older pediatric age, multiple locations of pain, increased hospitalization, and presence of depression[88] • Level of pain acceptance, catastrophizing and other cognitive distortions, and functional disability all strongly correlate to manifestation of depression[91]	• Psychological therapies have moderate beneficial effects on reducing pain intensity, small benefit on pain-related disability, and variable benefit for depression, with particular benefits seen in youth with musculoskeletal pain and depression[90] • CBT, acceptance and commitment therapy are efficacious for pediatric chronic pain and depression in which pain impairment beliefs and pain reactivity are mediating psychological factors affecting treatment outcomes[90,92] • Dose-dependent psychotherapeutic improvements in headache are seen, whereas dose effects are not seen in other pain-related presentations[90] • Youth with SCD often receive suboptimal treatment of comorbid depression, with up to 80% never receiving antidepressant medication[89] 　o SSRIs more commonly used in this population, with SNRIs being used at an increasing rate for potential dual benefit in targeting neuropathic pain[89]
Transplant	35[93]	• Youth with liver transplant show worse total physical, emotional, social, and school functioning than healthy controls or peers with diabetes or cancer[94] • Poor medication adherence in solid organ transplant recipients associated with depression, anxiety, and posttraumatic stress[95,96] • Depression can worsen quality of life and adherence to immunosuppressive therapies, and result in youth engaging in high-risk behaviors directly affecting pretransplant and posttransplant course, including tobacco use, illicit drug use, poor adherence to dietary regimens, and poor exercise[97]	• CBT, social support groups, exercise, and music therapy are all beneficial in youth with end-stage renal disease and transplant[98] • SSRIs are safe with cautious dosing because of absorption and end-organ effects[98,99] 　o In liver failure, drug bioavailability may increase because of portosystemic shunting and doses may need to be decreased 　o In peripheral edema with increased volume distribution, dosages may need to be increased 　o Hepatic and renal metabolism may disrupt clearance of drugs, often requiring downward titration of dosing 　o Citalopram and escitalopram have least risk of drug-drug interactions, but carry higher risk of QT prolongation[99,100]

Abbreviations: CA, cancer; CBT, cognitive behavior therapy; CNS, central nervous system; DM, diabetes mellitus; HPA, hypothalamic-pituitary-adrenal; IBD, inflammatory bowel disease; IMPACT, improving mood promoting access to collaborative treatment; IQ, intelligence quotient; OR, odds ratio; PAT, psychosocial assessment tool; SCD, sickle cell disease; SNRIs, serotonin norepinephrine reuptake inhibitors; SSRIs, selective serotonin reuptake inhibitors.

Box 1
Core components to effective education in care for medically ill youth with depression

Youth
- Developmentally informed
- Collaborative
- Consistent
- Include relevant medical and mental health providers
- Provided in time and setting when child comfortable and safe
- Use pictures, models, play, and toys to assist education delivery
- Language should be concrete, simple, succinct, familiar, nonthreatening

Families
- Can deliver simultaneously or independently to family depending on nature and complexity of communications
  - Avoid communications with significant uncertainty with patient alone because these communications often need to occur with the caregivers first before delivering to the patient and family
- Gear familial education to literacy level, language, culture, and level of understanding of the family
- Routinely check for caregiver understanding of child's physical disease and emotional state
  - Important to assess caregiver understanding of impact of disease on child's physical, social, and emotional functioning

Interdisciplinary team
- Highly important but often missed
- Many members of care team may have limited or differential understanding of interactions between child's mental health and medical illness
- Can be valuable to have routine multidisciplinary rounds or case conferences
- Education is an important component of mental health consultation to the primary medical team
- Highly encouraged to have regular interdisciplinary education to improve awareness of the complex interplay between medical and mental health needs

---

collaborative communication between mental health and medical providers, as well as flexibility in mental health treatment structure, planning, and goals. The psychotherapeutic relationship may be especially important in reinforcing patient and family values in biopsychosocial treatments, as well as supporting end-of-life discussions when medical treatment is ineffective in stemming disease.[102]

Treatment recommendations for medically ill depressed youth need to be tailored to the individual child and family's needs. Clinicians first need to determine the depression severity and potential biopsychosocial contributors because these will inform the types of treatments recommended. Psychotherapeutic interventions should be provided early and often, even during diagnostic evaluations. Beyond the importance of psychotherapy for depression treatment in general, there is added importance in medically ill youth because psychopharmacologic interventions may not be indicated or tolerated because of young age, medical comorbidities, and/or serious drug-drug interactions.

In addition to addressing physical symptoms that may overlap with depression, stepwise psychotherapeutic approaches include supporting and building adaptive coping skills, psychoeducation, and recommending specific individual, familial, environmental, educational, and recreational supports. Nonpharmacologic interventions include teaching patients simple, concrete, and actionable behavioral strategies and coping skill activities targeting disease, pain, discomfort, and associated distorted cognitions, strong emotions, and maladaptive behaviors. This process usually involves challenging negative cognitive distortions that perpetuate pain or adverse experiences, thus promoting emotional self-regulation. These interventions can include deep breathing, muscle relaxation, and guided imagery.[103] Self-hypnosis and biofeedback to dampen aversive arousal can be particularly beneficial for youth with somatization and pain.[103,104] In medically ill youth, evidence is greatest for the use of supportive-expressive talk therapy and cognitive behavior therapies that include behavioral activation, problem solving, interpersonal therapy, and mindfulness-based therapy.[84,103,105,106]

Spirituality can be a powerful adaptive coping strategy in medically ill youth. Spiritual coping can be enhanced through hospital chaplaincy services or partnering with community-based spiritual resources.[107] Furthermore, family and marital therapy may be indicated given the nature of the chronic stress on the family system.[103] Addressing stressors, such as school difficulties, is an important component of depression management. Thoughtful, interdisciplinary, and collaborative communications between mental health providers, medical professionals, and school personnel can aid in limiting disruptions to schooling, easing transitions between school and health systems, and making strategic use of school-based and homebound instruction to enhance child autonomy, improve functionality, and preserve school engagement.[108] Psychotherapeutic interventions must comprehensively consider the whole person, family, school, and the community to mitigate the effects of physical disease on psychological health.

Pharmacologic and Somatic Treatments

There is a scarcity of randomized controlled depression treatment trials in medically ill youth because most studies exclude patients with medical illness. Psychiatric treatment is informed by standard depression treatment guidelines in children, evidence from the general pediatric population and medically ill adults, level 4 expert consensus publications, and clinical experience.[6,15–21,109]

Pharmacologic treatment: initiation, maintenance, and termination
Integrative primary care models for depressed medically ill youth have shown improvements in both physical and mental health outcomes.[110] Psychiatric care is needed when a patient shows recurrent or treatment-resistant depression; significant behavioral dysregulation, including life-threatening nonadherence; history of suicide attempts or ideations; substance abuse; other severe psychiatric comorbidities; or an unsafe family environment.

Approach to psychopharmacology in medically ill youth
- Careful evaluation of all home-prescribed medications, including over-the-counter, alternative, and dietary products.
- Polypharmacy should be avoided to reduce potential drug-drug interactions and mitigate risk for overdose.
- Barbiturates and benzodiazepines should be avoided, when possible, in severely depressed medically ill youth because of risk for serious respiratory and cardiovascular suppression.
- To monitor for drug-drug interactions, several pharmacologic resources and Web sites can be helpful in addition to individual medical institution–based drug databases and pharmacy consultation.
- Antidepressants should be started at low doses and slowly titrated to therapeutic effect.
  - Baseline laboratory tests are not routinely recommended before starting antidepressants but should be obtained when clinically relevant.

- Common laboratory and diagnostic testing with a fasting lipid panel, complete blood count with differential, electrolyte studies, thyroid studies, renal and liver function tests, and electrocardiogram may be considered.
- Reassess tolerability, safety, and response to intervention no more than 2 weeks after starting medication with follow-up every 2 to 4 weeks.[111]
- If failure to show improvement, further dose increases should take place at small increments every 2 to 4 weeks.
  - Provide enough time to evaluate effectiveness of dose adjustments.
- Adherence and tolerability to antidepressant must be assessed regularly.
  - Medically ill youth often struggle with compliance because of competing medical needs, poor oral intake, or worsening physical disease.[112]
- In treatment-resistant depression, conduct thorough review of biopsychosocial factors and their changes, including a diagnostic assessment reevaluation.

Further genotyping of cytochrome P450 genes may be used as part of a broader assessment.[113]

Selective serotonin reuptake inhibitors (SSRIs) are considered first-line treatment of medically ill youth with depression.[112] Although generic antidepressants are safe and effective, the pharmacokinetic bioequivalence of generic compounds ranges from 80% to 125% compared with brand-name drugs.[111] Thus, switching between brand and generic medication can change the efficacy or produce side effects, particularly in medically ill youth who may be more sensitive to these changes. There are no specific recommendations for the first-choice antidepressant because the differences between the individual medications are small.[111] Antidepressant selection should involve understanding patient-specific psychiatric and medical needs, past antidepressant experience, potential drug interactions, and prescriber expertise (**Box 2**).

There are no specific guidelines for the duration of antidepressant treatment in medically ill youth after achieving symptomatic remission, therefore general population treatment guidelines are recommended.[6,109] Antidepressant discontinuation should be gradual unless required otherwise by unfavorable medical illness course or its treatment. Abrupt discontinuation of antidepressants with shorter duration of action, particularly paroxetine, may be associated with a withdrawal syndrome characterized by flulike symptoms, insomnia, dizziness, paresthesias, tiredness, nausea, visual disturbances, abnormal movements, and headaches.[115] These symptoms

---

Box 2
Clinical pearls in psychopharmacologic management of depression in medically ill youth

- Patients with sleep disturbance may benefit from mirtazapine or trazodone, but beneficial sleep effects must be balanced against potential daytime sedation[111]

- Mirtazapine is frequently used in youth with cancer and cystic fibrosis because it can stimulate appetite, potentiate weight gain, has few drug-drug interactions, and is a 5-hydroxytryptamine receptor antagonist with antiemetic properties[81,114]

- In youth with pronounced pain, duloxetine or serotonin norepinephrine reuptake inhibitors (SNRIs) can be considered[81]

- Fluoxetine's long half-life and inhibition of cytochrome P450 2D6 make it less useful in medically ill youth[113]

- Stimulant medications, such as products based on methylphenidate or amphetamine, can improve motivation, energy, and appetite, especially in palliative care patients, because of their potentiation of opiate analgesics[81]

Table 3	
Side effect considerations in antidepressant treatment of medically ill youth	
Neurologic	• Seizure risk with antidepressant treatment very low (>0.1%)[116] • Seizure risk highest for clomipramine, then amitriptyline, venlafaxine, citalopram, sertraline, trazodone, mirtazapine, paroxetine, bupropion, and escitalopram[116] • Negligible seizure risk for fluoxetine and duloxetine[116] • Movement disorders, myoclonus, and extrapyramidal signs, particularly with abrupt discontinuation of treatment, reported with use of fluoxetine, paroxetine, fluvoxamine, and sertraline[117–119] • Dose-related, reversible frontal lobe–like amotivational syndrome, characterized by apathy, indifference, and disinhibition, has been reported in youth[120] • SSRIs can alter sleep architecture and quality[121] • Fluoxetine increases REM latency and suppresses REM sleep[121]
Hematologic	• SSRIs can inhibit platelet aggregation by altering platelet serotonin receptors, reduce platelet counts, and increase gastrointestinal bleeding risk[112] • Bupropion has least bleed risk, followed by SNRIs and SSRIs[122] • Bleed risk may be doubled with concomitant use of nonsteroidal antiinflammatory agents[123] • Antidepressants should be used cautiously with platelet disorders, thrombocytopenia, undergoing surgery, and in patients taking antiepileptic drugs • Recommended that platelet level be greater than 100,000 cubic milliliter of blood before initiating SSRI treatment[113]
Cardiovascular	• SSRI use, especially high doses of citalopram and escitalopram, should be carefully monitored in patients with arrhythmias, heart failure, and other cardiovascular disorders, because of dose-dependent QT prolongation and TdP[124] • TdP often idiosyncratic, and association with antidepressant dose and QTc prolongation remain unclear[125] • Sertraline has the least risk of QT prolongation of the SSRIs[100] • Caution should be taken in assessing for other agents that may prolong QT interval, electrolyte disturbances that may affect QT, and SSRI dose escalation in youth with history of prolonged QT
Metabolic	• Weight changes and fluid shifts affect serum drug concentrations, especially in patients with hepatic and renal insufficiency • Dosing adjusted according to patient's evolving weight and volume to prevent drug toxicity and subtherapeutic treatment[81]

Abbreviations: REM, rapid eye movement; TdP, torsades de pointes.

may be misinterpreted as worsening medical illness and lead to unnecessary interventions.

Neurostimulation treatment

Although rarely used, electroconvulsive therapy (ECT) can be an effective treatment of severe, life-threatening depression when more conservative treatments have been unsuccessful or when depression is associated with psychosis, unremitting suicidality, catatonia, neuroleptic malignant syndrome, intolerance of oral antidepressants, or rapidly deteriorating physical status.[128,129] ECT has been safely used in adults with medical illnesses, including central nervous system disease.[130] Pediatric data are still emerging but it seems promising as a potential treatment option in select cases.[129]

Repetitive transcranial magnetic stimulation has been effective in adults with epilepsy and stroke, but evidence-based data in medically ill youth are lacking.[131,132] Similarly, the evidence base regarding use of other neuromodulatory therapies, such as transcranial direct current stimulation, magnetic seizure therapy, vagus nerve stimulation, and deep brain stimulation, for depression in medically ill youth is just emerging.[133,134]

Special Considerations for Adverse Effects

Consultation with subspecialty pediatric providers may be warranted in youth at higher risk for specific side effects because of potential interaction between an antidepressant and medical illness or treatment (**Table 3**).

Serotonin syndrome/toxicity

Serotonin toxicity and adrenergic adverse effects have been reported in the concomitant use of SSRIs with other serotonergic drugs, including ondansetron, muscle relaxants, opioids, tricyclic antidepressants (commonly used for functional pain or headaches), and sumatriptan.[126] In particular, the antibiotic linezolid, a reversible monoamine oxidase inhibitor, is commonly used to treat patients with treatment-resistant gram-positive bacterial infections and leads to serotonin syndrome with concomitant SSRI use.[127]

LEVELS OF CARE

Integrated and collaborative care models provide opportunities for simultaneous care of medical and psychiatric concerns. The value of psychiatric consultation is significant and is associated with reductions in hospital length of stay and health care use in hospitalized medically ill youth.[135] Most medically ill youth with depression receive mental health care in outpatient settings. This care may be with their PCP, a mental health provider, or embedded as part of pediatric subspecialty care. The criteria for treatment of depression in medically ill youth in more intense outpatient treatment settings or inpatient psychiatric units are similar to those for youth without medical illness. In medically ill children, additional criteria that may warrant inpatient psychiatric admission include:

- Somatization resulting in severe impairment and decompensation in functioning
- Severe treatment nonadherence posing high risk of imminent harm
- Further diagnostic assessment for complex presentations with significant medical and psychiatric overlay

Care of medically ill children in the inpatient psychiatric unit requires access to medical staffing and acute medical support when needed, close communication with involved medical providers, and routine review of potential drug-drug and medical-psychiatric disease interactions.

The transition from higher levels of psychiatric care to less restrictive outpatient environments is equally important. Careful disposition planning is important to prevent recidivism and to coordinate care with multiple outpatient providers. PCPs, key pediatric subspecialists, and outpatient mental health providers should be contacted early during inpatient psychiatric admission and provided a summary report of the patient's stay. Partial hospital day treatment models, particularly with a family-based focus, allow for intensive intervention in complex pediatric illness in which clinicians can address family illness beliefs and relationships to improve health outcomes.[136]

OUTCOMES AND PROGNOSIS

Pediatric medical illness increases the risk of adult depression.[137] In a large systematic review and meta-analysis of 34 studies of 45,358 patients, there was an association of childhood chronic physical illness and adult depression (odds ratio, 1.31; 95% confidence interval, 1.12–1.54).[138] When separately assessing childhood medical illness by disease type, cancer, more than asthma or type 1 diabetes mellitus, is significantly associated with adult depression.[138] This finding is particularly relevant given increasing cancer survival in youth. Adult depression in the setting of previous childhood medical illness often presents with more intense symptoms and is more impairing than in the general population.[139] Psychosocial adjustment can also be impaired in adults who experience chronic medical illness in youth.[139] This impairment is compounded by missed developmental, academic, social, and work-related opportunities in youth with medical illness, which can cause increased purposelessness and lower functionality at the critical transitional period to adulthood.[140,141] Childhood depression also increases the risk of physical disease in adulthood, increasing risk of both physical morbidity and mortality.[137,142,143] Therefore, early identification and management of depression in medically ill youth, along with effective medical treatment, is important for future adult physical and emotional health.

SUMMARY

Medically ill youth are at higher risk of developing depression because of complex interactions between biological, psychosocial, developmental, and environmental factors. Early identification and prevention of depression require a proactive approach with early awareness, interdisciplinary collaboration, and a thoughtful diagnostic evaluation. Depression management is driven by a sound diagnostic formulation routinely revised based on emerging information regarding both medical illness and psychiatric symptoms. With a coordinated approach and an understanding of the delicate interface of physical disease and depressive illness, clinicians can ameliorate physical and emotional difficulties, enhance patient functioning, and improve quality of life during a critical period in their patients' lives and futures.

REFERENCES

1. Van Cleave J, Gortmaker SL, Perrin JM. Dynamics of obesity and chronic health conditions among children and youth. JAMA 2010;303(7):623–30.
2. Russell CJ, Simon TD. Care of children with medical complexity in the hospital setting. Pediatr Ann 2014;43(7):e157–62.
3. Maneta E, DeMaso D. Depression in medically ill children. In: Barsky A, Silbersweig D, editors. Depression in medical illness. New York: McGraw Hill Education; 2017. p. 325–34.
4. Pinquart M, Shen Y. Depressive symptoms in children and adolescents with chronic physical illness: an updated meta-analysis. J Pediatr Psychol 2011; 36(4):375–84.
5. Popp JM, Robinson JL, Britner PA, et al. Parent adaptation and family functioning in relation to narratives of children with chronic illness. J Pediatr Nurs 2014;29:58–64.
6. Birmaher B, Brent D, AACAP Work Group on Quality Issues. Practice parameter for the assessment and treatment of children and adolescents with depressive disorders. J Am Acad Child Adolesc Psychiatry 2007;46(11):1503–26.
7. Snell C, Fernandes S, Bujoreanu IS, et al. Depression, illness severity, and healthcare utilization in cystic fibrosis. Pediatr Pulmonol 2014;49(12):1177–81.
8. Clark JG, Srinath AI, Youk AO, et al. Predictors of depression in youth with Crohn disease. J Pediatr Gastroenterol Nutr 2014;58(5):569–73.

9. Kim J, Szigethy EM, Melhem NM, et al. Inflammatory markers and the pathogenesis of pediatric depression and suicide: a systematic review of the literature. J Clin Psychiatry 2014;75(11):1242–53.

10. Brzozowski B, Mazur-Bialy A, Pajdo R, et al. Mechanisms by which stress affects the experimental and clinical inflammatory bowel disease (IBD): role of brain-gut Axis. Curr Neuropharmacol 2016;14(8):892–900.

11. Smith HR. Depression in cancer patients: pathogenesis, implications and treatment (Review). Oncol Lett 2015;9(4):1509–14.

12. Pinquart M. Systematic review: bullying involvement of children with and without chronic physical illness and/or physical/sensory disability- a meta-analytic comparison with health/nondisabled peers. J Pediatr Psychol 2017;42(3):245–59.

13. Quittner AL, Goldbeck L, Abbott J, et al. Prevalence of depression and anxiety in patients with cystic fibrosis and parent caregivers: results of the International Depression Epidemiological Study across nine countries. Thorax 2014;69: 1090–7.

14. Incledon E, Williams L, Hazell T, et al. A review of factors associated with mental health in siblings of children with chronic illness. J Child Health Care 2015;19(2): 182–94.

15. DeMaso DR, Martini DR, Cahen LA. Practice parameter for the psychiatric assessment and management of physically ill children and adolescents. J Am Acad Child Adolesc Psychiatry 2009;48(2):213–33.

16. Forman-Hoffman V, McClure E, McKeeman J, et al. Screening for major depressive disorder in children and adolescents: a systematic review for the U.S. Preventive services Task Force. Ann Intern Med 2016;164(5):342–9.

17. Farraye FA, Melmed GY, Lichtenstein GR, et al. ACG clinical guideline: preventative care in inflammatory bowel disease. Am J Gastroenterol 2017;112(2): 241–58.

18. Quittner AL, Abbott J, Georgiopoulos AM, et al. International committee on mental health in cystic fibrosis: cystic fibrosis foundation and European cystic fibrosis society consensus statements for screening and treating depression and anxiety. Thorax 2016;71(1):26–34.

19. Siu AL. Screening for depression in children and adolescents: US Preventative services Task Force recommendation statement. Pediatrics 2016;137:1–8.

20. American Diabetes Association. Standards of medical care in diabetes 2016. Diabetes Care 2016;39(supplement 1):S1–12.

21. Hauser W, Moser G, Klose P, et al. Psychosocial issues in evidence-based guidelines on inflammatory bowel diseases: a review. World J Gastroenterol 2014;20:3663.

22. Richardson LP, McCauley E, Grossman DC, et al. Evaluation of the Patient Health Questionairre-9 Item for detecting major depression among adolescents. Pediatrics 2010;126(6):1117–23.

23. Nomura Y, Wickramaratne PJ, Warner V, et al. Family discord, parental depression, and psychopathology in offspring: ten-year follow-up. J Am Acad Child Adolesc Psychiatry 2002;41(4):402–9.

24. Allgaier A, Fruhe B, Pietsch K, et al. Is the Children's Depression Inventory Short version a valid screening tool in pediatric care? A comparison to its full-length version. J Psychosom Res 2012;73:369–74.

25. White D, Leach C, Sims R, et al. Validation of the hospital anxiety and depression scale for use with adolescents. Br J Psychiatry 1999;175:452–4.

26. Russell CE, Bouffet E, Beaton J, et al. Balancing grief and survival: experiences of children with brain tumors and their parents. J Psychosoc Oncol 2016;34(5): 376–99.

27. Benton T, Staab J, Evans DL. Medical co-morbidity in depressive disorders. Ann Clin Psychiatry 2007;19(4):289–303.

28. Safa M, Boroujerdi FG, Talischi F, et al. Relationship of coping styles with suicidal behavior in hospitalized asthma and chronic obstructive pulmonary disease patients: substance abusers versus non-substance abusers. Tanaffos 2014;13(3):23–30.

29. Lu Y, Mak KK, van Bever HP, et al. Prevalence of anxiety and depressive symptoms in adolescents with asthma: a meta-analysis and meta-regression. Pediatr Allergy Immunol 2012;23(8):707–15.

30. Van Lieshout RJ, MacQueen GM. Relations between asthma and psychological distress: an old idea revisted. Chem Immunol Allergy 2012;98:1–13.

31. Mineur YS, Picciotto MR. Nicotine receptors and depression: revisiting and revising the cholinergic hypothesis. Trends Pharmacol Sci 2010;31(12):580–6.

32. Shanahan L, Copeland WE, Worthman CM, et al. Children with both asthma and depression are at risk for heightened inflammation. J Pediatr 2013;163(5): 1443–7.

33. Ferro MA, Van Lieshout RJ, Scott JG, et al. Condition-specific associations of symptoms of depression and anxiety in adolescents and young adults with asthma and food allergy. J Asthma 2016;53(3):282–8.

34. Booster GD, Oland AA, Bender BG. Psychosocial factors in severe pediatric asthma. Immunol Allergy Clin North Am 2016;36(3):449–60.

35. Gobin V, Van Steendam K, Denys D, et al. Selective serotonin reuptake inhibitors as a novel class of immunosuppressants. Int Immunopharmacol 2014;20(1): 148–56.

36. Brown ES, Sayed N, Van Enkevort E, et al. A randomized, double-blind, placebo-controlled trial of escitalopram in patients with asthma and major depressive disorder. J Allergy Clin Immunol Pract 2018. https://doi.org/10.1016/j.jaip. 2018.01.010.

37. Garcia G, Snell C, Sawicki G, et al. Mental health screening of medically-admitted patients with cystic fibrosis. Psychosomatics 2018;59(2):158–68.

38. Iturralde E, Adams RN, Barley RC, et al. Implementation of depression screening and global health assessment in pediatric subspecialty clinics. J Adolesc Health 2017;61(5):591–8.

39. Awaad MI, Darahim KE. Depression and anxiety in adolescents with congenital heart disease. Middle East Current Psychiatry 2015;22(1):2–8.

40. Areias ME, Pinto CI, Vieira PF, et al. Long term psychosocial outcomes of congenital heart disease (CHD) in adolescents and young adults. Transl Pediatr 2013;2(3):90–8.

41. DeMaso DR, Calderon J, Taylor GA, et al. Psychiatric disorders in adolescents with single ventricle congenital heart disease. Pediatrics 2017;139(3): e20162241.

42. Jackson JL, Misiti B, Bridge JA, et al. Emotional functioning of adolescents and adults with congenital heart disease: a meta-analysis. Congenit Heart Dis 2015; 10(1):2–12.

43. Karsdorp PA, Everaerd W, Kindt M. Psychological and cognitive functioning in children and adolescents with congenital heart disease: a meta-analysis. J Pediatr Psychol 2007;32(5):527–41.

44. Lane DA, Millane TA, Lip GY. Psychological interventions for depression in adolescents and adults with congenital heart disease. Cochrane Database Syst Rev 2013;(10):CD004372.

45. Dunn DW, Besag F, Caplan R, et al. Psychiatric and behavioral disorders in children with epilepsy (ILAE Task Force Report): anxiety, depression and childhood epilepsy. Epileptic Disord 2016. https://doi.org/10.1684/epd.2016.0813.

46. Kwong KL, Lam D, Tsui S, et al. Anxiety and depression in adolescents with epilepsy. J Child Neurol 2016;31(2):203–10.

47. Camfield P, Camfield C. Incidence, prevalence and aetiology of seizures and epilepsy in children. Epileptic Disord 2015;17(2):117–23.

48. Kanner AM. Most antidepressant drugs are safe for patients with epilepsy at therapeutic doses: a review of the evidence. Epilepsy Behav 2016;61:282–6.

49. Brown KM, Crouch BI. Bupropion overdose: significant toxicity in pediatrics. Clin Pediatr Emerg Med 2017;18(3):212–7.

50. Buchberger B, Huppertz H, Krabbe L, et al. Symptoms of depression and anxiety in youth with type 1 diabetes: a systematic review and meta-analysis. Psychoneuroendocrinology 2016;70:70–84.

51. Hood KK, Beavers DP, Yi_Frazier J, et al. Psychosocial burden and glycemic control during the first 6 years of diabetes: results from the SEARCH for Diabetes in Youth study. J Adolesc Health 2014;55(4):498–504.

52. Butwicka A, Frisen L, Almqvist C, et al. Risks of psychiatric disorders and suicide attempts in children and adolescents with type 1 diabetes: a population-based cohort study. Diabetes Care 2015;38(3):453–9.

53. Plener PL, Molz E, Berger G, et al. Depression, metabolic control, and antidepressant medication in young patients with type 1 diabetes. Pediatr Diabetes 2015;16(1):58–66.

54. Sarkar S, Balhara YPS. Diabetes mellitus and suicide. Indian J Endocrinol Metab 2014;18(4):468–74.

55. Markowitz S, Gonzalez JS, Wilkinson JL, et al. Treating depression in diabetes: emerging findings. Psychosomatics 2011;52(1):1–18.

56. Georgiades A, Zucker N, Friedman KE, et al. Changes in depressive symptoms and glycemic control in diabetes mellitus. Psychosom Med 2007;69:235–41.

57. Goodnick PJ. Use of antidepressants in treatment of comorbid diabetes mellitus and depression as well as in diabetic neuropathy. Ann Clin Psychiatry 2001;13: 31–4.

58. Morrison KM, Shin S, Tarnopolsky M, et al. Association of depression and health related quality of life with body composition in children and youth with obesity. J Affect Disord 2015;172:18–23.

59. Quek Y, Tam WW, Zhang MWB, et al. Exploring the association between childhood and adolescent obesity and depression: a meta-analysis. Obes Rev 2017; 18(7):742–54.

60. Reeves GM, Postolache TT, Snitker S. Childhood obesity and depression: connection between these growing problems in growing children. Int J Child Health Hum Dev 2008;1(2):103–14.

61. Anderson SE, Cohen P, Naumova EN, et al. Adolescent obesity and risk for subsequent major depressive disorder and anxiety disorder: prospective evidence. Psychosom Med 2007;69:740–7.

62. Dockray S, Susman EJ, Dorn LD. Depression, cortisol reactivity, and obesity in childhood and adolescence. J Adolesc Health 2009;45:344–50.

63. Goosens L, Braet C, Van Vlierberghe L, et al. Loss of control over eating in over-weight youngsters: the role of anxiety, depression and emotional eating. Eur Eat Disord Rev 2009;17(1):68–78.

64. Mihalopoulos NL, Spigarelli MG. Comanagement of pediatric depression and obesity: a clear need for evidence. Clin Ther 2015;37(9):1933–7.

65. Allison DB, Newcomer JW, Dunn AL, et al. Obesity among those with mental dis-orders: a National Institute of Mental Health meeting report. Am J Prev Med 2009;36:341–50.

66. Expert Panel on Integrated Guidelines for Cardiovascular Health and Risk Reduction in Children and Adolescents, National Heart, Lung, and Blood Insti-tute. Expert panel on integrated guidelines for cardiovascular health and risk reduction in children and adolescents: summary report. Pediatrics 2011; 128(Suppl 5):S213–56.

67. Raeder MB, Bjelland I, Emil Vollset S, et al. Obesity, dyslipidemia, and diabetes with selective serotonin reuptake inhibitors: the Hordaland Health Study. J Clin Psychiatry 2006;67:1974–82.

68. Mavrides N, Pao M. Updates in paediatric psycho-oncology. Int Rev Psychiatry 2014;26(1):63–73.

69. Coughtrey A, Millington A, Bennett S, et al. The effectiveness of psychosocial interventions for psychological outcomes in pediatric oncology: a systematic re-view. J Pain Symptom Manage 2018;55(3):1004–17.

70. Kurtz BP, Abrams AN. Psychiatric aspects of pediatric cancer. Child Adolesc Psychiatr Clin N Am 2010;19:401–21.

71. Kaye EC, Brinkman TM, Baker JN. Development of depression in survivors of childhood and adolescent cancer: a multi-level life course conceptual frame-work. Support Care Cancer 2017;25(6):2009–17.

72. Kazak AE, Brier M, Alderfer MA, et al. Screening for psychosocial risk in pedi-atric cancer. Pediatr Blood Cancer 2012;59(5):822–7.

73. Kazak AE. Pediatric Psychosocial Preventative Health Model (PPPHM): research, practice and collaboration in pediatric family systems medicine. Fam Syst Health 2006;24:381–95.

74. Li M, Fitzgerald P, Rodin G. Evidence-based treatment of depression in patients with cancer. J Clin Oncol 2012;30:1187–96.

75. Strong VR, Waters R, Hibberd C, et al. Management of depression for people with cancer (SMaRT oncology 1): a randomised trial. Lancet 2008;372:40–8.

76. Kissane DW, Levin T, Hales S, et al. Psychotherapy for depression in cancer and palliative care. In: Kissane DW, Maj M, Sartorius N, editors. Depression and can-cer. Chichester (United Kingdom): Wiley-Blackwell; 2011. p. 177–206.

77. Breitbart W, Rosenfeld B, Gibson C, et al. Meaning-centered group psychother-apy for patients with advanced cancer: a pilot randomized controlled trial. Psy-chooncology 2010;19:21–8.

78. Chochinov HM, Hack T, Hassard T, et al. Dignity therapy: a novel psychothera-peutic intervention for patients near the end of life. J Clin Oncol 2005;23:5520–5.

79. Ando MT, Morita T, Akechi T, et al. The efficacy of mindfulness-based meditation therapy on anxiety, depression, and spirituality in Japanese patients with can-cer. J Palliat Med 2009;12:1091–4.

80. Hemeryck A, Belpaire FM. Selective serotonin reuptake inhibitors and cyto-chrome P-450 mediated drug-drug interactions: an update. Curr Drug Metab 2002;3:13–37.

81. Rackley S, Bostwick JM. Depression in medically ill patients. Psychiatr Clin North Am 2012;35:231–47.

82. Keethy D, Mrakotsky C, Szigethy E. Pediatric IBD and depression: treatment implications. Curr Opin Pediatr 2014;26(5):561–7.

83. Szigethy EM, Youk AO, Benhayon D, et al. Depression subtypes in pediatric inflammatory bowel disease. J Pediatr Gastroenterol Nutr 2014;58(5):574–81.

84. Szigethy E, Bujoreanu SI, Youk AO, et al. Randomized efficacy trial of two psychotherapies for depression in youth with inflammatory bowel disease. J Am Acad Child Adolesc Psychiatry 2014;53(7):726–35.

85. Loftus EV, Guerin A, Yu AP, et al. Increased risks of developing anxiety and depression in young patient with Crohn's disease. Am J Gastroenterol 2011; 106:1670–7.

86. Mikocka-Walus A, Knowles SR, Keefer L, et al. Controversies revisited: a systematic review of the comorbidity of depression and anxiety with inflammatory bowel diseases. Inflamm Bowel Dis 2016;22:752–62.

87. McLafferty L, Craig A, Levine A, et al. Thematic analysis of physical illness perceptions in depressed youth with inflammatory bowel disease. Inflamm Bowel Dis 2011;17(supplement 1):S54.

88. Zernikow B, Wager J, Hechler T. Characteristics of highly impaired children with severe chronic pain: a 5-year retrospective study on 2249 pediatric pain patients. BMC Pediatr 2012;12:54.

89. Jerrell JM, Tripathi A, McIntyre RS. Prevalence and treatment of depression in children and adolescents with sickle Cell disease: a retrospective cohort study. Prim Care Companion CNS Disord 2011;13(2). https://doi.org/10.40088/PCC.10m01063.

90. Fisher E, Heathcote L, Palermo TM, et al. Systematic review and meta-analysis of psychological therapies for children with chronic pain. J Pediatr Psychol 2014;39(8):763–82.

91. Weiss KE, Hahn A, Wallace DP, et al. Acceptance of pain: associations with depression, Catastrophizing, and functional disability among children and adolescents in an interdisciplinary chronic pain rehabilitation program. J Pediatr Psychol 2013;38(7):756–65.

92. Wicksell RK, Olsson GL, Hayes SC. Mediators of change in acceptance and commitment therapy for pediatric chronic pain. Pain 2011;152(12):2792–801.

93. Kirk AD, Knechtle SJ, Larsen CP, et al. Textbook of organ transplantation. West Sussex, UK: Wiley; 2014. p. 1482.

94. Fredricks EM, Lopez MJ, Magee JC, et al. Psychological functioning, nonadherence and health outcomes after pediatric liver transplantation. Am J Transplant 2007;7(8):1974–83.

95. McCormick King ML, Mee LL, Gutierrez-Colina AM, et al. Adherence in pediatric transplant recipients. J Pediatr Psychol 2014;39(3):283–93.

96. Killian MO, Schuman DL, Mayersohn GS, et al. Psychosocial predictors of medication non-adherence in pediatric organ transplantation: a systematic review. Pediatr Transplant 2018;22(4):e13188.

97. Dobbels F, Decorte A, Roskams A, et al. Health-related quality of life, treatment adherence, symptom experience and depression in adolescent renal transplant patients. Pediatr Transplant 2010;14:216–23.

98. Cohen SD, Norris L, Acquaviva K, et al. Screening, diagnosis, and treatment of depression in patients with end-stage renal disease. Clin J Am Soc Nephrol 2007;2(6):1332–42.

99. Crone CC, Gabriel GM. Treatment of anxiety and depression in transplant patients: pharmacokinetic considerations. Clin Pharmacokinet 2004;43(6):361–94.

100. Beach SR, Celano CM, Sugrue AM, et al. QT prolongation, torsades de pointes, and psychiatric medication medications: a 5-year update. Psychosomatics 2018;59(2):105–22.

101. Pao M, Ballard ED, Rosenstein DL. Growing up in the hospital. JAMA 2007; 297(24):2752–5.

102. Pao M, Mahoney MR. "Will you remember me?": talking with adolescents about death and dying. Child Adolesc Psychiatr Clin N Am 2018;27(4):511–26.

103. Balon R. Cognitive-behavioral therapy, psychotherapy and psychosocial interventions in the medically ill. Psychother Psychosom 2009;78(5):261–4.

104. Thrabrew H, Ruppeldt P, Sollers JJ. Systematic review of biofeedback interventions for addressing anxiety and depression in children and adolescents with long-term physical conditions. Appl Psychophysiol Biofeedback 2018;43(3): 179–92.

105. Eccleston C, Palermo TM, Fisher E, et al. Psychological interventions for parents of children and adolescents with chronic illness. Cochrane Database Syst Rev 2012;(8):CD009660.

106. Schwab A, Rusconi-Serpa S, Schechter DR. Psychodynamic approaches to medically ill children and their traumatically stressed parents. Child Adolesc Psychiatr Clin N Am 2013;22(1):119–39.

107. Reynolds N, Mrug S, Hensler M, et al. Spiritual coping and adjustment in adolescents with chronic illness: a 2-year prospective study. J Pediatr Psychol 2014;39(5):542–51.

108. Shaw SR, McCabe PC. Hospital-to-school transition for children with chronic illness: meeting the new challenges of an evolving health care system. Psychol Sch 2008;45(1):74–87.

109. Cheung AH, Zuckerbrot RA, Jensen PS, et al. Guidelines for adolescent depression in primary care (GLAD-PC): II. Treatment and ongoing m5rttanagement. Pediatrics 2007;120(5):e1313–26.

110. Woltmann E, Grogan-Kaylor A, Perron B, et al. Comparative effectiveness of collaborative chronic care models for mental health conditions across primary, specialty, and behavioral health care settings: systematic review and meta-analysis. Am J Psychiatry 2012;169(8):790–804.

111. Kennedy SH, Lam RW, McIntyre RS, et al. Canadian Network for Mood and Anxiety Treatments (CANMAT) 2016 clinical guidelines for the management of adults with major depressive disorder: section 3. Pharmacological treatments. Can J Psychiatry 2016;61(9):540–60.

112. Bursch B, Forgey M. Psychopharmacology for medically ill adolescents. Curr Psychiatry Rep 2013;15:395.

113. Boland JR, Duffy B, Myer NM. Clinical utility of pharmacogenetics-guided treatment of depression and anxiety. Pers Med Psychiatry 2018;7-8:7–13.

114. Kast RE, Foley KF. Cancer chemotherapy and cachexia: mirtazapine and olanzapine are 5-HT3 antagonists with good anti-nausea effects. Department Medical Laboratory and Radiation Sciences, University of Vermont, Burlington, VT, USASearch for more papers by this author. Eur J Cancer Care 2007;16(4): 351–4.

115. Renoir T. Selective serotonin reuptake inhibitor antidepressant treatment discontinuation syndrome: a review of the clinical evidence and the possible mechanisms involved. Front Pharmacol 2013;4:45.

116. Steinert T, Fröscher W. Epileptic seizures under antidepressive drug treatment: systematic review. Pharmacopsychiatry 2018;51:121–35.

117. Hamilton MS, Opler LA. Akathisia, suicidality, and fluoxetine. J Clin Psychiatry 1992;53(11):401–6.
118. Nicholson SD. Extra pyramidal side effects associated with paroxetine. West Engl Med J 1992;107(3):90–1.
119. Opler LA. Sertraline and akathisia. Am J Psychiatry 1994;151(4):620–1.
120. Opler LA, Ramirez PM, Lee SK. Serotonergic agents and frontal lobe syndrome. J Clin Psychiatry 1994;55(8):362–3.
121. Rush AJ, Armitage R, Gillin JC, et al. Comparative effects of nefazadone and fluoxetine on sleep in outpatients with major depressive disorder. Biol Psychiatry 1998;44(1):3–14.
122. Bixby AL, Vandenberg A, Bostwick JR. Clinical management of bleeding risk with antidepressants. Ann Pharmacother 2018. https://doi.org/10.1177/1060028018794005.
123. Anglin R, Yuan Y, Moayyedi P, et al. Risk of upper gastrointestinal bleeding with selective serotonin reuptake inhibitors with or without concurrent nonsteroidal anti-inflammatory use: a systematic review and meta – analysis. Am J Gastroenterol 2014;109:811–9.
124. Waring WS, Graham A, Gray J, et al. Evaluation of a QT nomogram for risk assessment after antidepressant overdose. Br J Clin Pharmacol 2010;70(6):881–5.
125. Viewing WV, Hasnain M, Howland RH, et al. Citalopram, QTc interval prolongation, and torsade de pointes. How should we apply the recent FDA ruling? Am J Med 2012;125(9):859–68.
126. Kawai Y, DeMonbrun AG, Chambers RS, et al. A previously healthy adolescent with acute encephalopathy and decorticate posturing. Pediatrics 2017;139(1):e20153779.
127. Ramsey TD, Lau TT, Ensom MH. Serotonergic and adrenergic drug interactions associated with linezolid: a critical review and practical management approach. Ann Pharmacother 2013;47(4):543–60.
128. Ghaziuddin N, Kutcher SP, Knapp P, The Work Group on Quality Issues. Practice parameter for use of electroconvulsive therapy with adolescents. J Am Acad Child Adolesc Psychiatry 2004;43(12):1521–39.
129. Shoirah H, Hamoda HM. Electroconvulsive therapy in children and adolescents. Expert Rev Neurother 2011;11(1):127–37.
130. Rasmussen KG, Rummans TA, Richardson JW. Electroconvulsive therapy in the medically ill. Psychiatr Clin North Am 2002;25(1):177–93.
131. Fregni F, Pascual-Leone A. Transcranial magnetic stimulation for the treatment of depression in neurologic disorders. Curr Psychiatry Rep 2005;7(5):381–90.
132. Muszkat D, Polanczyk GV, Costa Dias TG, et al. Transcranial direct current stimulation in child and adolescent psychiatry. J Child Adolesc Psychopharmacol 2016;26(7):590–7.
133. Croarkin PE, Rotenberg A, Wall CA, et al. Magnetic resonance imaging-guided, open –label, high frequency repetitive transcranial magnetic stimulation for adolescents with major depressive disorder. J Child Adolesc Psychopharmacol 2016;26(7):582–9.
134. Croarkin PE, Rotenberg A. Pediatric neuromodulation comes of age. J child Adolesc Psychopharmacol 2016;26(7):578–81.
135. Bujoreanu S, White MT, Gerber B, et al. Effect of timing of psychiatry consultation on length of pediatric hospitalization and hospital charges. Hosp Pediatr 2015;5(5):269–75.

136. Rickerby ML, DerMarderosian D, Nassau J, et al. Family-based integrated care (FBIC) in a partial hospital program for complex pediatric illness: fostering shifts in family illness beliefs and relationships. Child Adolesc Psychiatr Clin N Am 2017;26(4):733–59.

137. Fryers T, Brugha T. Childhood determinants of adult psychiatric disorder. Clin Pract Epidemiol Ment Health 2013;9:1–50.

138. Secinti E, Thompson EJ, Richards M, et al. Research review: childhood chronic physical illness and adult emotional health- a systematic review and meta-analysis. J Child Psychol Psychiatry 2017;58(7):753–69.

139. LeBlanc LA, Goldsmith T, Patel DR. Behavioral aspects of chronic illness in children and adolescents. Pediatr Clin North Am 2003;50(4):859–78.

140. Nathan PC, Henderson TO, Kirchhoff AC, et al. Financial hardship and the economic effect of childhood cancer survivorship. J Clin Oncol 2018;36(21): 2198–205.

141. Stabile M, Allin S. The economic costs of childhood disability. Future Child 2012; 22(1):65–96.

142. Archer G, Kuh D, Hotopf M, et al. Adolescent affective symptoms and mortality. Br J Psychiatry 2018;213(1):419–24.

143. Hayes BD, Klein-Schwartz W, Clark RF, et al. Comparison of toxicity of acute overdoses with citalopram and escitalopram. J Emerg Med 2010;39(1):44–8.

Depression among Youth Living with HIV/AIDS

Tami D. Benton, MD[a],*, Warren Yiu Kee Ng, MD, MPH[b,1], Denise Leung, MD[c],
Alexandra Canetti, MD[d], Niranjan Karnik, MD, PhD[e]

KEYWORDS

- Depression • Pediatric HIV/AIDS • Behaviorally acquired HIV
- Vertically acquired HIV • Congenital HIV • Adolescent HIV

KEY POINTS

- Despite advances in the detection and treatment of human immunodeficiency virus/AIDS globally, adolescents continue to be disproportionately affected, with human immunodeficiency virus becoming increasingly a disease of adolescence.
- Depression is prevalent among human immunodeficiency virus-positive youths, serving as a risk factor for nonadherence, risky sexual behaviors, low viral suppression, and progression to AIDS.
- Depression is a risk factor for becoming human immunodeficiency virus positive, affecting decision making about sexual encounters, adherence to safe sex practices, and use of substances during sexual contacts.
- Current evidence-based pharmacotherapies and psychotherapies for depression are effective for depression for human immunodeficiency virus-positive youth, but medications may require attention to drug interactions.

Human immunodeficiency virus (HIV) disease is increasingly a disease of adolescence. The most recent estimates by the Centers for Disease Control and Prevention (CDC) indicate that 25% of new HIV diagnoses in the United States occurred

Disclosure Statement: The authors have nothing to disclose.
[a] Children's Hospital of Philadelphia, Perelman School of Medicine at the University of Pennsylvania, 3440 Market Street, Suite 400, Philadelphia, PA 19104, USA; [b] Division of Child and Adolescent Psychiatry, Columbia University Irving Medical Center, New York Presbyterian Hospital/Columbia University Medical Center, 635 W 165th St, #EI 610, New York, NY 10032, USA; [c] Child and Adolescent Pediatric Psychiatry Community Services, Division of Child and Adolescent Psychiatry, Columbia University Irving Medical Center, 3959 Broadway, MSCH 6N 615A, New York, NY 10032, USA; [d] Special Needs Clinic and School Based Mental Health Program, Columbia University Irving Medical Center, 622 West 168th St, VC4 East, New York, NY 10032, USA; [e] Department of Psychiatry & Behavioral Sciences, Rush Medical College, Rush University Medical Center, 1645 West Jackson Blvd., Suite 600, Chicago, IL 60612, USA
[1] Present address: 635 West 165th Street, EI#610, New York, NY 10032.
* Corresponding author.
E-mail address: bentont@email.chop.edu

Abbreviations	
ART	Antiretroviral therapy
ATN	Adolescents trials network
CBT	Cognitive-behavioral therapy
CDC	Centers for disease control and prevention
COMB	Combination treatment of cognitive-behavioral therapy and medication management algorithm
HIV	Human immunodeficiency virus
PHIV-	Youth born without HIV from HIV-infected mothers
PHIV+	Perinatally infected persons with HIV
YLWHA	Youth living with HIV and AIDS.

among 13- to 24-year-olds.[1] Fortunately, with advances in antiretroviral treatments (ART), youth living with HIV and AIDS (YLWHA) can live long healthy lives, provided that they have effective medications and adhere to treatment guidelines. Without consistent and effective ART use, YLWHA are at risk for poor viral control, increased risk of viral transmission, poor medical outcomes, and decreased quality of life.[2,3] YLWHA have high rates of psychiatric disorders, including depression. Therefore treating depression is critical to physical health and preventing HIV disease progression and transmission.[3] Depression among YLWHA has been associated with decreased adherence to ART, decreased treatment engagement, increased substance use, unsafe sex practices, and poor viral suppression.[4–6] Furthermore, the presence of depression among adolescents, both YHWHA and HIV uninfected, increases the risks for sexually transmitted infections including HIV. In this article, we review the complex interplay between youth, HIV, and depression, and how child and adolescent psychiatrists can best care for this vulnerable population through prevention and interventions.

PREVALENCE OF HUMAN IMMUNODEFICIENCY VIRUS AMONG YOUTH

Progress in HIV detection and treatments have transformed an infection, once considered fatal, into a chronic disease. Those who acquire HIV disease either congenitally or behaviorally, are much more likely to die of illnesses related to aging, rather than those related to AIDS. ARTs have significantly improved the quality of life and health status of youths infected with HIV. Although HIV continues to be pandemic worldwide, efforts in the United States have been successful in reducing new cases of HIV infections. The CDC estimates that annual HIV infections have decreased by 24% among youth overall from 2010 through 2015. Although incident cases of HIV infection decreased by 19% in the United States over the last decade, there was an 87% increase in new infections among subsets of 13- to 24-year-olds[1] who currently account for 21% of all new HIV infections.[7] Among those newly infected cases identified in 2016, sexual and ethnic minority groups were disproportionally represented, with 81% of those new infections occurring among gay/bisexual men who classified themselves as African American (54%) or Hispanic/Latino (25%).[8]

A further analysis of the data provided by the CDC from 2011 through 2015 for YLWHA are alarming. Of the 60,300 known cases of adolescents living with HIV in the United States, 51% of those individuals were undiagnosed, the highest rate of undiagnosed HIV infection among any age group. Of those diagnosed, only 41% received any treatment for HIV disease, and only 31% were retained in HIV care. Viral suppression, the key requirement for the prevention of progression of HIV disease to

AIDS, was achieved in only 27% of those receiving care—the lowest rate of viral suppression for any age group. YYLWHA accounted for 8% of new AIDS diagnosis and 100 deaths in 2015.[1,8]

DEPRESSION AS A RISK FACTOR FOR HUMAN IMMUNODEFICIENCY VIRUS INFECTION

Behaviors typically initiated during adolescence such as sexual and substance use experimentation are factors imposing risk for sexually transmitted diseases for youths, including HIV disease. Adolescence is also the developmental phase during which the rates of mood disorders, specifically depression, begin to increase, creating the perfect storm for HIV risk. Recent epidemiologic data from the National Comorbidity Survey found lifetime prevalence rates of depression among adolescents of 11% and 12 month prevalence rates of 7.5%.[9] Furthermore, evidence suggests that youth with mental health conditions are more likely to have a history of early sexual debut and higher rates of sexually transmitted diseases than youths without psychiatric conditions.[10] It is well-documented that depression increases risk for acquiring HIV disease because youth who are depressed engage in risk behaviors, including unsafe sexual practices, are less likely to use condoms[11] and more likely to use substances.[12] Depression and low self-esteem have been associated with low contraceptive use, sexually active peers, permissive sexual attitudes, and high pregnancy risks.[13,14] Internalizing symptoms associated with depression have been linked to limited ability to make decisions about safe sex with partners, decreased assertiveness, and low perceived self-efficacy in sexual relationships.[15] Personal attributes have also been implicated in adolescent HIV risk behaviors including cognitions about HIV/AIDS, affect dysregulation, mental health conditions, sexual abuse, and personality traits.[16]

In a recent study examining how depression and substance use interacted to predict risky sexual behaviors and sexually transmitted diseases among a population of African American female adolescents, investigators found that 40% of the 701 youths between the ages of 14 and 20 years reported significant depression on the Center for Epidemiologic Studies Depression Scale screener, and that 64% had reported substance use in the 90 days before the assessment.[17] In this study, depression was associated with recently incarcerated partner involvement, sexual sensation seeking, unprotected sex, and an incident sexually transmitted infection over the study period, suggesting that this population might benefit from future prevention efforts targeting the intersection of depression and substance use.

DEPRESSION AMONG YOUTH LIVING WITH HUMAN IMMUNODEFICIENCY VIRUS/ACQUIRED IMMUNE DEFICIENCY SYNDROME

Depression is more prevalent among HIV+ youth (21%–50%) compared with their peers, regardless of their mode of infection (congenital or behavioral).[18,19] Although there are similarities between the mental health needs of both populations, there are also significant differences that impact their psychosocial environments, treatment experiences, and treatment needs.

BEHAVIORALLY ACQUIRED HUMAN IMMUNODEFICIENCY VIRUS

Depression contributes to increased morbidity and mortality for YLWHA. Depression is a risk factor for HIV infection and interferes with adherence to medical treatments and safe sex practices that prevent further transmission of the virus.[20–22] Depression is associated with increased health care costs and poor health outcomes for these youth[23]

In one multisite study examining a sample of YLWHA receiving medical care through adolescent medicine clinics as part of the Adolescents Trials Network (ATN), a sample of 2032 YLWHA (ages 12–24 years) were assessed across 20 sites using a computerized audio assisted self-interview and the Brief Symptom Inventory to assess mental health symptoms. These assessments were administered to youths who had acquired HIV congenitally and behaviorally. The sample was composed of 33% females and 67% males with mean age of 20.3 years. Overall, 18% of youth reported clinically significant symptoms on the Brief Symptom Inventory. YLWHA with behaviorally acquired infection compared with congenital infection had twice the odds (21% vs 10.8%) of reporting clinically significant symptoms. Psychological symptoms were significantly higher for those who acquired HIV behaviorally (21%) compared with congenitally (10.8%).[24]

Pao and colleagues[18] studied YLWHA in an adolescent clinic using the Structured Clinical Interview for Axis I Disorders in the *Diagnostic and Statistical Manual of Mental Disorders*, 4th edition, to evaluate 34 HIV+ adolescents (mean age, 18.5 years) attending an urban clinic for current and lifetime rates of psychiatric disorders. High prevalence rates of lifetime psychiatric disorders among the sample were identified, with 68% having met criteria for depression during their lifetimes in addition to high rates of substance abuse (59%) and conduct disorder (29%). The investigators found that 44% met criteria for major depression and that the majority of the sample had a psychiatric diagnosis before their HIV diagnosis. In another study examining 147 HIV+ young women ages 13 to 24 years (mean age, 20.6) using the National Institutes of Mental Health diagnostic interview schedule to assess specifically for depression, investigators found that 10% met the criteria for a major depressive disorder.[25]

Another study examined 174 HIV+ youths ages 13 to 24 years old receiving medical treatment in a primary care clinic, using a diagnostic questionnaire adapted for the primary care setting to screen for mental health conditions and violence, followed by a clinical diagnostic interview (*Diagnostic and Statistical Manual of Mental Disorders*, 4th edition). Among that sample, 15% met criteria for a major depressive disorder.[26] Other studies have reported high rates of depressive disorders using psychological symptom inventories.[20–23,25] Taken together, these studies suggest higher prevalence rates of depressive disorders among YLWHA than the general adolescent population.

In a more recent study, Walsh and colleagues,[27] in a retrospective review of a clinical database obtained through a subspecialty clinic studied 130 YLWHA who were screened for depression with the 9-item Patient Health Questionnaire 9/Patient Health Questionnaire A and substance use with the CRAFFT (Car, Relax, Alone, Forget, Friends, Trouble) screening tool. Twenty-four percent of the sample screened positive for depression risk. Those youths who acquired HIV behaviorally were more likely to endorse self-harm/suicidal thoughts than those with congenital transmission.

CONGENITALLY ACQUIRED HUMAN IMMUNODEFICIENCY VIRUS

Youth born with HIV congenitally are also called perinatally infected (PHIV+) and represent a population with unique characteristics related to the combined epidemics of HIV and substance use in the United States in the early 1980s and 1990s. PHIV+ were primarily from ethnic minority, socioeconomically disadvantaged families affected by the high prevalence of substance abuse, psychiatric disorders, and trauma within inner cities.[28] With the successful prevention of HIV infection from mother to infant (vertical) transmission, the administration of zidovudine, the use of elective caesarean sections, and the effective implementation of prenatal screening, the eradication of perinatal HIV infection has become a reality within the United States.[29],[30] These successes have led to a cohort that has aged into adolescence and early adulthood with new challenges and realities, including treatment adherence and psychiatric disorders.[31]

These youth and long-term survivors have contributed to our understanding of the developmental issues unique to HIV and the genetic, social, cultural, and environmental vulnerabilities and factors. Having grown up contributing to the development of pediatric HIV treatment guidelines, they experienced more illnesses, hospitalizations, and adversities. The stigma related to the societal climate surrounding HIV/AIDS early in the epidemic contributed to the psychosocial and psychological challenges. Given the unique experiences and risks, it is not surprising that PHIV+ youth had greater psychiatric disorders and vulnerabilities compared with their peers.[32]

Although adherence to ART is critical to life, health, and physical well-being, mental health issues are often adherence barriers. Nonadherence to ART and mental health problems were the most frequent combination of adherence challenges with 23% of PHIV+ youth in 1 study.[33] With the onset of adolescence, mood disorders and depression emerge, further complicating the developmental and psychosocial challenges. In another study, PHIV+ youth with depression had greater odds for nonadherence at different time points over 2 years.[34] Depression, a common barrier to adherence for adults living with HIV/AIDS, is also significant for PHIV+ youth. From the patient perspective, depression was identified as a barrier for more than 15% of participants across all age groups from children to adults. However, 26% of adolescents identified depression as a barrier in an international systematic review.[35]

Mellins and colleagues[36] compared PHIV+ youth and HIV-negative youth from households affected by an HIV-infected parent or caregiver and tried to isolate the unique contributions of HIV from the contextual factors of genetics, biology, environment and socioeconomic factors. Project (Child and Adolescent Self Awareness and Health Study) is one of the largest US-based longitudinal studies specifically examining the behavioral health outcomes of PHIV+ youth compared with youth born without HIV from HIV-infected mothers (PHIV- youth). A longitudinal cohort of 280 youth with 166 PHIV+ and 114 PHIV- youth aged 9 to 16 years at baseline in New York City has shed some light on the contributions of HIV to psychiatric sequelae.[36] The PHIV+ youth reported more use of mental health services (38% vs 23%; $P = .032$), but both groups had a high prevalence of psychiatric disorders, with 69% meeting criteria for at least 1 psychiatric disorder. Among these youth, 22% of youth had another psychiatric disorder. In this study, PHIV+ youth were three times more likely to report a mood disorder (odds ratio, 3.16; $P = .02$). PHIV+ youth with a psychiatric disorder including depression or dysthymia were more likely to use substances with an odds ratio of 4.0 ($P = .01$). The risk factors for behavioral health sequelae included family vulnerability for substance abuse and psychiatric disorders, bereavement, discrimination, poverty, inadequate housing, and exposure to trauma.[16],[36]

Another multisite study, IMPAACT (International Maternal Pediatrics Adolescent AIDS Clinical Trials Group), also found a high prevalence with 61% of PHIV+ and HIV-negative youth from HIV affected families having a psychiatric diagnosis. Among 319 PHIV+ youth and 256 controls aged 6 to 17 years, 17% of the PHIV+ youth were diagnosed with a mood disorder, including major depressive disorder, bipolar mood disorder, and dysthymia, with an odds ratio of 7.4. This study also demonstrated that PHIV+ youth were more likely to receive medication (23% vs 12%; $P<.001$)

and mental health treatment, including both behavior and medication interventions (37% vs 22%; $P<.001$) compared with the PHIV- youth.[37]

Another exacerbating factor to psychiatric disorders among PHIV+ youth was the severity of the HIV disease. HIV/AIDS disease progression is associated with a worsening of psychiatric and neurocognitive disorders. A study compared 81 PHIV+ youth with an AIDS-defining diagnosis using CDC class C classification, compared with youth with less severe HIV disease, 60% were more likely to have a psychiatric diagnosis compared with 37%. They were also more likely to receive psychiatric medication (31% vs 14%), have a mood disorder (42% vs 21%), or have a psychiatric hospitalization (26% vs 7%). PHIV+ youth with greater HIV disease severity with a CD4 count of less than 25% versus 25% or greater had a 19% probability of depression symptoms compared with 8%.[38] PHIV+ youth have a high prevalence of depression and other psychiatric disorders. Similar to peers who acquire HIV behaviorally, depression can impact the success of medical treatment and ART therapy, further worsening their health and mental health outcomes and quality of life.

TREATMENT FOR DEPRESSION IN THE CONTEXT OF HUMAN IMMUNODEFICIENCY VIRUS AND ACQUIRED IMMUNE DEFICIENCY SYNDROME

There is increasing recognition that the identification and treatment of depressive disorders is critical to effective medical outcomes for YLWHA. ARTs have effectively increased life expectancy for YLWHA, decreased new infections, and improved the quality of life for individuals impacted by HIV and their caregivers.[4,5,39] The importance of this recognition is further magnified by emerging evidence that depression is associated with an increase in the mortality rate among HIV+ women[40] and with disease progression in HIV+ men.[41] Making a diagnosis of depression, however, can be complicated by the complex developmental, biologic, psychological, and social circumstances associated with this illness in youth, resulting in psychiatric symptoms that are often unrecognized and untreated.[42]

In the context of HIV infection, the diagnosis of depressive disorders can be even more challenging because many vegetative symptoms of depression (eg, fatigue and insomnia most commonly, as well as pain and appetite loss) are observed in many patients throughout the course of their HIV illness, even when depression is not present. However, in both the early and late phases of HIV disease, these symptoms correlate more closely with a mood disorder (when present) than with clinical correlates of infection. The prominence of diminished mood in the morning coupled with anhedonia should alert clinicians to the presence of a major depressive disorder and should help to distinguish it from demoralization or an adjustment disorder. Clinical detection of depressive symptoms is even more important given a well-documented decrease in adherence to ARTs in the context of depression. Fortunately, recent studies have shown that the treatment of depressive symptoms in patients with HIV infection improves psychosocial functioning and quality of life.[43,44]

Adherence to ART is a complex health behavior that is influenced by the drug regimen, patient and family factors, and the patient–provider relationship.[35,45] There have been a dearth of studies examining effective treatment interventions for YLWHA[46] and strategies have been based on current practice guidelines for treating youth, adult studies, and previously used algorithms. Several studies have demonstrated that treatment addressing the issues unique to YLWHA—including stigma, medical symptoms, poverty, and alienation from families—are critical to treatment success.

It is important to be aware of the social determinants of mental health disparities that exist in the access for mental health care for YLHA. A study by Whiteley and colleagues[46] found that psychiatrically symptomatic black youth living with HIV were less likely than their symptomatic nonblack peers to receive mental health care and psychiatric medications.

USING MEDICATION AND PSYCHOTHERAPY TO TREAT DEPRESSION IN YOUTH LIVING WITH HUMAN IMMUNODEFICIENCY VIRUS/ACQUIRED IMMUNE DEFICIENCY SYNDROME

There is evidence to support combined treatment using psychotherapy and medication management to address the symptoms of depression in general. Evidence from the ATN has reinforced the efficacy of combined treatment for depressive symptoms in YLWHA. A study led by Brown and colleagues[2] at 4 ATN sites involving 44 participants showed the effectiveness of a structured approach to combination treatment of cognitive-behavioral therapy (CBT) and medication management algorithm (COMB) in significantly lowering depressive symptoms based on the Quick Inventory for Depression Symptoms scale compared with patients who were administered treatment as usual. Those in COMB were significantly more likely to respond (Quick Inventory for Depression Symptoms-SR >50% decrease from baseline; 85% vs 20%; $P<.001$) at 24 weeks with the pattern maintained at week 48 (88% vs 33%; $P<.001$).[2] In addition, those in COMB were more likely to receive psychotherapy than treatment as usual (95% vs 45%; $P<.001$) and to attend more sessions over the 24-week period (12.6 sessions vs 5.0 sessions; $P<.001$).[2]

In the ATN trials, a structured medication algorithm was formulated based on the current practice parameters for depression, data from adult and adolescent depression trials, and previously used algorithms. Of note, the CBT delivered during this trial was specifically tailored to YLWHA, addressing topics such as medical symptoms, poverty, stigma, and alienation from families. The ATN used health and wellness CBT to reduce depression, improve adherence, and promote mental health. A mixed deficits and strength model decreased negative mood and cognitions of youth while enhancing strengths, positive experience, mood, and cognitions.[47] Stage 1 of the treatment involved engagement in treatment, with psychoeducation being provided on the cooccurrence of depressive illness and HIV infection, treatment options, rapport building, and an explanation of the CBT model for treatment of depression. Motivational interviewing skills were also used to give patients insight, knowledge, and skills to strengthen their own motivation for change. Stage 2 emphasized a decrease in symptoms by teaching core CBT skills to target any remaining depressive symptoms. Stage 3 included achieving and maintaining wellness strategies and lifestyle changes to extend recovery. Other investigators have used multisystemic therapy, an intensive family- and community-based treatment program, to improve antiretroviral adherence and health outcomes in pediatric patients.[48]

The use of medications to treat depression in YLWHA continues to remain primarily empirical. Unlike the adult population, there are no studies comparing the efficacy of antidepressants including the selective serotonin reuptake inhibitors in YLWHA or how to proceed after only a partial or no response to medications.[2] Clinicians treating depression in YLWHA have generally followed current practice parameters on treating adults with HIV while incorporating adolescent depression treatment guidelines and being cognizant of drug-drug interactions (**Table 1**). Among the selective serotonin reuptake inhibitors, fluoxetine, imipramine, sertraline, and paroxetine have evidence from double-blind trials of being effective in treating major depressive disorder in

Table 1
Medication interactions with antiretroviral medications

Medication	Interactions with ARTs
Tricyclic antidepressants	The tricyclic antidepressants have been shown to have increased plasma levels when taken with ritonavir, sometimes requiring dosage adjustments. As such, it is recommended that tricyclic antidepressant blood levels should be monitored when being used concurrently with ritonavir.
Selective serotonin reuptake inhibitors	Ritonavir increase the levels of sertraline and citalopram. Fluoxetine and fluvoxamine are decreased by nevirapine. Fluoxetine and fluvoxamine increase the levels of amprenavir, delaviridine, efavirenz, indinavir, lopinavir/ritonavir, nelfinavir, ritonavir, and saquinavir.
Trazodone	Darunavir, indinavir, lopinavir/ritonavir, and ritonavir has the potential to increase the side effects of Trazodone which include nausea, dizziness, hypotension, and syncope.
St John's Wort (*Hypericum perforatum*)	Decreases in indinovir levels have been reported with the administration of St John's Wort.

Data from Dubé B, Benton T, Cruess DG, et al. Neuropsychiatric manifestations of HIV infection and AIDS. J Psychiatry Neurosci 2005;30(4):237–46.

adults with HIV.[49] **Table 2** lists the medications that have approval from the US Food and Drug Administration to treat major depression in children and adolescents[50] and **Table 3** lists those approved to treat bipolar 1 depression in children and adolescents. An important consideration in selecting an antidepressant medication is the side effect profile and drug-drug interactions with ART, because they can negatively impact the quality of life and medication adherence; conversely, medication side effects can also be used to mitigate HIV-related symptoms such as fatigue, insomnia, and weight loss.

Table 2
Medications approved by the US Food and Drug Administration to treat major depression in children and adolescents

Medication	Age (y)	Dosage (mg/d)	Metabolized	Antiretroviral Effects (Most Commonly Used Antiretrovirals)
Escitalopram	≥12	10–20	Liver extensively CYP450: 2C19 (primary), 2D6, 3A4 substrate	—
Fluoxetine	≥8	10–20	Liver, CYP450: 2C19 (primary) substrate	Levels decreased by nevirapine Fluoxetine increases levels of amprenavir, delaviridine, efavirenz, indinavir, lopinavir/ritonavir, nelfinavir, ritonavir, and saquinavir

Adapted from Centers for Medicare and Medicaid Services. Antidepressant Medications: U.S. Food and Drug Administration-approved indications and dosages for use in pediatric patients. Available at: https://www.cms.gov/Medicare-Medicaid-Coordination/Fraud-Prevention/Medicaid-Integrity-Education/Pharmacy-Education-Materials/Downloads/ad-pediatric-dosingchart.pdf. Accessed May 11 2016.

Table 3
Medications approved by the US Food and Drug Administration to treat bipolar depression

Medication	Age (y)	Dosage (mg/d)	Metabolized	Antiretroviral Effects (Most Commonly Used Antiretrovirals)
Olanzapine/ fluoxetine	≥10	3/25–12/50	Olanzapine: liver extensively; CYP450 1A2, 2D6 (minor), 2C19 (substrate) Fluoxetine: liver, CYP450: 2C19, (primary) substrate	Levels decreased by nevirapine Fluoxetine increases levels of amprenavir, delaviridine, efavirenz, indinavir, lopinavir/ritonavir, nelfinavir, ritonavir, and saquinavir

Adapted from Centers for Medicare and Medicaid Services. Antidepressant Medications: U.S. Food and Drug Administration-approved indications and dosages for use in pediatric patients. Available at: https://www.cms.gov/Medicare-Medicaid-Coordination/Fraud-Prevention/Medicaid-Integrity-Education/Pharmacy-Education-Materials/Downloads/ad-pediatric-dosingchart.pdf. Accessed May 11 2016.

It is also important to inquire about and monitor the use of nontraditional agents used to treat depressive symptoms such as St John's Wort owing to their impact on ART treatment efficacy.[6]

SUMMARY

Tremendous progress has been made in reducing new HIV/AIDS cases in the United States. Screening, early detection, rapid testing, and early ARTs have been effective in preventing transmission and prolonging health. HIV disease is now a chronic health condition and YLWHA who are receiving treatment are living longer and healthier lives. Although many youth are doing well, studies suggests that this is not true for all populations of adolescents affected by HIV, especially ethnic minority youth. Adolescents continue to have higher rates of undiagnosed and untreated infections and, for those in treatment, they have the lowest rates of viral suppression required to prevent the progression to AIDS.

YLWHA have a high prevalence of depression and other psychiatric conditions, and the presence of depression impacts the success of medical treatment and ART therapy, worsening both their physical health and mental health outcomes. Depression is also a risk for acquiring the HIV virus and for transmitting the virus to others. Child and adolescent psychiatrists play an important role in preventing new infections for adolescents with depression by identifying and treating the depression and other psychiatric conditions that place youth at risk. Child and adolescent psychiatrists are also ideally prepared to evaluate the adolescent's adherence to treatment recommendations, to assess for risky sexual practices and behaviors that place them at risk, to make recommendations about safe sex practices or treatments, and to connect them with appropriate physical health providers or other interventions.

The psychiatric evaluation of YLWHA requires a comprehensive biopsychosocial assessment that includes multiple informants involved in the youth's care, including caregivers, schools, and other agencies. Inclusion of this care team will contextualize the presenting symptoms and allow for the anticipation of health care challenges. A discussion and treatment plan at a developmentally appropriate level that includes the youth, care team, and supportive others acknowledges the importance of their sense of autonomy, independence, and confidentiality. The disclosure of the youth's

HIV status, when, to whom, and how the disclosure occurs is an important component unique to YLWHA. A comprehensive assessment must also include stressors that are common for YLWHA such as loss of family or friends who may be HIV infected, changes in health status, or other psychosocial challenges. A regular assessment of cognitive functioning, adherence to medications, lifestyle, and safer sex practices should be included. Alcohol and drug use should be assessed as risk factors for unsafe sexual activity and poor health outcomes.[51]

One potential challenge for child and adolescent psychiatrists treating YLWHA is acknowledging any discomfort with inquiring about sexual behaviors with high-risk teens, both HIV infected and uninfected. Direct questions should be asked about the adolescents' sexual behaviors, the role and meaning of sexual relationships, the use of condoms, the context for sexual activities and sexual attitudes, beliefs and behaviors of their peers, and the quality of their peer and partner relationships. The initiation of these discussion in the context of a therapeutic relationship conveys the importance of the adolescent's concerns and the therapists concerns about safety, and provides a forum for discussion that the adolescent might use to gain awareness of their own sexual practices, and to increase motivation for engaging in safer sexual practices.[52]

Treatment studies for YLWHA, suggest that interventions used to treat depression for all adolescents are effective for youth living with HIV, although the best outcomes occur when treatments are modified to recognize and integrate challenges unique to youth living with HIV/AIDS. YLWHA with their complex risks and vulnerabilities benefit from comprehensive and integrated psychiatric treatment coordinated with their HIV medical care. Integrated treatment teams can best address the multiple barriers and challenges that YLWHA encounter.

Despite considerable progress, HIV remains a significant health risk for adolescents, and depression heightens that risk. Child and adolescent psychiatrists have an important role to play in curbing this epidemic for youth by identification and treatment of depression and other mental health conditions to reduce risks for new infections and increase HIV treatment adherence, treatment success, safer sex practices, and overall quality of life.

REFERENCES

1. Centers for Disease Control and Prevention. HIV among youth. Available at: https://www.cdc.gov/hiv/group/age/youth/index.html. Accessed February 15, 2019.
2. Brown LK, Kennard BD, Emslie GJ, et al. Effective treatment of depressive disorders in medical clinics for adolescents and young adults living with HIV: a controlled trial. J Acquir Immune Defic Syndr 2016;71(1):38–46.
3. MacDonell K, Naar-King S, Huszti H, et al. Barriers to medication adherence in behaviorally and perinatally infected youth living with HIV. AIDS Behav 2013; 17(1):86–93.
4. Reisner SL, Mimiaga MJ, Skeer M, et al. A review of HIV antiretroviral adherence and intervention studies among HIV-infected youth. Top HIV Med 2009;17(1):14–25.
5. Murphy DA, Belzer M, Durako SJ, et al. Longitudinal antiretroviral adherence among adolescents infected with human immunodeficiency virus. Arch Pediatr Adolesc Med 2005;159(8):764–70.
6. Dubé B, Benton T, Cruess DG, et al. Neuropsychiatric manifestations of HIV infection and AIDS. J Psychiatry Neurosci 2005;30(4):237.
7. Centers for Disease Control and Prevention.STIs among young Americans 2013. Available at: https://www.cdc.gov/nchhstp/newsroom/2013/sam-2013.html. Accessed February 15, 2019.

8. National Center for HIV/AIDS VH, STD, and TB Prevention. National HIV prevention Conference in: Centers for Disease Control and Prevention, ed. 2017.

9. Avenevoli S, Swendsen J, He JP, et al. Major depression in the national comorbidity survey-adolescent supplement: prevalence, correlates, and treatment. J Am Acad Child Adolesc Psychiatry 2015;54(1):37–44.e2.

10. Baker DG, Mossman D. Potential HIV exposure in psychiatrically hospitalized adolescent girls. Am J Psychiatry 1991;148(4):528–30.

11. Brown LK, Hadley W, Stewart A, et al. Psychiatric disorders and sexual risk among adolescents in mental health treatment. J Consult Clin Psychol 2010; 78(4):590–7.

12. Aruffo JF, Gottlieb A, Webb R, et al. Adolescent psychiatric inpatients: alcohol use and HIV risk-taking behavior. Psychiatr Rehabil J 1994;17(4):150–6.

13. Dolcini MM, Adler NE. Perceived competencies, peer group affiliation, and risk behavior among early adolescents. Health Psychol 1994;13(6):496–506.

14. Rotheram-Borus MJ, Mahler KA, Rosario M. AIDS prevention with adolescents. AIDS Educ Prev 1995;7(4):320–36.

15. Brooks-Gunn J, Paikoff R. Sexuality and developmental transitions during adolescence. In: Schulenberg J, Maggs JL, Hurrelmann K, editors. Health risks and developmental transitions during adolescence. New York: Cambridge University Press; 1997. p. 190–219.

16. Donenberg GR, Pao M. Youths and HIV/AIDS: psychiatry's role in a changing epidemic. J Am Acad Child Adolesc Psychiatry 2005;44(8):728–47.

17. Jackson JM, Seth P, DiClemente RJ, et al. Association of depressive symptoms and substance use with risky sexual behavior and sexually transmitted infections among African American female adolescents seeking sexual health care. Am J Public Health 2015;105(10):2137–42.

18. Pao M, Lyon M, D'Angelo LJ, et al. Psychiatric diagnoses in adolescents seropositive for the human immunodeficiency virus. Arch Pediatr Adolesc Med 2000; 154(3):240–4.

19. Gaughan DM, Hughes MD, Oleske JM, et al. Psychiatric hospitalizations among children and youths with human immunodeficiency virus infection. Pediatrics 2004;113(6):e544–51.

20. Murphy DA, Roberts KJ, Martin DJ, et al. Barriers to antiretroviral adherence among HIV-infected adults. AIDS Patient Care STDS 2000;14(1):47–58.

21. Orban LA, Stein R, Koenig LJ, et al. Coping strategies of adolescents living with HIV: disease-specific stressors and responses. AIDS Care 2010;22(4):420–30.

22. Lam PK, Naar-King S, Wright K. Social support and disclosure as predictors of mental health in HIV-positive youth. AIDS Patient Care STDS 2007;21(1):20–9.

23. Stein JA, Rotheram-Borus MJ, Swendeman D, et al. Predictors of sexual transmission risk behaviors among HIV-positive young men. AIDS Care 2005;17(4): 433–42.

24. Brown LK, Whiteley L, Harper GW, et al. Psychological symptoms among 2032 youth living with HIV: a multisite study. AIDS Patient Care STDS 2015;29(4):212–9.

25. Clum G, Chung S-E, Ellen JM, Adolescent Medicine Trials Network for HIVAI. Mediators of HIV-related stigma and risk behavior in HIV infected young women. AIDS Care 2009;21(11):1455–62.

26. Martinez J, Hosek SG, Carleton RA. Screening and assessing violence and mental health disorders in a cohort of inner city HIV-positive youth between 1998-2006. AIDS Patient Care STDS 2009;23(6):469–75.

27. Walsh ASJ, Wesley KL, Tan SY, et al. Screening for depression among youth with HIV in an integrated care setting. AIDS Care 2017;29(7):851–7.

28. Havens J, Mellins CA, Ryan S. The mental health treatment of children and families affected by HIV/AIDS. In: Wicks LA, editor. Psychotherapy and AIDS: the human dimension. New York: Taylor & Francis; 1997.

29. Connor EM, Sperling RS, Gelber R, et al. Reduction of maternal-infant transmission of human immunodeficiency virus type 1 with zidovudine treatment. N Engl J Med 1994;331(18):1173–80.

30. Nesheim SR, FitzHarris LF, Lampe MA, et al. Reconsidering the number of women with HIV infection who give birth annually in the United States. Public Health Rep 2018;133(6):637–43.

31. Kang E, Mellins CA, Ng WYK, et al. Standing between two worlds in Harlem: a developmental psychopathology perspective of perinatally acquired human immunodeficiency virus and adolescence. J Appl Dev Psychol 2008;29(3):227–37.

32. Mellins CA, Malee KM. Understanding the mental health of youth living with perinatal HIV infection: lessons learned and current challenges. J Int AIDS Soc 2013; 16:18593.

33. Mellins CA, Tassiopoulos K, Malee K, et al. Behavioral health risks in perinatally HIV-exposed youth: co-occurrence of sexual and drug use behavior, mental health problems, and nonadherence to antiretroviral treatment. AIDS Patient Care STDS 2011;25(7):413–22.

34. Kacanek D, Angelidou K, Williams PL, et al. Psychiatric symptoms and antiretroviral nonadherence in US youth with perinatal HIV: a longitudinal study. AIDS 2015;29(10):1227–37.

35. Shubber Z, Mills EJ, Nachega JB, et al. Patient-reported barriers to adherence to antiretroviral therapy: a systematic review and meta-analysis. PLoS Med 2016; 13(11):e1002183.

36. Mellins CA, Elkington KS, Leu CS, et al. Prevalence and change in psychiatric disorders among perinatally HIV-infected and HIV-exposed youth. AIDS Care 2012;24(8):953–62.

37. Chernoff M, Nachman S, Williams P, et al. Mental health treatment patterns in perinatally HIV-infected youth and controls. Pediatrics 2009;124(2):627–36.

38. Wood SM, Shah SS, Steenhoff AP, et al. The impact of AIDS diagnoses on long-term neurocognitive and psychiatric outcomes of surviving adolescents with perinatally acquired HIV. AIDS 2009;23(14):1859–65.

39. Battles HB, Wiener LS. From adolescence through young adulthood: psychosocial adjustment associated with long-term survival of HIV. J Adolesc Health 2002;30(3):161–8.

40. Ickovics JR, Hamburger ME, Vlahov D, et al. Mortality, CD4 cell count decline, and depressive symptoms among HIV-seropositive women: longitudinal analysis from the HIV Epidemiology Research Study. JAMA 2001;285(11):1466–74.

41. Leserman J, Petitto JM, Gu H, et al. Progression to AIDS, a clinical AIDS condition and mortality: psychosocial and physiological predictors. Psychol Med 2002; 32(6):1059–73.

42. Evans DL, Charney DS. Mood disorders and medical illness: a major public health problem. Biol Psychiatry 2003;54(3):177–80.

43. Lyketsos CG, Treisman GJ. Mood disorders in HIV infection. Psychiatr Ann 2001; 31(1):45–9.

44. Ammassari A, Antinori A, Aloisi MS, et al. Depressive symptoms, neurocognitive impairment, and adherence to highly active antiretroviral therapy among HIV-infected persons. Psychosomatics 2004;45(5):394–402.

45. Elliott AJ, Russo J, Roy-Byrne PP. The effect of changes in depression on health related quality of life (HRQoL) in HIV infection. Gen Hosp Psychiatry 2002;24(1): 43–7.

46. Whiteley LB, Brown LK, Swenson R, et al. Disparities in mental health care among HIV-infected youth. J Int Assoc Provid AIDS Care 2014;13(1):29–34.

47. Kennard B, Brown L, Hawkins L, et al. Development and implementation of health and wellness CBT for individuals with depression and HIV. Cogn Behav Pract 2014;21(2):237–46.

48. Ellis DA, Naar-King S, Cunningham PB, et al. Use of multisystemic therapy to improve antiretroviral adherence and health outcomes in HIV-infected pediatric patients: evaluation of a pilot program. AIDS Patient Care STDS 2006;20(2): 112–21.

49. Yanofski J, Croarkin P. Choosing antidepressants for HIV and AIDS patients: insights on safety and side effects. Psychiatry (Edgmont) 2008;5(5):61–6.

50. Antidepressant Medications: U.S.. Food and drug administration-approved indications and dosages for use in pediatric patients 2015. Available at: https://www. cms.gov/Medicare-Medicaid-Coordination/Fraud-Prevention/Medicaid-Integrity-Education/Pharmacy-Education-Materials/Downloads/ad-pediatric-dosingchart. pdf. Accessed May 11, 2016.

51. Benton TD. Psychiatric considerations in children and adolescents with HIV/ AIDS. Child Adolesc Psychiatr Clin N Am 2010;19(2):387–400, x.

52. Brown LK, Lourie KJ. Motivational interviewing and the prevention of HIV among adolescents. Adolescents, alcohol, and substance abuse: Reaching teens through brief interventions. New York: Guilford Press; 2001. p. 244–74.

Integrated Treatment of Adolescents with Co-occurring Depression and Substance Use Disorder

Jesse D. Hinckley, MD, PhD*, Paula Riggs, MD

KEYWORDS

- Substance use disorders • Co-occurring disorders • Adolescents • SBIRT
- Motivational interviewing • MET/CBT • Fluoxetine

KEY POINTS

- Substance use disorders (SUDs) are commonly co-occurring in adolescents with depression; all adolescents should be screened for substance use.
- Screening, Brief Intervention, and Referral to Treatment (SBIRT) is an efficient method for detecting co-occurring SUD and engaging the adolescent in treatment.
- Motivational enhancement therapy/cognitive behavioral therapy is an evidence-based treatment modality for treatment of co-occurring depression and SUD.
- Fluoxetine is well-tolerated in substance-involved adolescents with depression and should be considered if there is no improvement in depression symptoms with psychotherapy.
- Adolescents with severe SUD should be referred to evidence-based SUD treatment, with concurrent management of depression.

INTRODUCTION

Adolescence is a vital neurodevelopmental period characterized by maturation of the brain that continues into young adulthood.[1] This period poses a vulnerable time for the onset of psychiatric disorders, including depressive disorders and substance use disorders (SUDs), 2 of the most common psychiatric disorders diagnosed in adolescence that often co-occur. Among adolescents with major depressive disorder (MDD), substance use is twice as common compared with the general population.[2] Similarly,

Disclosure statement: Dr J.D. Hinckley had received grants from National Institute of Health (NIH K12 DA000357 and NIH U10 DA013720).
Division of Substance Dependence, Department of Psychiatry, University of Colorado School of Medicine, 13001 East 17th Place, MS F570, Aurora, CO 80045, USA
* Corresponding author.
E-mail address: jesse.hinckley@ucdenver.edu

Child Adolesc Psychiatric Clin N Am 28 (2019) 461–472
https://doi.org/10.1016/j.chc.2019.02.006
1056-4993/19/© 2019 Elsevier Inc. All rights reserved.

childpsych.theclinics.com

among adolescents with SUD, the prevalence of comorbid depression is estimated to be 3 to 6 times higher than the general population.[3] High rates of comorbidity may be attributable to significant overlap of environmental factors, including family disruption, poor parental monitoring, early childhood loss, and personal trauma.[4–6] Multiple shared neurophysiologic changes have been also identified, including serotonin levels, monoamine oxidase, activity, and dopamine-2 receptor expression and hypothalamus-pituitary-adrenal axis-mediated neuroendocrine response to stress.[7]

Adolescents with SUD and comorbid MDD often start using substances at a younger age, use more frequently and at higher levels, and use more chronically than nondepressed adolescents with SUD.[8,9] In most adolescents with co-occurring disorders, symptoms of depression manifest at a younger age than the onset of SUD.[6,10,11] However, when substance use precedes the onset of depression, it should not be assumed that the depression is substance-induced.[12] Further, the sequence of onset is not predictive of response to depression treatment.[10]

The severity of substance-related impairment is associated with more severe depression.[2] Similarly, depression severity is associated with greater SUD severity.[13] Adolescents with comorbid disorders also report higher levels of family or home dysfunction, interpersonal difficulties, school and legal problems, and sexual or physical abuse.[8,9] Perhaps of greatest concern, comorbid SUD is associated with an increased incidence of suicidal ideation and suicide attempts and is an independent risk factor that differentiates adolescents that attempt suicide from adolescents with suicidal ideation.[14–17]

There are also several treatment implications of comorbid depression and SUD, including increased treatment dropout, poorer treatment outcomes for both depression and SUD, and earlier time to relapse of substance use.[18–20] Previous studies indicate that treating depression alone does not significantly reduce substance use,[21] and SUD treatment alone does not result in remission of depression.[12,22] Taken together, these findings suggest treatment of co-occurring MDD and SUD should be integrated. However, the National Survey on Drug Use and Health from 2004 to 2010 found 48% received any form of depression treatment, 10% received any form of SUD treatment, and fewer than 8% received treatment for depression and SUD in the past year.[23]

Despite increasing awareness and a growing clinical consensus supporting integrated treatment, many barriers to progress remain, including inadequate third-party payer reimbursement for integrated treatment and a critical workforce shortage of clinicians with dual training in mental health and addiction. There is also a lack of research to inform development of effective integrated treatment models. Herein we review evidence-based recommendations for screening, brief intervention, and treatment of SUD, as well as randomized controlled trials (RCTs) of co-occurring depression and SUD and research-derived principles of integrated treatment.

SCREENING, BRIEF INTERVENTION, AND REFERRAL TO TREATMENT

The Substance Abuse and Mental Health Services Administration (SAMHSA) and the American Academy of Pediatrics recommend universal substance use screening, brief intervention, and referral to treatment (SBIRT) as part of routine adolescent health care starting at 12 years old.[24] In adolescents with depression, screening for substance use is a selective intervention vital to the detection of comorbid SUD and engagement in treatment. Efficient screening tools for substance use should be brief, with high sensitivity and specificity to discriminate levels of substance use risk.[24] Validated screening tools in adolescents include the National Institute on Alcohol Abuse and Alcoholism (NIAAA) Youth Screen,[25] Brief Screener for Tobacco, Alcohol and Other Drugs,[26] and Screening to Brief Intervention (S2BI)[27] (**Box 1**). The S2BI is uniquely structured to discriminate between no SUD (used once or twice), mild or moderate SUD (monthly use), or severe SUD (weekly use or more). Other assessment tools, including the CRAFFT (Car, Relax Alone, Friends/Family, Forget, Trouble), have been validated to screen for substance use risk.[28] However, such tools may be more useful to evaluate substance-related problems than for initial substance screening and risk stratification.[24]

Brief Intervention: Responding to Screening

Brief intervention (BI) is a 5-minute to 15-minute conversation designed to deliver timely feedback regarding substance use screening results determined by the frequency of reported use and encompasses a range of responses. It is founded in principles of motivational interviewing (MI), using open-ended questions, statements of affirmation, and reflections and summaries to explore and resolve ambivalence to change to encourage healthy choices (eg, treatment compliance) and reduce risky behaviors (eg, substance use).[29] Multiple online resources have been developed to provide training and to assist with implementation of MI and SBIRT (**Box 2**). The National Institute on Drug Abuse has also produced "Facts for Teens" and other resources to provide accessible, medically based health advice.

It is important to tailor feedback and BI to the individual. For adolescents who report no substance use, offer praise to positively reinforce good decisions and to prevent or

---

Box 1
Brief screening tools for adolescent substance use

National Institute on Alcohol Abuse and Alcoholism (NIAAA) Youth Screen

- Two-question alcohol screen that asks about past-year personal use and friends' use
- Level of risk is determined by the youth's age and number of days of drinking
- Incorporates principles of screening, brief intervention, and referral to treatment
- Self-administered or clinician-administered and compatible with electronic medical records (EMR)
- Available online: https://pubs.niaaa.nih.gov/publications/Practitioner/YouthGuide/YouthGuide.pdf

Brief Screener for Tobacco, Alcohol, and Other Drugs (BSTAD)

- Expands on NIAAA Youth Screen to include tobacco, marijuana, other illicit drugs, prescription drugs and over-the-counter medications, and inhalants
- If past-year drug use is endorsed quantify the number of days used in the past year for each substance
- Self-administered or clinician-administered and compatible with EMR
- Available online: https://www.drugabuse.gov/ast/bstad/#/

Screening to Brief Intervention (S2BI)

- Asks one frequency of use question for each substance for tobacco, alcohol, marijuana, and other illicit drug use
- Discriminates risk categories of adolescent substance and the likelihood of mild, moderate, or severe substance use disorder
- Self-administered or clinician-administered and compatible with EMR
- Available online: https://www.drugabuse.gov/ast/s2bi/#/

Box 2
Online resources for motivational interviewing and SBIRT

Motivational interviewing

- National Institute on Drug Abuse (NIDA) continuing medical education course: https://www.drugabuse.gov/blending-initiative/cme-ce-simulation
- Motivational Interviewing Network of Trainers: https://motivationalinterviewing.org/
- American Addiction Center: https://drugabuse.com/library/motivational-interviewing/

SBIRT

- Substance Abuse and Mental Health Services Administration: https://www.integration.samhsa.gov/clinical-practice/SBIRT, https://www.samhsa.gov/sbirt
- Institute for Research, Education, and Training in Addictions (IRETA) training: https://ireta.org/resources/sbirt-for-adolescents-2/
- IRETA toolkit: https://ireta.org/resources/sbirt-toolkit/
- NIDA resources: https://www.drugabuse.gov/children-and-teens

---

delay onset of problem use. Also provide feedback that most peers do not use substances regularly. Adolescents who report occasional use (once or twice), but no regular use, likely do not meet criteria for SUD. Offer brief advice that includes praising the adolescent's honesty, recognizing patient strengths, providing brief medically based advice about substance use, and encouraging questions.

When substance is at least monthly, the adolescent typically meets criteria for a mild to moderate SUD. BI should be thoughtfully implemented and individualized with the objectives of providing feedback about use, empowering the adolescent to be responsible for change, advising on how to change, offering a menu of treatment options, and conveying empathy to further engage the adolescent in treatment.[30] For adolescents who screen positive for both depression and risky substance use, it is important for clinicians to explore the connections between substance use and depression, provide medically based advice regarding the interactions between substance use and depression, and recommend concurrent treatment for both disorders. Borus and colleagues[31] provide additional information on SBIRT and sample intervention conversations provided for each level of intervention.

Referral to Treatment for Adolescent Substance Use Disorder

Adolescents who report at least weekly substance use are likely to meet criteria for severe SUD and should be referred to SUD treatment. BI should be initiated with the goals of guiding the adolescent to recognize problems related to their substance use and using an MI approach to facilitate substance treatment referral and engagement (**Box 3**). Treatments for SUD include psychosocial and pharmacologic interventions. Psychosocial interventions are categorized as family-based therapy and individual or group behavioral therapy, which is founded in operant conditioning and social learning (**Table 1**). The primary behavioral therapy modalities are motivational enhancement therapy (MET),[32,33] cognitive behavioral therapy (CBT),[34] and contingency management[35,36] (CM; **Box 4**). Although varied in modality, studies of psychosocial interventions for SUD have demonstrated comparable reductions in days of substance use.[37–39]

Pharmacotherapy for SUD is most often used adjunctively with psychosocial interventions. Medications targeting tobacco, alcohol, opioid, and cannabis use disorders

> **Box 3**
> **Finding local substance use disorder treatment programs**
>
> The availability of treatment programs varies regionally, and access to care is often limited by insufficient third-party payer coverage and a paucity of child and adolescent psychiatrists with training in addiction. SAMHSA offers an online treatment service locator and national help line to identify local treatment programs:
>
> - https://findtreatment.samhsa.gov
> - 1 to 800 to 662-HELP

have been evaluated via RCTs in adolescents with mixed results (**Table 2**). Reduction in days or amount of substance use have been replicated for nicotine patch[40–42] and bupropion SR[43–45] for tobacco use disorder and buprenorphine[46,47] for opioid use disorder. Single studies has demonstrated efficacy of varenicline[48] for tobacco use disorder and N-acetylcysteine[49] for cannabis use disorder.

In adolescents with co-occurring depression, it is important to recognize that current evidence-based interventions for SUD have not been specifically designed to

Table 1
Evidence-based psychosocial interventions for adolescent substance use disorder

Intervention	Description
Adolescent Community Reinforcement Approach (A-CRA)[53]	Combination of 10 weekly individual, manual-standardized motivational enhancement therapy (MET)/cognitive behavior therapy (CBT) sessions, 2 parent training sessions, and 2 family therapy sessions delivered by certified master's-level therapists.
Community reinforcement approach and family training (CRAFT)[54,55]	Combination of individual MET/CBT sessions, parent or "concerned significant others" training, and family therapy delivered by master's-level therapists. CRAFT has been implemented in individual and group settings and is typically delivered weekly over a period of 3–4 mo.
Functional family therapy (FFT)[56]	Strength-based family therapy delivered by certified therapists, typically in 12–14 weekly sessions over 3–5 mo.
MET/CBT[38,57,58]	Weekly, manual-standardized MET/CBT delivered by master's-level therapists and has been adapted to be delivered as individual and group therapy over a period of 6–12 sessions.
MET/CBT + contingency management (CM)[36]	Twelve weekly individual, manual-standardized MET/CBT sessions delivered by master's-level therapists. CM is implemented using the "fishbowl" method for abstinence confirmed by urine drug screen.
Multidimensional family therapy (MDFT)[59]	Family-based intervention typically delivered by master's-level therapists in 12–16 individual and family therapy sessions over 4–6 mo.
Multisystemic therapy (MST)[60,61]	Family-based intervention that is typically delivered by master's-level therapists in once-weekly to twice-weekly family therapy sessions over a period of 3–6 mo.

Box 4
Behavioral therapies for substance use

Motivational enhancement therapy

Brief therapeutic implemented over 2 to 4 sessions that consists of a comprehensive diagnostic assessment, feedback regarding assessment, and 1 to 2 individual therapy sessions founded in principles of motivational interviewing to facilitate identification of problematic behavior, develop discrepancies, and increase and reinforce motivation to change. Motivational enhancement therapy (MET) is often used in combination with cognitive behavioral therapy (CBT) or other treatment modality.

Cognitive behavioral therapy

CBT is a structured, often manual-standardized, intervention that uses in-session modeling and practice, with extra-session practice, to teach new skills and problem-solving strategies. Primary substance use topics include patterns of use, coping with cravings, planning for high-risk situations, and identifying barriers to sobriety. As with CBT for depression, typical affective modules include addressing cognitive distortions, enhancing behavioral activation, interpersonal communication, and managing thoughts of self-harm. CBT is implemented in individual and group formats to reduce substance use, target affective disorders, and address other comorbid problems.

Contingency management

Contingency management (CM) is an abstinence-based behavioral intervention program that provides incentives to increase positive reinforcement. As described by Stanger and colleagues,[36] the "fishbowl" method allows adolescents to draw from a bowl containing non-prize slips (positive encouragement, n = 250) and prize slips composed of small (n = 209), medium (n = 40), and large (n = 1) prizes. Draws are typically earned for confirmed abstinence by urine drug screen and therapy session attendance. CM is most commonly used in conjunction with other therapeutic modalities, including MET/CBT, to reinforce participation in treatment and abstinent behaviors.

---

integrate treatment of co-occurring depression, and secondary psychiatric disorder outcomes are rarely reported. There is broad variability among substance treatment programs in approach to evaluation and management of co-occurring psychiatric disorders. In substance treatment programs in which there is not a clinician to evaluate and treat co-occurring psychiatric disorders, it is important for the referring psychiatrist to coordinate care, which may include medication management for depression during substance treatment.

INTEGRATED TREATMENT OF DEPRESSION AND SUBSTANCE USE DISORDER: REVIEW OF RANDOMIZED CONTROLLED TRIALS

Three RCTs have been conducted in adolescents with co-occurring MDD and SUD using fluoxetine or placebo and concurrent therapy for SUD. Riggs and colleagues[50] conducted the largest RCT in adolescents meeting *Diagnostic and Statistical Manual (DSM)-IV* criteria for MDD and at least 1 non-tobacco SUD (N = 126). Participants were randomized to fluoxetine 20 mg daily or matching placebo, and all adolescents received weekly individual MET/CBT for SUD throughout the 16-week trial. Results showed fluoxetine was superior to placebo in reducing depression symptom severity. Clinically significant reductions in symptoms of depression in both treatment groups suggest that MET/CBT for SUD may have contributed to improvement in depression.

Table 2
Randomized controlled trials of medications for substance use disorder in adolescents

SUD Indication	Medication	Number of Studies (N)	Dosing	Safety and Tolerability	SUD Outcomes
Tobacco use disorder	NRT[40–42,62]	4 (517)	Variable	Positive	Increased rates of abstinence for nicotine patch compared with placebo Variable outcomes for nicotine gum and nasal spray
	Bupropion SR[43–45]	3 (659)	150–300 mg daily	Positive	Increased rates of abstinence at bupropion SR 300 mg daily compared with 150 mg daily and placebo
	Varenicline[48]	1 (29)	1 mg BID	Positive	Increased rates of abstinence compared with placebo
Alcohol use disorder	Naltrexone[63,64]	2 (156)	25–50 mg daily	Positive	Mixed results for rates of heavy drinking and days of drinking
Opioid use disorder	Buprenorhpine[46,47]	2 (188)	Variable dosing based on weight and opioid use	Positive	Increased rates of abstinence and retention in treatment compared with control condition (clonidine or 14-d buprenorphine/naloxone detox)
Cannabis use disorder	N-acetylcysteine[49]	1 (116)	1200 mg BID	Positive	Increased rate of abstinence compared with placebo
	Topiramate[65]	1 (66)	200 mg daily	High dropout due to side effects	Reduction in amount used but not abstinence

Abbreviations: BID, twice a day; NRT, nicotine replacement therapy; SUD, substance use disorder.
Courtesy of Gray KM, MD, Charleston, SC.

Reductions in days of substance use were significant in both groups, with no significant difference between groups. Overall, fluoxetine was well tolerated and, despite ongoing substance use in most participants, adverse side effects were similar to those reported in non–substance-involved depressed youth.

Subsequently, Cornelius and colleagues[51] conducted an RCT of adolescents with co-occurring MDD and alcohol use disorder (N = 50), randomized to fluoxetine 20 mg daily or matching placebo. All adolescents received 9 individual sessions of MET/CBT for the treatment of MDD and alcohol use disorder over the 12-week trial. Cornelius and colleagues[52] completed a second RCT of similar design in adolescents with co-occurring MDD and cannabis use disorder (N = 70). There was significant improvement in depressive symptoms in the fluoxetine and placebo treatment arms of both studies There was also a significant reduction in *DSM-IV* criteria for alcohol or cannabis use disorders, respectively, although reduction in days of alcohol use or cannabis use were not statistically significant. Overall, fluoxetine was not shown to be superior to placebo in reducing symptoms of depression or SUD, nor days of alcohol or cannabis use. As observed by Riggs and colleagues,[50] fluoxetine was well-tolerated in adolescents with MDD and alcohol or cannabis use disorder.

SUMMARY: BEST PRACTICES FOR CO-OCCURRING DEPRESSION AND SUBSTANCE USE DISORDER

In adolescents, depressive disorders and SUD are frequently co-occurring. Given the psychosocial consequences, treatment implications, and increased rates of suicidal ideation and suicide attempts, it is essential to screen all adolescents with depression for substance use as part of the comprehensive diagnostic evaluation. Through more widespread implementation of SBIRT, it is anticipated the number of adolescents receiving treatment for depression and SUD will increase. Many adolescents with co-occurring MDD and mild to moderate SUD may be managed in a general child and adolescent psychiatry outpatient setting. Review of RCTs in adolescents with co-occurring disorders suggest the following evidence-based approach to integrating depression and substance use treatment:

- MET/CBT may be the most effective intervention for adolescents with co-occurring depression and SUD. However, the impact of family-based interventions on depression has not been evaluated by RCT.
- Monitor depression symptoms regularly using validated psychiatric measures (eg, Patient Health Quesionnaire-9, Beck Depression Inventory, Children's Depression Rating Scale-Revised) and monitor substance use at each visit using self-report and urine drug screen.
- If there is no reduction in depression symptoms in the first month of treatment, consider initiating fluoxetine 20 mg daily. The efficacy and safety of other antidepressants have not been studied in adolescents with SUD and should be carefully considered and monitored at the provider's discretion.
- If there is no improvement in SUD, consider increased family involvement or referral to more intensive substance use treatment.

Adolescents with severe SUD should be referred to specific substance use treatment. The primary treatment modalities for SUD include family-based therapy and individual or group behavioral psychosocial interventions, including MET, CBT, and CM. It is important for the referring provider to be familiar with local substance use treatment programs and coordinate care, as it may be necessary to continue to manage depression treatment concurrent with SUD treatment.

REFERENCES

1. Casey BJ, Jones RM, Hare TA. The adolescent brain. Ann N Y Acad Sci 2008; 1124:111–26.
2. Goldstein BI, Shamseddeen W, Spirito A, et al. Substance use and the treatment of resistant depression in adolescents. J Am Acad Child Adolesc Psychiatry 2009;48(12):1182–92.
3. Kaminer Y, Connor DF, Curry JF. Comorbid adolescent substance use and major depressive disorders: a review. Psychiatry (Edgmont) 2007;4(12):32–43.
4. Kendler KS, Jacobson KC, Prescott CA, et al. Specificity of genetic and environmental risk factors for use and abuse/dependence of cannabis, cocaine, hallucinogens, sedatives, stimulants, and opiates in male twins. Am J Psychiatry 2003; 160(4):687–95.
5. Volkow ND. The reality of comorbidity: depression and drug abuse. Biol Psychiatry 2004;56(10):714–7.
6. Libby AM, Orton HD, Stover SK, et al. What came first, major depression or substance use disorder? Clinical characteristics and substance use comparing teens in a treatment cohort. Addict Behav 2005;30(9):1649–62.
7. Brady KT, Sinha R. Co-occurring mental and substance use disorders: the neurobiological effects of chronic stress. Am J Psychiatry 2005;162(8):1483–93.
8. Grella CE, Hser YI, Joshi V, et al. Drug treatment outcomes for adolescents with comorbid mental and substance use disorders. J Nerv Ment Dis 2001;189(6): 384–92.
9. Rowe CL, Liddle HA, Greenbaum PE, et al. Impact of psychiatric comorbidity on treatment of adolescent drug abusers. J Subst Abuse Treat 2004;26(2):129–40.
10. Bukstein OG, Glancy LJ, Kaminer Y. Patterns of affective comorbidity in a clinical population of dually diagnosed adolescent substance abusers. J Am Acad Child Adolesc Psychiatry 1992;31(6):1041–5.
11. Hodgins S, Tengstrom A, Bylin S, et al. Consulting for substance abuse: mental disorders among adolescents and their parents. Nord J Psychiatry 2007;61(5): 379–86.
12. Riggs PD, Baker S, Mikulich SK, et al. Depression in substance-dependent delinquents. J Am Acad Child Adolesc Psychiatry 1995;34(6):764–71.
13. Whitmore EA, Mikulich SK, Thompson LL, et al. Influences on adolescent substance dependence: conduct disorder, depression, attention deficit hyperactivity disorder, and gender. Drug Alcohol Depend 1997;47(2):87–97.
14. Kandel DB, Raveis VH, Davies M. Suicidal ideation in adolescence: depression, substance use, and other risk factors. J Youth Adolesc 1991;20(2):289–309.
15. Garrison CZ, McKeown RE, Valois RF, et al. Aggression, substance use, and suicidal behaviors in high school students. Am J Public Health 1993;83(2):179–84.
16. Negron R, Piacentini J, Graae F, et al. Microanalysis of adolescent suicide attempters and ideators during the acute suicidal episode. J Am Acad Child Adolesc Psychiatry 1997;36(11):1512–9.
17. Gould MS, King R, Greenwald S, et al. Psychopathology associated with suicidal ideation and attempts among children and adolescents. J Am Acad Child Adolesc Psychiatry 1998;37(9):915–23.
18. Cornelius JR, Maisto SA, Martin CS, et al. Major depression associated with earlier alcohol relapse in treated teens with AUD. Addict Behav 2004;29(5): 1035–8.

19. White AM, Jordan JD, Schroeder KM, et al. Predictors of relapse during treatment and treatment completion among marijuana-dependent adolescents in an intensive outpatient substance abuse program. Subst Abus 2004;25(1):53–9.

20. Hersh J, Curry JF, Becker SJ. The influence of comorbid depression and conduct disorder on MET/CBT treatment outcome for adolescent substance use disorders. Int J Cogn Ther 2013;6(4):325–41.

21. Schmitz JM, Averill P, Stotts AL, et al. Fluoxetine treatment of cocaine-dependent patients with major depressive disorder. Drug Alcohol Depend 2001;63(3): 207–14.

22. Brown SA, Schuckit MA. Changes in depression among abstinent alcoholics. J Stud Alcohol 1988;49(5):412–7.

23. Dicola LA, Gaydos LM, Druss BG, et al. Health insurance and treatment of adolescents with co-occurring major depression and substance use disorders. J Am Acad Child Adolesc Psychiatry 2013;52(9):953–60.

24. Levy SJ, Williams JF, Committee on Substance Use and Prevention. Substance use screening, brief intervention, and referral to treatment. Pediatrics 2016; 138(1) [pii:e20161211].

25. National Institute on Alcohol Abuse and Alcoholism. Alcoholism NIoAAa. Alcohol screening and brief intervention for youth: a practitioner's guide. Bethesda (MD): National Institute on Alcohol Abuse and Alcoholism; 2011.

26. Kelly SM, Gryczynski J, Mitchell SG, et al. Validity of brief screening instrument for adolescent tobacco, alcohol, and drug use. Pediatrics 2014;133(5):819–26.

27. Levy S, Weiss R, Sherritt L, et al. An electronic screen for triaging adolescent substance use by risk levels. JAMA Pediatr 2014;168(9):822–8.

28. Knight JR, Shrier LA, Bravender TD, et al. A new brief screen for adolescent substance abuse. Arch Pediatr Adolesc Med 1999;153(6):591–6.

29. Miller WR, Rollnick S. Motivational interviewing: preparing people for change. 2nd edition. New York: Guilford Press; 2002.

30. Miller WR, Rollnick S. Motivational interviewing: helping people change. 3rd edition. New York: Guilford Press; 2013.

31. Borus J, Parhami I, Levy S. Screening, brief intervention, and referral to treatment. Child Adolesc Psychiatr Clin N Am 2016;25(4):579–601.

32. Marijuana Treatment Project Research Group. Brief treatments for cannabis dependence: findings from a randomized multisite trial. J Consult Clin Psychol 2004;72(3):455–66.

33. Tevyaw TO, Monti PM. Motivational enhancement and other brief interventions for adolescent substance abuse: foundations, applications and evaluations. Addiction 2004;99(Suppl 2):63–75.

34. Carroll KM. Behavioral therapies for co-occurring substance use and mood disorders. Biol Psychiatry 2004;56(10):778–84.

35. Kamon J, Budney A, Stanger C. A contingency management intervention for adolescent marijuana abuse and conduct problems. J Am Acad Child Adolesc Psychiatry 2005;44(6):513–21.

36. Stanger C, Ryan SR, Scherer EA, et al. Clinic- and home-based contingency management plus parent training for adolescent cannabis use disorders. J Am Acad Child Adolesc Psychiatry 2015;54(6):445–53.e2.

37. Kaminer Y, Burleson JA, Goldberger R. Cognitive-behavioral coping skills and psychoeducation therapies for adolescent substance abuse. J Nerv Ment Dis 2002;190(11):737–45.

38. Dennis M, Godley SH, Diamond G, et al. The Cannabis Youth Treatment (CYT) Study: main findings from two randomized trials. J Subst Abuse Treat 2004; 27(3):197–213.

39. Liddle HA, Rowe CL. Adolescent substance abuse: research and clinical advances. New York: Cambridge University Press; 2006.

40. Hanson K, Allen S, Jensen S, et al. Treatment of adolescent smokers with the nicotine patch. Nicotine Tob Res 2003;5(4):515–26.

41. Moolchan ET, Robinson ML, Ernst M, et al. Safety and efficacy of the nicotine patch and gum for the treatment of adolescent tobacco addiction. Pediatrics 2005;115(4):e407–14.

42. Scherphof CS, van den Eijnden RJ, Engels RC, et al. Short-term efficacy of nicotine replacement therapy for smoking cessation in adolescents: a randomized controlled trial. J Subst Abuse Treat 2014;46(2):120–7.

43. Killen JD, Robinson TN, Ammerman S, et al. Randomized clinical trial of the efficacy of bupropion combined with nicotine patch in the treatment of adolescent smokers. J Consult Clin Psychol 2004;72(4):729–35.

44. Muramoto ML, Leischow SJ, Sherrill D, et al. Randomized, double-blind, placebo-controlled trial of 2 dosages of sustained-release bupropion for adolescent smoking cessation. Arch Pediatr Adolesc Med 2007;161(11):1068–74.

45. Gray KM, Carpenter MJ, Baker NL, et al. Bupropion SR and contingency management for adolescent smoking cessation. J Subst Abuse Treat 2011;40(1): 77–86.

46. Marsch LA, Bickel WK, Badger GJ, et al. Comparison of pharmacological treatments for opioid-dependent adolescents: a randomized controlled trial. Arch Gen Psychiatry 2005;62(10):1157–64.

47. Woody GE, Poole SA, Subramaniam G, et al. Extended vs short-term buprenorphine-naloxone for treatment of opioid-addicted youth: a randomized trial. JAMA 2008;300(17):2003–11.

48. Gray KM, Carpenter MJ, Lewis AL, et al. Varenicline versus bupropion XL for smoking cessation in older adolescents: a randomized, double-blind pilot trial. Nicotine Tob Res 2012;14(2):234–9.

49. Gray KM, Carpenter MJ, Baker NL, et al. A double-blind randomized controlled trial of N-acetylcysteine in cannabis-dependent adolescents. Am J Psychiatry 2012;169(8):805–12.

50. Riggs PD, Mikulich-Gilbertson SK, Davies RD, et al. A randomized controlled trial of fluoxetine and cognitive behavioral therapy in adolescents with major depression, behavior problems, and substance use disorders. Arch Pediatr Adolesc Med 2007;161(11):1026–34.

51. Cornelius JR, Bukstein OG, Wood DS, et al. Double-blind placebo-controlled trial of fluoxetine in adolescents with comorbid major depression and an alcohol use disorder. Addict Behav 2009;34(10):905–9.

52. Cornelius JR, Bukstein OG, Douaihy AB, et al. Double-blind fluoxetine trial in comorbid MDD-CUD youth and young adults. Drug Alcohol Depend 2010;112(1–2): 39–45.

53. Godley SH, Smith JE, Passetti LL, et al. The Adolescent Community Reinforcement Approach (A-CRA) as a model paradigm for the management of adolescents with substance use disorders and co-occurring psychiatric disorders. Subst Abus 2014;35(4):352–63.

54. Meyers RJ, Roozen HG, Smith JE. The community reinforcement approach: an update of the evidence. Alcohol Res Health 2011;33(4):380–8.

55. Manuel JK, Austin JL, Miller WR, et al. Community reinforcement and family training: a pilot comparison of group and self-directed delivery. J Subst Abuse Treat 2012;43(1):129–36.
56. Waldron HB, Slesnick N, Brody JL, et al. Treatment outcomes for adolescent substance abuse at 4- and 7-month assessments. J Consult Clin Psychol 2001;69(5): 802–13.
57. Wagner EF, Brown SA, Monti PM, et al. Innovations in adolescent substance abuse intervention. Alcohol Clin Exp Res 1999;23(2):236–49.
58. Kaminer Y, Burleson JA, Blitz C, et al. Psychotherapies for adolescent substance abusers: a pilot study. J Nerv Ment Dis 1998;186(11):684–90.
59. Liddle HA, Rowe CL, Dakof GA, et al. Multidimensional family therapy for young adolescent substance abuse: twelve-month outcomes of a randomized controlled trial. J Consult Clin Psychol 2009;77(1):12–25.
60. Henggeler SW, Pickrel SG, Brondino MJ, et al. Eliminating (almost) treatment dropout of substance abusing or dependent delinquents through home-based multisystemic therapy. Am J Psychiatry 1996;153(3):427–8.
61. Henggeler SW, Clingempeel WG, Brondino MJ, et al. Four-year follow-up of multisystemic therapy with substance-abusing and substance-dependent juvenile offenders. J Am Acad Child Adolesc Psychiatry 2002;41(7):868–74.
62. Rubinstein ML, Benowitz NL, Auerback GM, et al. A randomized trial of nicotine nasal spray in adolescent smokers. Pediatrics 2008;122(3):e595–600.
63. Miranda R, Ray L, Blanchard A, et al. Effects of naltrexone on adolescent alcohol cue reactivity and sensitivity: an initial randomized trial. Addict Biol 2014;19(5): 941–54.
64. O'Malley SS, Corbin WR, Leeman RF, et al. Reduction of alcohol drinking in young adults by naltrexone: a double-blind, placebo-controlled, randomized clinical trial of efficacy and safety. J Clin Psychiatry 2015;76(2):e207–13.
65. Miranda R Jr, Treloar H, Blanchard A, et al. Topiramate and motivational enhancement therapy for cannabis use among youth: a randomized placebo-controlled pilot study. Addict Biol 2017;22(3):779–90.

Depression in African American and Black Caribbean Youth and the Intersection of Spirituality and Religion

Clinical Opportunities and Considerations

Lisa M. Cullins, MD[a],*, Martine M. Solages, MD[b],
Shalice McKnight, DO[c]

KEYWORDS

- Depression • Children and adolescents • African American • Black Caribbean
- Spirituality • Religion • Culture

KEY POINTS

- Major risk factors for depression in African American and black Caribbean youth are lower socioeconomic status, substance use, family history, and exposure to violence, as well as overt racism, perceived racial discrimination, microaggressions/macroaggressions, and implicit bias.
- Community connectedness, spirituality/religion, and family cohesion are protective factors for depression in African American and black Caribbean youth and their families.
- Forging a healthy provider-patient alliance with a culturally sensitive lens is essential in effective service delivery models for the treatment of depression in African American and black Caribbean youth and their families.

Similar to any other illness, depression can seize any individual, child, or family and does not discriminate against age, socioeconomic class, race, or ethnicity. However, the risk factors, presentation, and diagnostic and treatment variables may differ in ethnic minorities. Just like their Latino peers, African American and black Caribbean children and adolescents continue to experience disparities in access to and quality

Disclosures: None.
[a] George Washington University School of Medicine, Washington, DC, USA; [b] 10903 New Hampshire Avenue, Silver Spring, MD 20904, USA; [c] Fort Belvoir Community Hospital, 9300 DeWitt Loop, Fort Belvoir, VA 22060, USA
* Corresponding author. 4000 Blackburn Lane, Suite 260, Burtonsville, MD 20866.
E-mail address: lisacullins@yahoo.com

of mental health services compared with non-Latino white peers. Exploring how depression affects African American and black Caribbean youth and their families and current barriers to treatment may assist in closing this mental health disparity and gap, which is imperative. This article examines risk and protective factors, unique clinical presentation, and the poignant interface of spirituality and religion affecting depression in this population of youth.

Mental health within the African American community has reached a point of crisis, with increased chronicity and severity.[1] Depression rates, although lower than in other ethnic and racial counterparts, have resulted in greater lifetime functional impairment and association with serious sequelae, such as suicide.[1] However, African American youth have been unable to escape this daunting reality, as shown by an increased suicide rate among children 5 to 11 years old from 1993 to 1997 compared with 2008 to 2012.[1] This increase is concerning because, during the same time frame, there was a decreased rate among white children of the same ages. This age-related racial disparity highlights the need to explore hidden factors that are contributing to suicide and depression in African American youth, not readily captured through the standard assessment tools, measures, and processes.

Within the African American community, depression is often viewed as a great masquerader, leading to poor identification and misdiagnosis. Classic signs and symptoms are not always evident and may manifest through unconventional means, such as aggression, violence, irritability, frustration, and trauma. Although traditional risk factors, not limited to lower socioeconomic status, substance use, family history, and exposure to violence, do predispose African Americans to depression, there are additional systemic stressors and biases that increase vulnerability within this population. As times continue to evolve, it is important to understand how factors such as overt racism, perceived racial discrimination, implicit bias, social injustice, police brutality, and microaggressions/macroaggressions affect African American youth. In the absence of early interventions, the constant exposure to the aforementioned factors could result in insults to identity, self-esteem, confidence, and happiness. It is therefore important to identify depression early on and engage youth and families in order to mitigate adverse outcomes.

The basic signs and symptoms of depression are consistent in all children and adolescents. Along with irritability and/or depressed mood, there may be changes in sleep, appetite, energy level, interests, attention, concentration, and motivation. However, when integrating and fully acknowledging culture, race, and ethnicity in African American youth, differences do emerge in belief systems and perception of illness, adaptability, risk factors, protective factors, help-seeking behaviors, and the perceptions of the medical community that must be considered.

There are key risk and protective factors for depression to consider in African American youth. Risk factors may include poverty (ie, food, housing, and financial insecurities/instabilities), community trauma (ie, witnessing violence both at home and in the community), polyvictimization, neighborhood social disorganization, repeated experiences of discrimination, and chronic exposure to racism.[2] Many of these identifiable risk factors disproportionately affect minority children and their families. Parental conflict and/or lower levels of family cohesion and adaptability are associated with higher rates of suicide attempts in African American adolescents.[3] Albeit multifaceted, bullying could be understood as a traumatic event, given its impact on children and adolescents' wellbeing, and is an important risk factor to consider. Sexual minority youth in particular are exposed to heightened levels of bullying.[4] They also are more likely to have been victims of both physical and sexual abuse and may feel less social connectedness to their communities, their churches, and even family, despite these all serving as protective factors in the traditional African American culture. Thus, ethnic minority gay, lesbian, bisexual, and transgender youth have higher risk levels for depression.[4]

Protective factors may include community connectedness. Ethnic enclaves may provide mental health benefits by enhancing resident collective identity and reducing exposure to discrimination. These benefits may attenuate some of the socioeconomic disadvantages that typically characterize racially segregated communities and facilitate psychosocial adjustment.[5] Links to the church, close interpersonal relationships, and family cohesion have been found to be protective factors for African American youth. Research has suggested that religion has a positive impact as a protective factor to suicide. In particular, involvement in the church can encourage social connection, improve self-esteem, and may provide a sense of meaning to the person's life.[3] Individual factors such as active coping or dynamic and adaptive response to stress can be features in African American culture that may serve as protective factors.[6] Similar to the known benefits of social and community supports, positive early teacher interactions have been found to enhance resilience, adaptability, and self-esteem, ameliorating mental health risks and other psychosocial stressors.[7]

There are numerous elements that influence help-seeking behaviors, perceptions of illness, and adaptive coping strategies. In African American families, early identification and intervention for depression in youth relies on the family's perception and understanding of illness. The association of changes in mood, sleep, appetite, interests, and energy level may not be understood as symptoms of depression. Instead, these changes could be viewed as a typical and normative response to psychosocial stressors, which African American families disproportionately experience, with greater intensity, frequency, and chronicity in their communities. There are many instances in which opportunities for early identification and intervention are missed, simply because the youth and the caregiver do not assign their feelings, thoughts, and behaviors to symptoms of depression. Previous research supports this notion by indicating that African American youth do not recognize depression as a medical disease but view it as a concern that can be controlled through strong will and religious faith.[8]

It has also been shown that not only are these opportunities to intervene missed by youth and caregivers, they may also be missed by medical professionals. African American children are less likely to be referred for mental health services by their primary care provider compared with white children.[9,10]

Even after both the child and caregiver embrace the possibility of depression and the primary care provider has referred them for mental health services, factors such as stigma, structural barriers, faith-based cultural attributions, and mistrust of the medical community may emerge as impediments to pursuing and accessing care, especially quality care. With regard to stigma, African American families may fear that a diagnosis of mental illness might adversely label their child and disadvantage their child throughout life in educational, social, financial, and vocational realms.[9]

Systemic barriers to the pursuit and acquisition of quality mental health care for African American families are overwhelming. Population-level barriers include socioeconomic disparities, stigma, poor health education, and lack of activism/advocacy; provider factors include deficits in cross-cultural knowledge, skills, patient orientation, attitudinal sensitivity, and language, and a dearth of bicultural providers; systemic factors include services location, cost, convenience, wait times, depth and breadth of clinical training, and culturally competent care.[10,11]

In addition, the notion that African American families may delay recommended receipt of mental health care for their children because of their mistrust of the medical community is not farfetched. It has both historical and contemporary roots. In the

Tuskegee Experiment, which lasted for more than 40 years, investigators failed to obtain informed consent from the participants and withheld readily available syphilis treatment from African American men.[12] African American and Hispanic/Latino youth are more likely to be diagnosed with psychotic disorders and behavioral problems, whereas white youth are more likely to be diagnosed with depressive disorders and bipolar disorder.[13] Such trends have been shown in both pediatric inpatient and outpatient settings. This diagnostic trend in ethnic minority children and adolescents was consistent with previous research that found that African American adult patients were diagnosed at higher rates with psychotic disorders and at lower rates of mood disorders; white adult patients were diagnosed with higher rates of mood disorders and lower rates of psychotic disorders across mental health settings.[13] This stark contrast may be caused by a possible delay in treatment, with African American families presenting to psychiatric emergency services once the child had significantly declined only after community and family supports were ineffective. These contrasts could have also been secondary to provider bias, cultural variations in clinical presentations, stress adaptation, clinical misperceptions, and stereotypes of mental disorder leading to diagnostic errors and misdiagnosis.[13] Further, these clinical diagnostic disparities have led African American youth to be more likely to receive treatment in more restrictive environments. Therefore, even now, mistrust of the medical community continues to be fueled by costly diagnostic errors, misdiagnosis, and greater restrictive dispositions for African American youth.

The term community connectedness is intended to describe strength-based properties of neighborhoods, including social cohesion, collective efficacy, social capital, and social support.[2] Community connectedness may increase an individual's motivation and ability to adaptively respond to adversity. Greater community connectedness may provide adolescents with coping resources outside their homes, including having additional adults to talk with, persons to provide aid in times of need, and feelings of protection. These protective factors may guard against depression and other problem behaviors.[13]

Once depression is diagnosed in an African American youth, effective treatments exist. The presence and engagement of a culturally sensitive and competent provider fosters a therapeutic alliance with both the child and the family.[14] If this therapeutic alliance is absent it is extremely difficult for any meaningful treatment to ensue even with medications, because this omission could lead to missed appointments and medication noncompliance. As a component of both the therapeutic alliance and treatment process, psychoeducation is essential to treatment adherence and success. There are numerous evidence-based treatments that are effective in this population of youth. Of note, African American families may be more likely to explore and use complimentary alternative medicine and approaches such as prayer, herbal remedies, and relaxation. These remedies may have been explored before seeking mental health care or concurrently. Providers should ask about this use and integrate this information into their clinical decision-making strategies and psychoeducation with the youth and their families.[14]

Research in this important area has outlined clear, attainable recommendations for prevention, early identification, and intervention for depression in African American children and adolescents. Social awareness and education of the signs and symptoms of depression in African American communities are paramount, especially in schools, faith-based institutions, and primary care clinics. Services need to be developed and implemented in natural settings that are in close proximity to the communities, with flexible hours that can accommodate caregivers who are employed in positions that do not provide flexible time off at varying hours. Pediatric medical homes and schools are excellent natural settings to house treatment services. Services also need to be delivered by culturally aware, sensitive, and competent providers open to listening to their patients' stories, validating, partnering, and learning from them. Services must be consistent and stable with limited turnover and disruptions. It is important to expand the treatment team to include supportive teachers, appropriate academic supports, coaches, and faith-based and community mentors. Extracurricular activities, faith-based youth groups, academic enrichment, and opportunities for African American youth to develop their passions and cultivate their strengths are protective factors. The roadmap exists, but it takes a collective, diverse global body surrounding the youth to actualize, mobilize, and maintain it.

APPRECIATING THE DIVERSITY OF BLACK YOUTH: BLACK CARIBBEAN YOUTH AND DEPRESSION

Clinical studies frequently represent the black American population as a monolith, with few attempts to examine the potential significance of the diverse spectrum of black identities. Black Caribbean American youth are a growing population whose mental health needs are poorly understood. Although migration from the Caribbean to the United States has occurred since the 1800s, changes in immigration policies in 1965 led to a significant increase in the numbers of Caribbean migrants. There are now 4 million Caribbean immigrants in the United States, 50% of whom identify as black. Fifty percent of black immigrants in the United States have origins in the Caribbean.[15,16] Only limited data exist about how black Caribbean Americans and other subgroups of the black American population may be distinct in terms of their experiences with mental health issues.

Black immigrant communities have described themselves as underrepresented or invisible in broader dialogues about immigration, but nonetheless contend with the stressors of immigration.[17,18] Within the black Caribbean population in the United States, the limited available data suggest that risk of psychiatric illness may vary across generations, genders, and socioeconomic classes. Greater length of stay in the United States may be associated with a higher risk of mental health problems.[19] Black Caribbean immigrant and second-generation youth may struggle with acculturation, language barriers, family separation, and discrimination, all of which can affect their risk of mood, anxiety, and posttraumatic disorders and inform the pivotal childhood task of identity formation. Idioms of distress from a youth's country of origin may persist, transmute, or dissipate during the process of immigration and acculturation, complicating psychiatric diagnosis and formulation. Immigration can powerfully shape parent-child relationship dynamics; for example, by shifting children into translator roles or other positions of authority within the family.[20]

Although immigration and acculturation stress may have adverse psychological impacts, more research is needed about factors that protect or buffer against the development of mental health problems. For example, a family's socioeconomic status or educational attainment before migration, family and community connectedness, and a strong sense of ethnic identity may be protective against the development of psychological or social difficulties. However, it is likely that the relationship between these factors and an immigrant or second-generation youth's mental health is nonlinear. For example, family connectedness may bolster resilience but may also slow a youth's integration into the community outside of the home.[20] In one study, high levels of identification with an ethnic identity seemed to protect against negative outcomes such as depression in US-born immigrant-origin youth but not in foreign-born youth.[21]

In addition to facing stressors related to the immigration and second-generation experience, black Caribbean American youth must navigate entry into the black American population as a whole. Notably, immigrants become exposed to race-based discrimination that they may not have encountered overtly in their countries of origin. Reports of discrimination seem to increase with the length of time in the United States, perhaps indicating that time in the United States increases both the likelihood of experiencing discrimination and recognition of discriminatory forces.[22] However, discrimination has been associated with depression in US born immigrant-origin youth, but not necessarily for foreign-born youth.[21] Further exploration into the complex process of racial group identification for black Caribbean youth is needed.

INTERSECTION OF SPIRITUALITY/RELIGION AND DEPRESSION IN AFRICAN AMERICAN YOUTH AND FAMILIES

The protective values and omnipresence of spirituality and religion has been a common theme deeply threaded in the black diaspora that warrants its own spotlight in the discourse pertaining to depression in African American children and adolescents. Failing to delve into and crystallize an understanding about its cultural underpinnings and influence would be a serious oversight and missed opportunity to further sharpen clinical acumen.

It is estimated that 84% of the world's population ascribes to a spiritual belief with guiding principles to govern their individual and communal practices.[23] These practices often help to shape these people's identities and worldviews. In some instances, this leads to revelation, enlightenment, or awakening, which in turn, has the ability to change a life for the better. In the United States, African Americans are reported to be markedly more religious on a variety of measures than the US population as a whole, with 79% versus 56% overall citing spirituality as a significant part of their lives.[24] Historically, African Americans have leaned on spiritual tenets to combat adverse experiences, believing that faith in God brings solace, hope, and healing, especially in times of peril and discord. Because spirituality has been a pillar of support within the African American community, it is important to explore ways in which to leverage this differentiating factor in the context of mental health assessment and treatment.

SPIRITUALITY: WHAT IS IT AND WHY SHOULD CLINICIANS CARE?

Spirituality has long been regarded as an integral part of people's composition: body, soul, and spirit. Here the spirit represents the intangible part of a person that connects with God/a higher power. It houses emotions and character, serves as the life-giving part of human beings, and through communion with God/higher power, allows self-reflection, conviction, and surrender. It is an internal force that is often overlooked or disregarded by the outside observer; however, many rely heavily on this spiritual sense to navigate the issues of life. According to the US Religious Landscape Survey, conducted by Pew Research in 2007, more than half of African Americans attended religious services regularly, at least once a week; 76% prayed at least daily; and nearly 90% were certain of God's existence.[20] Brown and Gary's[25] research found that religious involvement was inversely related to depressive symptoms among African American people. When it comes to religious practices and beliefs, studies have shown that there is a protective factor against the development and persistence of mental health conditions. This spiritual regard and subsequent benefit applies to the younger generations of this subpopulation.

SPIRITUALITY: ITS PROTECTIVE NATURE AND BENEFITS

Research posits that the protective nature of spirituality does extend to youth and often in a greater capacity compared with adults.[26] The search for meaning and purpose in life that typically occurs during adolescence drives many to seek religion for answers.[26] Ninety-five percent of youth 13 to 17 years of age currently believe in God, with 85% to 95% stating that spiritual/religious beliefs and practices play an important role in their lives.[27] Compared with other ethnic and racial groups, African American youth are more likely to identify with a religious affiliation and to rely on spiritual beliefs and practices to cope with life stressors.[28] Holder and colleagues[29] found that African American youth reporting greater importance of religion engaged less frequently in voluntary sexual activity. Additional research showed a decrease in substance use and abuse when adolescents had a personal experience with God and were socially integrated within a spiritual community. Furthermore, African American youth with serious or chronic medical conditions were more likely to use spiritual coping to address their concerns and find meaning. With approximately 70% of African Americans reporting an increased sense of spiritual peace and well-being with regular religious involvement, it is only natural to consider spirituality as an effective means to improve mental health within the African American community.[24,26,29]

SPIRITUALITY AND MENTAL HEALTH: AN UNCONVENTIONAL APPROACH TO TREATMENT

The interplay between spirituality and mental health presents a rich opportunity to reach African American youth and their families. Research has found that many African Americans rely on faith, family, and social communities for emotional support rather than turning to health care professionals. Spirituality within the African American community is deeply relational and community-oriented and naturally lends itself to community-based care as a viable service delivery model. For example, faith-based programs have been instrumental in identifying those at risk by raising health awareness through screenings and health-related activities, resulting in positive outcomes.[30] Although this has largely focused on diabetes, high blood pressure, cancer, weight loss, smoking cessation, and cardiovascular disease, there is reason to believe that such faith-based promotion and screening would be beneficial in the area of mental health. In 2015, Hankerson and colleagues[31] published the first study of depression screenings conducted among African American adults in predominately African American churches, finding that it is feasible to screen for mental health disorders while partnering with pastors and church stakeholders. More research is needed regarding how best to cultivate such partnerships to aid in the identification and engagement of African American youth.

Despite scant literature, the following should be considered when establishing collaborative community/faith-based initiatives to address depression in youth:

1. Forge a healthy provider-patient relationship: the success of a meaningful collaboration begins with the doctor-patient relationship. The relationship between provider and patient must be fortified and built on trust. It is imperative that providers are unbiased and possess a willingness to reach beyond levels of comfort to best support the patient, including being aware of their own beliefs, attitudes, and perceptions.
2. Assess the role of spirituality in the youth and family's life: understanding cultural dynamics and identity assists in accuracy of diagnosis and development of an appropriate treatment plan. Mathai and North[32] (2003) found that more than 50%

of parents indicated that not only was spirituality important to them but they thought it should be addressed in the treatment of their children. The Diagnostic and Statistical Manual of Mental Disorders, Fifth Edition, Cultural Formulation is an invaluable tool that provides an adaptable framework to support cultural dialogue between providers and patients.

3. Identify and consult appropriate community/faith-based services: it is critical to work with agencies or key stakeholders that reflect the cultural, linguistic, racial, and ethnic differences of the population they serve. This approach assists in facilitating access to and use of appropriate resources. When appropriately matched, there is a mutual benefit between provider and clergy where mental health providers are able to learn from spiritual leaders regarding their practices/beliefs, with clergy receiving educational and professional strategies to assist in the delivery of care.

4. Implement effective service delivery models: although strategies and models may vary, there are key considerations to keep in mind when devising a program. Research has found that intervention has been most effective when targeted toward specific subgroups.[33] Pearce and colleagues[34] highlighted 2 factors, interpersonal religious experience and considering oneself spiritual, as being associated with lower levels of depression, with interpersonal religious experience having the stronger association. Youth need to be and to feel connected. This connection provides a level of support and buffers the youth from negative social and peer influences. Positive examples include church youth groups, mentorship programs, as well as general support from a congregation or spiritual friends.[35] However, there exists a slippery slope in the quality of social connectedness because negative interpersonal religious experiences can lead to increased depressive symptoms among youth. Age and gender differences within African American youth warrant additional exploration to further customize intervention.

Spirituality is an integral part of the lives of almost all African American youth. It is a logical entry point to address mental health issues with notable benefits. With more than 90% of youth currently reporting a belief in God, it is vital that providers inquire as to the role this belief plays in their lives. Community/faith-based partnerships hold promise in combating stigma and reducing institutional mistrust, thereby increasing accessibility and early identification. Such partnerships are an effective way to engage African American youth and families in order to bridge the gap between spirituality and mental health.

SUMMARY

African American and black Caribbean youth and their families have rich, bountiful cultural origins. These cultural complexities and intricacies deserve understanding and should not be contrived or stereotyped. Every patient encounter can be an opportunity for the clinician to be open and objective, hear the voices, and learn the unique stories of the children, adolescents, and families they have the privilege to serve. Depression pervades all socioeconomic levels, race, and ethnicities. If left unrecognized and untreated, depression can be devastating to the life trajectory of any child or adolescent. The tools to detect, comprehensively assess, and treat depression in children and adolescents exist. Research has led to advancements for these clinical tools to be refined and integrate linguistic and cultural factors when treating children and adolescents and their families. However, significant health care disparities continue to prevail in the access and quality of care for African American and black Caribbean youth.

These children continue to experience inequities in the health care system. Progress has been made, but much more work needs to, and can, be done.

REFERENCES

1. Bridge JA, Horowitz LM, Fontanella CA, et al. Age-related racial disparity in suicide rates among U.S. youths between 2001 and 2015. JAMA Pediatr 2018; 172(7):697–9.
2. Matlin S, Molock SD, Tebes JK. Suicidality and depression among African American adolescents: the role of family and peer support and community connectedness. Am J Orthopsychiatry 2011;81(1):108–17.
3. Balis T, Postolache T. Ethnic differences in adolescent suicide in the United States. Int J Child Health Hum Dev 2008;1(3):281–96.
4. Cook S, Valera P, Calebs B, et al. Adult attachment as a moderator of the association between childhood I traumatic experiences and depression symptoms among young black gay and bisexual men. Cultur Divers Ethnic Minor Psychol 2017;23(3):388–97.
5. Alegría M, Molina K, Chen C. Neighborhood characteristics and differential risk for depressive and anxiety disorders across racial/ethnic groups in the United States. Depress Anxiety 2014;31(1):27–37.
6. Breland-Noble A, Bell C, Burriss A. "Mama just won't accept this": adult perspectives on engaging depressed African American teens in clinical research and treatment. J Clin Psychol Med Settings 2011;18(3):225–34.
7. Scott S, Wallander J, Cameron L. Protective mechanisms for depression among racial/ethnic minority youth: empirical findings, issues, and recommendations. Clin Child Fam Psychol Rev 2015;18:346–69.
8. Breland-Noble A, Burriss A, Poole HK. Engaging depressed African American adolescents in treatment: lessons from the AAKOMA PROJECT. J Clin Psychol 2010;66(8):868–79.
9. Alegría M, Chatterji P, Wells K, et al. Disparity in depression treatment among racial and ethnic minority populations in the United States. Psychiatr Serv 2008;59(11):1264–72.
10. Nestor B, Cheek S, Liu R. Ethnic and racial differences in mental health service utilization for suicidal ideation and behavior in a nationally representative sample of adolescents. J Affect Disord 2016;202:197–202.
11. Alegria M, Vallas M, Pumariega A. Racial and ethnic disparities in pediatric mental health. Child Adolesc Psychiatr Clin N Am 2010;19(4):759–74.
12. Department of Health and Human Services. Centers for disease Control and Prevention. U.S. Public health service Syphillis study at Tuskegee. Available at: www. cdc.gov. Accessed December 14, 2015.
13. Muroff J, Edelsohn G, Joe S, et al. The role of race in diagnostic and disposition decision-making in a pediatric psychiatric emergency service (PES). Gen Hosp Psychiatry 2008;30(3):269–76.
14. Barner J, Bohman T, Brown C, et al. Use of complementary and alternative medicine (CAM) for treatment among African-Americans: a multivariate analysis. Res Social Adm Pharm 2010;6(3):196–208.
15. Thomas KJA. A demographic profile of Black Caribbean immigrants in the United States. Washington, DC: Migration Policy Institute; 2012.
16. Zong J, Batalova J. Caribbean immigrants in the United States. Washington, DC: Migration Policy Institute; 2016. Available at: https://www.migrationpolicy.org.

17. Guy TC. Black immigrants of the Caribbean: an invisible and forgotten community. Adult Learning 2001;13(1):18–21.
18. Easter M. For Black immigrants here illegally, a battle against both fear and historic discrimination. Los Angeles Times 2018. Available at: www.latimes.com.
19. Williams DR, Haile R, González HM, et al. The mental health of Black Caribbean immigrants: results from the national Survey of American life. Am J Public Health 2007;97:52–9.
20. Rothe EM, Pumariega AJ, Sabagh D. Identity and acculturation in immigrant and second generation adolescents. Adolesc Psychiatry 2011;1(1):72–81.
21. Tummala-Narra P, Claudius M. Perceived discrimination and depressive symptoms among immigrant-origin adolescents. Cultur Divers Ethnic Minor Psychol 2013;19(3):257–69.
22. Gee GC. Self-reported discrimination and mental health status among African descendants, Mexican Americans, and other latinos in the New Hampshire REACH 2010 initiative: the added dimension of immigration. Am J Public Health 2006; 96(10):1821–8.
23. Pew Research Center Religion and Public Life. The global religious Landscape. 2012. Available at: http://www.pewforum.org/2012/12/18/global-religious-landscape-exec/. Accessed December 18, 2012.
24. Pew Research Center Religion and Public Life. A religious Portrait of African-Americans. 2009. Available at: http://www.pewforum.org/2009/01/30/a-religious-portrait-of-african-americans/. Accessed January 30, 2009.
25. Brown DR, Gary LE. Religious involvement and health status among African-American males. J Natl Med Assoc 1994;86:825–31.
26. Miller L, Davies M, Greenwald S. Religiosity and substance abuse among adolescents in the national comorbidity Survey. J Am Acad Child Adolesc Psychiatry 2000;39:1190–7.
27. Gallup GJ, Bezilla R. The religious life of young Americans. Princeton (NJ): The George H. Gallup International Institute; 1992.
28. Pearce MJ, Little TD, Perez JE. Religiousness and depressive symptoms among adolescents. J Clin Child Adolesc Psychol 2003;32(2):267–76.
29. Holder DW, Durant RH, Harris TL, et al. The association between adolescent spirituality and voluntary sexual activity. J Adolesc Health 2000;26(4):295–302.
30. DeHaven MJ, Irby B, Hunter MD, et al. Health programs in faith-based organizations: are they effective. Am J Public Health 2004;94:61030.
31. Hankerson SH, Lee YA, Brawley DK, et al. Screening for depression in african-american churches. Am J Prev Med 2015;49:526–33.
32. Mathai J, North A. Spiritual history of parents of children attending a child and adolescent mental health service. Australas Psychiatry 2003;11:172–4.
33. Cotton S, Zebracki K, Rosenthal SL, et al. Religion/spirituality and adolescent health outcomes: a review. J Adolesc Health 2006;38(4):472–80.
34. Pearce MJ, Little TD, Perez JE. Religiousness and depressive symptoms among adolescents. J Clin Child Adolesc Psychol 2003;32(2):267–76.
35. Cotton S, Larkin E, Hoopes A, et al. The impact of adolescent spirituality on depressive symptoms and health risk behaviors. J Adolesc Health 2005;36(6): 529.

Depression in Latino and Immigrant Refugee Youth
Clinical Opportunities and Considerations

Milangel T. Concepcion Zayas, MD, MPH[a,1],
Lisa R. Fortuna, MD, MPH[b], Lisa M. Cullins, MD[c],*

KEYWORDS

- Depression • Children and adolescents • Latino • Immigrant • Refugee • Culture

KEY POINTS

- Over the past decade there has been burgeoning research in the epidemiology, prevalence, and health disparities in the identification, clinical presentation, and treatment approaches in Latino and immigrant refugee children and adolescents.
- Policies that protect against parental deportation and promote family stability can assist in improving child mental health and development and reducing childhood depression in Latino and other immigrant refugee populations.
- Evidence-based research has increased regarding effective diagnostic and treatment approaches for Latino and immigrant refugee children and adolescents, but these recommendations have been sparsely and inadequately disseminated and implemented across the country, leading to ongoing and persistent suboptimal outcomes for this population of youth, which is unacceptable.
- Extensive and thoughtful efforts should be made to thread these pieces together to create a system of care that addresses the unmet mental health needs of all children and adolescents, especially for vulnerable populations such as Latino and immigrant refugee youth.

Depression carries one of the highest global disease burdens. Better understanding of signs, symptoms, and effective treatments for depression is of utmost importance.[1] Further, given that depression is one of the leading risk factors of suicide and that suicide is now the second foremost cause of death in adolescents and young adults,

Disclosures: None.
[a] Dartmouth Geisel School of Medicine, Dartmouth-Hitchcock Medical Center, West Central Behavioral Health; [b] Boston Medical Center, Boston University School of Medicine, Doctors Office Building, 720 Harrison Avenue, Room 907, Boston, MA 02118, USA; [c] George Washington University School of Medicine, Washington, DC, USA
[1] Present address: 3 Placid Square, Lebanon, NH 03766.
* Corresponding author. 4000 Blackburn Lane, Suite 260, Burtonsville, MD 20866.
E-mail address: lisacullins@yahoo.com

Child Adolesc Psychiatric Clin N Am 28 (2019) 483–495
https://doi.org/10.1016/j.chc.2019.02.013
1056-4993/19/© 2019 Elsevier Inc. All rights reserved.
childpsych.theclinics.com

comprehensively examining prevention, early identification, and intervention for depression in children and adolescents is critical.[2]

Latino children and youth are the fastest growing population in the United States.[3] Latino youth have the highest rates of depression among minority groups, but this population remains undertreated and has limited access to mental health services.[4] Child and adolescent mental health providers may not be equipped to provide the necessary mental health care unless the cultural and linguistic needs of this population are addressed. This article:

1. Describes risk and protective factors in the emergence of depressive symptoms in Latino and immigrant refugee children and adolescents
2. Elucidates the clinical presentation of depression, opportunities, barriers, and treatment considerations for Latino and immigrant refugee children and adolescents
3. Provides practical recommendations for clinicians assessing Latino and immigrant refugee youth

LATIN AMERICAN CHILDREN AND ADOLESCENTS

Latin American/Hispanic youth (herein referred to as Latino youth) are the fastest growing population segment, representing 25% of the total US pediatric population, with continued future growth projections.[5] Latino youth originate from more than 20 countries of Central America, South America, and the Caribbean arbitrarily grouped into a homogenous population. They are in fact a heterogeneous group with diverse nationalities, race, socioeconomic and educational levels, citizenship status, and geographic locations within the United States.[6]

Most Latino children and adolescents are US born, and some of their families have lived in the United States for several generations. However, some of these youth are foreign born and recently moved to the United States (first generation). More than half of Latino youth have a foreign-born parent (second generation), with different types of sociohistorical backgrounds depending on their country of origin and immigration experiences.[3] Regardless of the generation, the immigration process can be distressing, rendering Latino youth and their families vulnerable to adverse outcomes and mental health problems.[7]

Violence exposure and displacement, prominent factors in many migration experiences, can increase the risk for depression.[8,9] Frequently, migrants from countries such as Colombia, Venezuela, Honduras, and Guatemala have faced violence in the context of political and civil strife, including civil war, coup d'états, and genocides.[10] Displacement secondary to acts of violence continues to affect many countries in Latin America. In Mexico, Honduras, Nicaragua, and El Salvador this violence is often the catalyst behind the surge of unaccompanied minors that have entered the United States since 2014.[11] Natural disasters have also led to the displacement of entire families. Most recently, Hurricane Maria ravaged Puerto Rico and displaced countless families.[10]

DEPRESSION IN LATINO YOUTH

Depression, a chronic disease that can have an early onset and lead to substantial disability, often goes unrecognized in children and adolescents.[2] The Diagnostic and Statistical Manual, Fifth Edition (DSM 5), is the classification system for depression used in the United States. Although different DSM versions have been widely referenced, limitations exist in its integration of cultural attributions and cross-cultural validity in the criterion and disease process of depression in children and adolescents.[12]

Compared with non-Latino youth in the United States, Latino youth consistently reported higher levels of sadness and hopelessness,[13] both known as indicators for depression.[14] Studies have shown that Latino children and adolescents have higher rates of depression and suicide attempts compared with non-Latino white and African American youth.[15] Nativity also is an important factor: US-born Latino youth have higher rates of depression and are more likely to attempt suicide than their foreign-born Latino peers.[16] Latina (feminine version of Latino) women are reportedly twice as likely as Latino men to have suicidal ideation, have a suicide plan, and/or attempted suicide over a 12-month duration.[13]

Depression can have different manifestations based on ethnicity. Culturally related beliefs about the cause of depression, its clinical presentation, and its treatment can influence approaches to clinical interventions.[17] A recent study described variations in the manifestation of anxiety/depression in an adult Hispanic/Latino population from different ethnic groups.[18] Although these results could be extrapolated to apply to Latino children and adolescents, limited research has been done to corroborate these findings in a pediatric population. In a qualitative study of Mexican American youth that examined youth's attitudes about depression, participants were able to identify symptoms that are common to depression as per the DSM 5. Participants most often recognized social withdrawal as an early sign of depression. They thought that a nonsupportive family environment could be the cause of depression. Regarding treatment, most participants thought that they were exclusively responsible for their own recovery.[19]

A multimodal approach to treatment that includes psychoeducation, individual therapy, family interventions, and medications (when indicated) is the recommended treatment of depression in children and adolescents.[20] Cognitive behavior therapy and interpersonal psychotherapy are treatments with empirical support for depression in Latino youth.[21,22] Notably, both group and family interventions have shown positive benefits for Latino children and adolescents. It has been posited that group interventions may be as efficacious as individual therapy for Latino youth[23] and family interventions may decrease internalizing symptoms in high-risk Latino youth in particular.[24] In summary, devising a multimodal treatment approach that focuses on the individual child or adolescent and the family as a whole is essential. Family involvement and interactions have been extremely influential in the onset and prognosis of depression in this population of youth.

Latino children and adolescents with depression additionally experience inequities in health and health care access.[4] Studies have shown that Latino youth are less likely than non-Hispanic white youth to receive mental health services,[25] including being offered psychotherapy or receiving antidepressants.[26] Further, lack of insurance coverage disproportionately affects Latino youth and has been linked to their limited access to care.[27]

SOCIOCULTURAL VARIABLES AND DEPRESSION IN LATINO YOUTH

Understanding concepts such as acculturation, acculturative stress, and discrimination is essential when providing clinical care to Latino youth with depression. Several scholars have shown that variables such as poverty, the immigration experience, acculturation, discrimination, and acculturative stress may adversely affect children and adolescents' psychological well-being and lead to depression in Latino youth.[28–30]

Acculturation, the process whereby individuals from one cultural group learn and adopt elements of another cultural group and integrate them into their original culture,[31] is a known risk factor of depression for Latino youth. Acculturative stress, the level of psychosocial strain experienced by immigrants and their descendants and their response to immigration-related challenges that they encounter as they adapt to the new country, can affect many aspects of the family unit.[32] Language barriers are also a component of acculturative stress that should be considered. Latino youth often must assume the role of language brokers for their parents or other adult family members. When adolescents perceive this role as a burden, it can transform into a risk factor for family-based acculturation stress, which can lead to an increase in alcohol and marijuana use in these adolescents.[33] Further, alcohol and marijuana use are known risk factors for depression. Language brokering at home for items such as housing, banking, and insurance forms can at times negatively affect the parent-child relationship, frequently altering the power of authority in the home. This shift in power can result in youth having more autonomy and parents having less control over their children's behavior.[34] Being a primary language broker in the family can lead to discrimination, another risk factor for depression.[35] Perceived discrimination can be detrimental to mental health outcomes and strongly associated with depression. Combined legal status of the parents or having family members with undocumented status can also increase the risk for depression.[36] In contrast, strong family values can serve as protective factors to mitigate acculturative stress in Latino youth. Values such as respeto (respect) and familismo (strong family connections, active coping strategies, and social supports) can minimize the detrimental influences of acculturative stress.[37] The following clinical case of an adolescent Latino youth with depression provides examples of some of these sociocultural variables (**Box 1**).

SUMMARY

Latino youth, the largest fastest growing minority group, are disproportionately affected by depression. Context and culturally related characteristics of depression

---

Box 1
Clinical case

Mercedes is a 16-year-old US-born Mexican American adolescent girl in 10th grade who presents after ingesting a bottle of her mother's blood pressure medication, with the intent to kill herself. She describes feelings of sadness and hopelessness. Although she enjoys listening to music and doing karate, she has lost interest in interacting with her friends and family, and complains of feeling tired, experiencing both problems with sleep initiation and hypersomnia. This clinical presentation has transpired over the past year in the context of multiple school stressors, including bullying. Mercedes has always been a good student, but since entering high school she has had some difficulties with peers and her grades have worsened. She identifies herself as a millennial. She lives at home with her parents, 2 siblings, and some extended family members. Both of her parents are first-generation immigrants from Mexico (father) and El Salvador (mother), and have limited English proficiency. Mercedes shares that there are some financial hardships at home and both her parents have 2 jobs. There have also been recent discussions with some family members around recent governmental policy changes that have them concerned. Mercedes' paternal grandmother recently died and since then her father has been isolative and drinks more frequently, refusing any type of help. In their household, her mother always goes to church and prays to "la Virgencita" whenever emotionally burdened. Her father always says that "Boys do not cry." The father often mentions his childhood hardships in Mexico.

are important given the different idiosyncrasies among and within ethnic groups in a globalized world. Misunderstandings of these variations can lead to incorrect diagnosis and treatment. Thus, the need to better understand these cultural variations is compelling. Researchers have posited that the development of instruments such as the DSM 5 Cultural Formulation Interview Fidelity Instrument offers an opportunity to explore how cultural competence improves mental health outcomes.[38,39] As this pivotal work proceeds, mental health clinicians should provide safe spaces and cultivate a level of trust with the children and adolescents they treat to foster the youth's sense of self, build on their family's strengths, and champion their cultural heritage. This step in treating depression in Latino youth is critical. If the richness of Latino culture is not appreciated and values of the dominant culture are imposed at any stage of treatment, it is possible that this special population of youth may feel marginalized and not fully benefit from the care they are receiving.

DEPRESSION IN IMMIGRANT REFUGEE YOUTH

Depression in the general, multifaceted, multicultural pediatric Latino population was discussed earlier. However, it is important to specifically and more comprehensively discuss how depression may emerge in Latino immigrant refugee youth to better comprehend this unique population. The immigrant population is projected to almost double in size and account for 18% of the US population by 2060; the health and mental health needs of this growing population are important to understand.[40–42] Population growth estimates only account for foreign-born children and do not take into account second-generation immigrants, which consist of another 38 million individuals. US births are expected to be a major factor for future population growth.[43] Immigrants face high levels of premigration and postmigration stressors that are expected to be detrimental to their mental health, including discrimination and acculturative stress.[44,45] However, despite these challenges, most research since the 1980s has shown that foreign-born immigrants may be less likely to develop mental disorders and more likely to be physically healthy than their US-born counterparts.[46,47] This finding is sometimes referred to as the healthy-immigrant paradox because, despite experiencing more stressors, which in turn usually increase the risk of mental and physical disorders, the first generation of immigrants seems to have reduced risk. However, across generations, the health advantage of immigrant children fades.[48] For example, researchers have found that the percentage of youth who are overweight or obese, a key indicator of physical health, is lowest for foreign-born youth.[49,50] The prevalence of mental health and substance use disorders is also lower for foreign-born youth compared with US-born counterparts. However, the prevalence of these problems grows larger for each generation, increasing as youth transition into adulthood.[51–53] Female gender, younger age, living in the United States for a longer period of time, and exposure to political violence in the country of origin are associated with developing depression.[54]

Both preimmigration-related and resettlement-related factors are associated with depression. Stressful migration and acculturation experiences of first-generation Latino youth negatively affect their psychological well-being. Potochnik and Perreira[7] conducted a study using the Latino Adolescent Migration, Health, and Adaptation (LAMHA) study, which surveyed 281 first-generation Latino immigrant youth, aged 12 to 19 years. They evaluated how migration stressors (ie, traumatic events, choice of migration, discrimination, and documentation status) and postmigration supports (ie, family and teacher support, acculturation, and personal motivation) were associated with mental health and well-being. The investigators found that migration stressors, including acculturative stress, poverty, and displacement, increased the risk of both depression and anxiety.[7] This study and others have found that receiving support from family and teachers reduces the risk for both depressive symptoms and anxiety. Immigration status also significantly influences the risk for depression. Compared with documented adolescents, undocumented adolescents were found to be at greater risk of developing anxiety disorder, and children in mixed-status families were also at greater risk of anxiety and depression.[7]

Refugee youth and families migrate to the United States fleeing wars, mass disasters, and political unrest. Because of trauma exposure, the more common mental health diagnoses associated with refugee populations include posttraumatic stress disorder (PTSD), major depressive disorder (MDD), generalized anxiety disorder, panic disorder, adjustment disorder, and somatization disorders.[55] Different studies have shown rates of PTSD and MDD in settled refugees to range from 10% to 40% and 5% to 15%, respectively. Children and adolescents exposed to psychological trauma have been found to have higher levels of PTSD compared with adults with similar exposure. Studies have revealed rates of PTSD from 50% to 90% and MDD from 6% to 40% among youth exposed to severe traumatic experiences.[55] Risk factors for PTSD and depression include the number of traumatic exposures, delayed asylum application processes, detention and traumatic separations, and the loss of culture and support systems. Interpersonal conflict, especially family conflict regarding expectations for cultural norms and behaviors, are other potential risk factors for depression and suicidal ideation.[51] Perceived discrimination represents an obstacle to community integration, especially for second-generation immigrants, and perceived discrimination is directly associated with lower psychological well-being and depression.[56]

Similar to immigrant youth, traditionally the refugee experience is divided into 3 categories: preflight, flight, and resettlement. The preflight phase may include, for example, physical and emotional trauma to the individual or family, the witnessing of murder, and social upheaval. Adolescents may also have participated in violence, voluntarily or not, as child soldiers or militants. Flight involves an uncertain journey from the host country to the resettlement site and may involve arduous travel, refugee camps, and/or detention centers. Children and adolescents are often separated from their families and at the mercy of others for care and protection. The resettlement process includes challenges such as the loss of culture, community, and language as well as the need to adapt to a new and foreign environment.[57] Children often straddle the old and new cultures because they learn new languages and cultural norms more quickly than their elders. Adolescent well-being is significantly affected by caregiver mental health, including depression in this refugee context.[57,58] However, opportunities to integrate child behavioral health programming with prevention and treatment of caregivers' mental health symptoms are limited.

There are many challenges in the detection and effective treatment of depression in immigrant and refugee youth. Often language and cultural barriers, and biases, whether of the refugee or the provider, can hinder identification of problems and the development of a therapeutic relationship.[59] Furthermore, there is little evidence for the efficacy of any particular treatment strategy. Much work remains to be done to develop culturally competent means of screening immigrant and refugee youth for depression and then implementing evidence-based interventions. Interventions designed to address prevention, treatment, and recovery from depression among Latino, immigrant, and refugee youth in the United States need to consider the importance of supportive communities and relationships; improving access to mental health care through expanded services, like behavioral health care integration in primary care, and overcoming cultural and systematic barriers to care are essential for addressing depression among youth in all of these groups.

While these challenges in the assessment process and lack of evidence-based interventions for Latino and immigrant refugee youth are being elucidated, individual clinicians have a unique opportunity to advocate for and to provide a space of healing for these children and adolescents and their families within their systems. Some practical clinical recommendations when assessing Latino and immigrant refugee youth are provided here.

PRACTICAL RECOMMENDATIONS

Recognizing the cultural diversity within Latino and immigrant refugee youth and their context is an essential first step when assessing these youth and their families. As with any child or adolescent psychiatric evaluation, Latino youth assessment should occur within the frame of reference of the ecosystem (family, school, community, culture) and the presenting concerns should be appraised within a developmental context with a biopsychosocial approach.

- Explore English language proficiency in the family. Parents of Latino youth and some first-generation Latino youth themselves may have limited English proficiency.
  - Before the appointment, arrange for the use of medical interpreters when needed.[60] Refrain from using the youth or any other family member as interpreters.
  - At the appointment, assess whether the youth is used as a language broker.
  - Integrate linguistic sensitivity when eliciting symptoms and in the evaluation, diagnostic formulation, and intervention recommendations in order to develop comprehensive and effective treatment plans.
  - Consider an extended appointment time when using interpreters.
- Build trust with the youth and the family member. The family is a significant part of the Latino youth culture.[61,62]
  - Before the appointment, prepare the office for multiple persons.
  - Offer to bring all the family members to the office for a formal introduction and openly explore the youth and the family preference for visits.
  - Explore family values, belief systems, and level of connectedness.
  - Family interventions that improve communication among the parent-child dyad are encouraged.
- Clinicians should learn about the immigration status of the family and listen to their unique story and strive to understand how their life experiences have affected their mental health and well-being. Most importantly, clinicians must be open to their patients and families educating them about their cultural similarities and differences.
  - Inquire about the country of origin and cultural identification.
  - Respect and validate the family's possible political and historical experiences.
  - Explore exposure to violence that the family (or individual members of the family) may have experienced.
  - Explore intergenerational trauma.
  - Explore possible fears of deportation.
- Clinicians should develop an understanding of how acculturative stress threatens the emotional well-being of the child.
  - Explore gender roles and perceptions in the family. This point is particularly important for adolescent girls in the context of safety planning for suicide attempts.

- ○ Inquire about number of generations in the United States and explore challenges related to intergenerational conflicts, social supports, and available resources for the family.
- ○ Explore and screen for polyvictimization. This information becomes critically important for sexual minority Latino youth because the risks of depression and suicide are even higher. These populations of youth are more likely to have been physically or sexually abused and/or bullied and may have more limited social supports and community connectedness.[63]
- Explore beliefs around mental illness, reasons for seeking treatment, and expectations of the doctor-patient relationship.
  - ○ Explore the idioms of distress, such as decaimiento, agitamiento, locura, and ataque de nervios (nerve attack).[61,64] In female Latino youth, researchers have contrasted the suicide attempt phenomenon in female Latino youth to ataque de nervios and hypothesize whether the attempts are a developmental or cultural variant of el ataque de nervios.[65]
  - ○ Inquire about idioms of distress when inquiring about the family history of psychiatric illness.
  - ○ Explore how stigma might play a role in their approach to mental health treatment and services.
  - ○ Explore the use of other family members, religion/spirituality, and/or the use of healers as alternative mental health supports in the family.
- Actively collaborate with primary care providers. Studies of Latino populations have found that they show more somatic complaints and will discuss them with their primary care providers.
- Engage Latino youth and their families in activities that promote resilience.
  - ○ Activities that promote social support at home and school can improve the effects of acculturation.
  - ○ Encourage the use of all forms of media to increase awareness, educate, and promote mental health and well-being, and also engage Latino youth and their families in psychiatric care, when indicated. For example, a recent study used entertainment-education to increase depression literacy, decrease stigma, and increase help-seeking knowledge and behavior in Latino youth. The intervention showed improvements in depression knowledge, self-efficacy to identify the need for treatment, and decreased stigma.[66]

SUMMARY

Over the past decade there has been burgeoning research in the epidemiology, prevalence, and health disparities in the identification, clinical presentation, and treatment approaches in Latino and immigrant refugee children and adolescents. This research has enlightened clinicians about opportunities, challenges, and substantive service deliveries and effective treatment modality recommendations for this population of youth that intricately integrate sociocultural factors.

At the policy level, the evidence has identified opportunities as well. One recent study found that mothers' Deferred Action for Child Arrivals eligibility significantly decreased adjustment and anxiety disorder diagnosis among their children.[67] Policies that protect against parental deportation and promote family stability can assist in improving child mental health and development. Advocacy for immigration policies that protect child and family well-being are important to consider in reducing childhood depression in Latino and other immigrant refugee populations.

Evidence-based research has increased regarding effective diagnostic and treatment approaches for Latino and immigrant refugee children and adolescents, but these recommendations have been sparsely and inadequately disseminated and implemented across the country, leading to ongoing and persistent suboptimal outcomes for this population of youth, which is unacceptable. Extensive and thoughtful efforts should be made to thread these pieces together to create a system of care that addresses the unmet mental health needs of all children and adolescents, especially for vulnerable populations such as Latino and immigrant refugee youth. Child and adolescent psychiatrists and mental health clinicians have an opportunity and responsibility to enhance service delivery with advocacy and clinical excellence for this population of youth.

REFERENCES

1. Kessler RC. The costs of depression. Psychiatr Clin North Am 2012;35(1):1–14.
2. Thapar A, Collishaw S, Pine DS, et al. Depression in adolescence. Lancet 2012; 379(9820):1056–67.
3. Bureau UC. Hispanic heritage month 2018. Available at: https://www.census.gov/newsroom/facts-for-features/2018/hispanic-heritage-month.html. Accessed September 7, 2018.
4. Alegria M, Vallas M, Pumariega A. Racial and ethnic disparities in pediatric mental health. Child Adolesc Psychiatr Clin N Am 2010. https://doi.org/10.1016/j.chc.2010.07.001.
5. Interagency Forum on Child F, Statistics F. America's children: key national indicators of well-being, 2017 2017. Available at: https://www.childstats.gov/pdf/ac2017/ac_17.pdf. Accessed September 18, 2018.
6. Foxen P, Mather M, Foxen P, et al. Towards a more equitable future the trends and challenges facing America's Latino children population. Washington D.C., National Council of La Raza 9-2016. Washington, DC. 2016. Available at: www.nclr.org. Accessed March 7, 2018.
7. Potochnick SR, Perreira KM. Depression and anxiety among first-generation immigrant Latino youth: key correlates and implications for future research NIH public access. J Nerv Ment Dis 2010;198(7):470–7.
8. Lê F, Tracy M, Norris FH, et al. Displacement, county social cohesion and depression after a large-scale traumatic event. Soc Psychiatry Psychiatr Epidemiol 2013. https://doi.org/10.1007/s00127-013-0698-7.
9. Fazel M, Reed RV, Panter-Brick C, et al. Mental health of displaced and refugee children resettled in high-income countries: risk and protective factors. Lancet 2012;379(9812):266–82.
10. Rodríguez J, De La Torre A, Miranda CT. Mental health in situations of armed conflict. Biomedica 2002;22(Suppl 2):337–46 [in Spanish]. Available at: http://www.ncbi.nlm.nih.gov/pubmed/12596454. Accessed August 16, 2018.
11. Boehner N, Goldberg P, Schmidt S, et al. Children on the run: unaccompanied children leaving Central America and Mexico and the need for international protection. Washington, DC: The United Nations High Commissioner For Refugees Regional Office For The United States and Caribbean; 2014.
12. Canino G, Alegría M. Psychiatric diagnosis - is it universal or relative to culture? J Child Psychol Psychiatry 2008;49(3):237–50.
13. Kann L, McManus T, Harris WA, et al. Youth risk behavior surveillance — United States, 2017. MMWR Surveill Summ 2018;67(8):1–114.

14. Horwitz AG, Berona J, Czyz EK, et al. Positive and negative expectations of hopelessness as longitudinal predictors of depression, suicidal ideation, and suicidal behavior in high-risk adolescents. Suicide Life Threat Behav 2017;47(2):168–76.
15. Guzmán Á, Koons A, Postolache T. Suicidal behavior in latinos: focus on the youth. Int J Adolesc Med Health 2009;21(4):431–40.
16. Fortuna LR, Perez DJ, Canino G, et al. Prevalence and Correlates of Lifetime suicidal ideation and attempts among Latino Subgroups in the United States NIH Public access. J Clin Psychiatry 2005;68:572–81. Available at: https://www.ncbi.nlm.nih.gov/pmc/articles/PMC2774123/pdf/nihms154115.pdf. Accessed February 8, 2019.
17. Jimenez DE, Bartels SJ, Cardenas V, et al. Cultural beliefs and mental health treatment preferences of ethnically diverse older adult consumers in primary care. Am J Geriatr Psychiatry 2012. https://doi.org/10.1097/JGP.0b013e318227f876.
18. Camacho Á, Gonzalez P, Buelna C, et al. Anxious-depression among hispanic/latinos from different backgrounds: results from the hispanic community health study/study of latinos (HCHS/SOL). Soc Psychiatry Psychiatr Epidemiol 2015. https://doi.org/10.1007/s00127-015-1120-4.
19. Fornos LB, Seguin Mika V, Bayles B, et al. A qualitative study of Mexican American adolescents and depression. J Sch Health 2005;75(5):162–70.
20. Birmaher B, Brent D, AACAP Work Group on Quality Issues, Bernet W, et al. Practice parameter for the assessment and treatment of children and adolescents with depressive disorders. J Am Acad Child Adolesc Psychiatry 2007;46(11):1503–26.
21. Huey SJ Jr, Polo AJ. Evidence-based psychosocial treatments for ethnic minority youth. J Clin Child Adolesc Psychol 2008;37(1):262–301. Available at: https://www.ncbi.nlm.nih.gov/pmc/articles/PMC2413000/pdf/nihms51473.pdf. Accessed February 8, 2019.
22. Rosselló J, Bernal G, Rivera-Medina C. Individual and group CBT and IPT for Puerto Rican adolescents with depressive symptoms. Cultur Divers Ethnic Minor Psychol 2008;14(3):234–45.
23. Cumba-Avilés E. Cognitive-behavioral group therapy for Latino youth with type 1 diabetes and depression: a case study. Clin Case Stud 2017;16(1):58–75.
24. Perrino T, Brincks A, Howe G, et al. Reducing internalizing symptoms among high-risk, hispanic adolescents: mediators of a preventive family intervention HHS public access author manuscript. Prev Sci 2016;17(5):595–605.
25. Marrast L, Himmelstein DU, Woolhandler S. Racial and ethnic disparities in mental health care for children and young adults. Int J Health Serv 2016;46(4):810–24.
26. Olfson M, He J-P, Merikangas KR. Psychotropic medication treatment of adolescents: results from the national comorbidity survey-adolescent supplement. J Am Acad Child Adolesc Psychiatry 2013;52(4):378–88.
27. Kirby JB, Hudson J, Miller GE. Explaining racial and ethnic differences in antidepressant use among adolescents. Med Care Res Rev 2010;67(3):342–63.
28. Goodman E, Slap GB, Huang B. The public health impact of socioeconomic status on adolescent depression and obesity. Am J Public Health 2003;93(11):1844–50. Available at: http://www.ncbi.nlm.nih.gov/pubmed/14600051. Accessed February 8, 2019.
29. Denavas-Walt C, Proctor BD. Income and poverty in the United States: 2014 current population reports. 2015. Available at: https://www.census.gov/content/dam/

Census/library/publications/2015/demo/p60-252.pdf. Accessed September 8, 2018.

30. Ornelas IJ, Perreira KM. The role of migration in the development of depressive symptoms among Latino immigrant parents in the USA. Soc Sci Med 2011; 73(8):1169–77.

31. Schwartz SJ, Unger JB, Zamboanga BL, et al. Rethinking the concept of acculturation: implications for theory and research. Am Psychol 2010;65(4):237–51.

32. Revollo H-W, Qureshi A, Collazos F, et al. Acculturative stress as a risk factor of depression and anxiety in the Latin American immigrant population. Int Rev Psychiatry 2011;23(1):84–92.

33. Kam JA, Lazarevic V. The stressful (and not so stressful) nature of language brokering: identifying when brokering functions as a cultural stressor for Latino immigrant children in early adolescence. J Youth Adolesc 2014;43(12): 1994–2011.

34. Roche KM, Lambert SF, Ghazarian SR, et al. Adolescent language brokering in diverse contexts: associations with parenting and parent-youth relationships in a new immigrant destination area. J Youth Adolesc 2015;44(1):77–89.

35. Benner AD, Graham S. Latino adolescents' experiences of discrimination across the first 2 years of high school: correlates and influences on educational outcomes. Child Dev 2011;82(2):508–19.

36. Arbona C, Olvera N, Rodriguez N, et al. Acculturative stress among documented and undocumented Latino immigrants in the United States. Hisp J Behav Sci 2010;32(3):362–84.

37. Lorenzo-Blanco EI, Unger JB, Baezconde-Garbanati L, et al. Acculturation, enculturation, and symptoms of depression in Hispanic youth: the roles of gender, Hispanic cultural values, and family functioning. J Youth Adolesc 2012;41(10): 1350–65.

38. Aggarwal NK, Glass A, Tirado A, et al. The development of the DSM-5 cultural formulation interview-fidelity instrument (CFI-FI): a pilot study. J Health Care Poor Underserved 2014;25(3):1397–417.

39. Lewis-Fernández R, Aggarwal NK, Bäärnhielm S, et al. Culture and psychiatric evaluation: operationalizing cultural formulation for DSM-5. Psychiatry 2014; 77(2):130–54.

40. Howe Hasanali S, De Jong GF, Roempke Graefe D. Hispanic-asian immigrant inequality in perceived medical need and access to regular physician care. J Immigr Minor Health 2016;18(1):219–27.

41. Colby SL, Ortman JM. Population estimates and Projections Current population Reports. 2015. Available at: www.census.gov. Accessed September 8, 2018.

42. Faq E, Costa D, Cooper D, et al. Economic policy institute answers to frequently asked questions the immigrant population 1. How many immigrants reside in the United States?. 2014. Available at: http://www.fiscalpolicy.org/FPI_NewAmericansOnLongIsland_20120119.pdf. Accessed September 8, 2018.

43. Pew Research Center. Modern immigration Wave brings 59 million to U.S., driving population growth and change through 2065: View of Immigration's impact on U.S. Society Mixed. 2015. Available at: www.pewresearch.org. Accessed September 8, 2018.

44. Pumariega AJ, Rothe E, Pumariega JB. Mental health of immigrants and refugees. Community Ment Health J 2005;41(5):581–97.

45. George U, Thomson MS, Chaze F, et al. Immigrant mental health, a public health issue: looking back and moving forward. Int J Environ Res Public Health 2015; 12(10):13624–48.

46. Burnam MA, Hough RL, Karno M, et al. Acculturation and lifetime prevalence of psychiatric disorders among Mexican Americans in Los Angeles. J Health Soc Behav 1987;28(1):89–102. Available at: http://www.ncbi.nlm.nih.gov/pubmed/3571910. Accessed February 8, 2019.
47. Vega WA, Kolody B, Aguilar-Gaxiola S, et al. Lifetime prevalence of DSM-III-R psychiatric disorders among urban and rural Mexican Americans in California. Arch Gen Psychiatry 1998;55(9):771–8. Available at: http://www.ncbi.nlm.nih.gov/pubmed/9736002. Accessed February 8, 2019.
48. Marks AK, Ejesi K, García Coll C. Understanding the U.S. Immigrant paradox in childhood and adolescence. Child Dev Perspect 2014;8(2):59–64.
49. Crosnoe R, Ramos-Wada A, Bonazzo C. Paradoxes in physical health. Fac Publ - Dep World Lang Sociol Cult Stud. 2015. Available at: https://digitalcommons.georgefox.edu/lang_fac/23. Accessed February 8, 2019.
50. McCullough MB, Marks AK. The immigrant paradox and adolescent obesity: examining health behaviors as potential mediators. J Dev Behav Pediatr 2014;35(2):138–43.
51. Fortuna LR, Álvarez K, Ramos Ortiz Z, et al. Mental health, migration stressors and suicidal ideation among Latino immigrants in Spain and the United States. Eur Psychiatry 2016;36:15–22.
52. Porche MV, Fortuna LR, Lin J, et al. Childhood trauma and psychiatric disorders as correlates of school dropout in a national sample of young adults. Child Dev 2011;82(3):982–98.
53. Alegría M, Canino G, Shrout PE, et al. Prevalence of mental illness in immigrant and non-immigrant U.S. Latino groups. Am J Psychiatry 2008;165(3):359–69.
54. Wong EC, Miles JNV. Prevalence and correlates of depression among new U.S. Immigrants. J Immigr Minor Health 2014;16(3):422–8.
55. Silove D, Ventevogel P, Rees S. The contemporary refugee crisis: an overview of mental health challenges. World Psychiatry 2017;16(2):130–9.
56. Giuliani C, Tagliabue S, Regalia C. Psychological well-being, multiple identities, and discrimination among first and second generation immigrant muslims. Eur J Psychol 2018;14(1):66–87.
57. Betancourt TS, Abdi S, Ito BS, et al. We left one war and came to another: resource loss, acculturative stress, and caregiver-child relationships in Somali refugee families. Cultur Divers Ethnic Minor Psychol 2015;21(1):114–25.
58. Meyer SR, Steinhaus M, Bangirana C, et al. The influence of caregiver depression on adolescent mental health outcomes: findings from refugee settlements in Uganda. BMC Psychiatry 2017;17(1):405.
59. Lincoln AK, Lazarevic V, White MT, et al. The impact of acculturation style and acculturative hassles on the mental health of Somali adolescent refugees. J Immigr Minor Health 2016;18(4):771–8.
60. Leng JCF, Changrani J, Tseng C-H, et al. Detection of depression with different interpreting methods among Chinese and Latino primary care patients: a randomized controlled trial. J Immigr Minor Health 2010;12(2):234–41.
61. Zayas LH, Pilat AM. Suicidal behavior in Latinas: explanatory cultural factors and implications for intervention. Suicide Life Threat Behav 2008;38(3):334–42.
62. Shetgiri R, Kataoka SH, Ryan GW, et al. Risk and resilience in Latinos. Am J Prev Med 2009;37(6):S217–24.
63. Cook SH, Valera P, Calebs BJ, et al. Adult attachment as a moderator of the association between childhood traumatic experiences and depression symptoms among young Black gay and bisexual men. Cultur Divers Ethnic Minor Psychol 2017;23(3):388–97.

64. Lewis-Fernández R, Gorritz M, Raggio GA, et al. Association of trauma-related disorders and dissociation with four idioms of distress among Latino psychiatric outpatients. Cult Med Psychiatry 2010;34(2):219–43.
65. Zayas LH, Gulbas LE. Are suicide attempts by young Latinas a cultural idiom of distress? Transcult Psychiatry 2012;49(5):718–34.
66. Hernandez MY, Organista KC. Entertainment-education? A fotonovela? A new strategy to improve depression literacy and help-seeking behaviors in at-risk immigrant Latinas. Am J Community Psychol 2013;52(3–4):224–35.
67. Hainmueller J, Lawrence D, Martén L, et al. Protecting unauthorized immigrant mothers improves their children's mental health. Science 2017;357(6355): 1041–4.

No Indians to Spare
Depression and Suicide in Indigenous American Children and Youth

Richard Livingston, MD[a],*, Rebecca Susan Daily, MD[b],
Anthony P.S. Guerrero, MD[c], John T. Walkup, MD[d],
Douglas K. Novins, MD[e]

KEYWORDS

- American Indian • Native hawaiian • Alaska native • Child psychiatry • Adolescent
- Depression • Suicide • Indigenous child

KEY POINTS

- The children of indigenous Americans demonstrate significant health disparities from the general population, including physical and mental health (depressive disorders among the issues) and general development.
- Although they are very heterogeneous, indigenous children overall have a higher risk of death by suicide and in some tribes for depressive illness, posttraumatic stress disorder, substance use disorders, and learning difficulties.
- This article reviews these data as well as indigenous American–specific studies on treatment and prevention, and offers clinical recommendations.

Disclosure Statement: Dr R. Livingston, Dr R.S. Daily, Dr A.P.S. Guerrero, and Dr J.T. Walkup have no disclosures. Dr D.K. Novins has research funding from the National Institutes of Health and the Administration for Children and Families.
[a] University of Arkansas College of Medicine, Little Rock, AR, USA; [b] St Elizabeth's Hospitals, 920 Stanton L. Young Boulevard, WP3470, Oklahoma City, OK 73104, USA; [c] Department of Psychiatry, Child and Adolescent Psychiatry Division, University of Hawai'i, John A. Burns School of Medicine, 1356 Lusitana Street, 4th Floor, Honolulu, HI 96813, USA; [d] Child and Adolescent Psychiatry, Northwestern University Feinberg School of Medicine, Ann & Robert H. Lurie Children's Hospital of Chicago, 225 East Chicago Avenue, Chicago, IL 60611, USA; [e] Division of Child & Adolescent Psychiatry, Department of Psychiatry, Pediatric Mental Health Institute, Children's Hospital Colorado, University of Colorado School of Medicine, Centers for American Indian & Alaska Native Health, Colorado School of Public Health, 13123 East 16th Avenue, Box 130, Aurora, CO 80045, USA
* Corresponding author. 4301 West Markham, slot 654, Little Rock AR 72205.
E-mail addresses: rllivingston@uams.edu; drlip78@gmail.com

Child Adolesc Psychiatric Clin N Am 28 (2019) 497–507
https://doi.org/10.1016/j.chc.2019.02.015
1056-4993/19/© 2019 Elsevier Inc. All rights reserved.

childpsych.theclinics.com

Abbreviations

AI	American indian
CBT	Cognitive-behavioral therapy
GSMS	The great smoky mountains study
HTR	historical trauma response
NSSI	nonsuicidal self-injury.

Sixteenth-century physicians believed the "humors" or bodily fluids—black bile, yellow bile, phlegm, and blood—control our natures. After careful examination of the physiognomy of a single indigenous American (synonymous with American Indian), one writer proclaimed that the American Indian (AI) is typically controlled primarily by the black bile, and hence melancholic in temperament.[1] AIs, Alaska Natives, Canadian First Nations peoples, and native Hawaiians all will be considered together as AI and, if specified, it will be with a particular referent.

Which ethnic group, after all, would have more reason to be under thrall to the "black bile"? AIs constitute the smallest US ethnic group, but have the greatest disparities in health care. At the 2010 census, 5.2 million Americans described themselves as AI/Alaska Native; 2.9 million designated that as our only ethnicity. Thirty-two percent are younger than 18, compared with 24% of the overall population, so AIs are young.

AIs are distributed among more than 500 recognized tribal entities that have some things culturally in common ("pan-Indian") but differ in language and in cultural particulars. Each tribe is sovereign and thus decides who is eligible for citizenship in that tribe; however, the US government insists on having a role in the process. Being an AI, therefore, involves some complex legal and procedural issues, with psychosocial enculturation factors and extreme minority status to provide layers of complexity.

Some AIs live on reservations, but most do not. Some speak and understand their tribal languages fluently; many do not. Many tribes have federally recognized sovereignty; each federally recognized tribe has both shared responsibility for its people's health and some sort of access to the Indian Health Service. Thus, it is that access to services, varying degrees of cultural participation and engagement, and a host of psychosocial issues—always to include a traumatic colonial history—contribute to the difficulties of growing up indigenous.

AIs are significantly more likely, at any age, to die at their own hand than any other ethnic group in the United States. Furthermore, accidental deaths and liver disease have added to suicide, such that the overall mortality rate for younger AI people is increasing.[2] The primary role of depressive illness in completed suicide is well-established for the majority culture, but studies are lacking for the AI, and the available data are somewhat inconsistent.

In this article, extant studies about depression and suicide and their risk and protective factors were reviewed. Compared with other ethnic groups, differences and similarities are noted and described. Preventive interventions, as well as pharmacologic and psychosocial treatments for this population, are described.

The overall picture of AI health is not a positive one. At birth, an AI child has a life expectancy about 10 years less than Hispanics and 7 years less than non-Hispanic whites. Poverty, adverse childhood experiences, diabetes, alcohol, and other drugs of abuse all contribute significantly. Despite treaties that included health care as part of the exchange for land, the Indian Health Service per capita expenditure for AI averages $3668, compared with a health care per capita cost of $9523 for the overall US population.[2]

PREVALENCE OF DEPRESSIVE DISORDERS IN AMERICAN INDIAN YOUTH

Two large epidemiologic studies included significant numbers of indigenous young people. Beals and her colleagues[3] studied the lifetime and 12-month prevalence of major disorders in samples from 2 tribes, including those ages 15 to 54, and compared the results with those of the National Comorbidity Survey. Surprisingly, depressive disorders were less prevalent in these 2 tribal samples, across the age ranges, than in the National Comorbidity Survey. The authors noted that the diagnostic criteria required several symptoms that must co-occur during a certain period of time, and suggested that the AI sample either did not experience that or responded differently to questions about it; hence, "Indian time" perception or memory issues may have altered interview responses. It was also possible, if counterintuitive, that these AI youth simply experienced fewer depressive episodes.

In older studies that measured depression on scales rather than using criteria from the *Diagnostic and Statistical Manual of Mental Disorders*, AI youth demonstrated high rates of depressive symptomatology. For example, in The Great Smoky Mountains Study (GSMS), the prevalence of depression was measured in AI youth in each of several waves of interviews, such that results were less dependent on the perception of simultaneity of symptoms during a single interview. In the GSMS overall, depressive disorders were comparable in prevalence between AI and non-AI participants.[4]

Native Hawaiians, compared with nonnative residents of Hawai'i, are at increased risk for suicide attempts (12.9% vs 9.6%, respectively), as well as diagnoses of depression, conduct disorder, substance abuse, anxiety, and obsessive-compulsive disorder.[5–7] As reviewed by Goebert and coworkers,[7] Native Hawaiian compared with Caucasian youth and young adults were 2.3 times more likely to die by suicide and 2 times more likely to have made a suicide attempt in the last year. Furthermore, since Hawaii began collecting suicide data in 1908, it seems that suicide rates for Native Hawaiians have been increasing. According to Yuen and colleagues,[8] Hawaiian cultural affiliation has been predictive of suicide attempts in youth, as have been depression, substance abuse, and socioeconomic status. Those authors also hypothesized that cultural tension and conflict may contribute specifically to suicidal behavior.

Else and colleagues[9] noted the spikes in suicidal behaviors in young Native Hawaiians, and discussed the similarity of these suicide patterns to those of indigenous peoples in the United States, Canada, and New Zealand. In reviewing other US-affiliated Pacific Islands, notably in the region of Micronesia, they also discussed the postwar disintegration of traditional family systems and its association with high rates of suicide completion. Guerrero and coworkers[10] listed other possible environmental and cultural risk factors, including the impact of colonization and genocide, extinction of the indigenous language, poverty, loss of homeland (including global warming and resource depletion), geographic isolation, and lack of mental health care availability.

COMPLEX ASSOCIATIONS OF RISK MARKERS

Particular groups at risk did emerge in the GSMS. Six percent of AI girls were identified as having very low birth weights, and 38% of those experienced a major depressive episode by age 16. The association with very low birth weight may be a marker for a broader condition or may represent a risk factor in itself.

From the earliest days' discussions of theoretic and clinical aspects of young people experiencing depression,[11] it has been posited that dysphoria and irritability should be considered cardinal signs of childhood depression. Robust sample size in GSMS allowed for careful examination of that possibility, and it seemed not to have been true of these particular depressed AI youth.[12]

The broad incidence and prevalence data for depressive disorders in AI youth are very limited. The data that are available in the 2 studies discussed herein suggest that the prevalence rates are not higher than those of the majority culture, despite the clearly increased suicide risks.

Substance abuse is apparently more prevalent among AI youth and may exercise its suicidal influences via a simple (general risk, with disinhibition and altered judgment) or more complex pathways. For example, inhalant abuse including gasoline is overrepresented among native children, and tetraethyl lead toxicity may be a specific marker for suicide risk in certain First Nations.

There may be risks associated with certain other health issues, as well; unhealthy behaviors of the sort that are called "obesogenic" seem to correlate positively with depressive symptoms, and negatively with self-efficacy, in AI populations. Poor nutrition, specifically with obesity or diabetes, could be part of a complex and overdetermined "hot mess" of risk factors.

AI youth are at high risk for diabetes; diabetes is associated with impaired metabolic functioning with increased levels of markers of inflammation including C-reactive protein and IL-6. Combined with symptoms of depression, as measured on the Center for Epidemiologic Studies Depression scale,[13] does this represent a coincidence or part of a complex of risk factors?

HISTORICAL TRAUMA AS A RISK FACTOR

Many AIs recall their elders telling stories of the bad things they experienced or heard about, and recall these stories being told with an air of intensity and immediacy, as if they had just happened. This could be part of the "historical trauma response (HTR),"[14] or may represent an AI style of narration. This phenomenon called HTR has been proposed and studies have begun, identifying the basic conditions from which arise the adversities that affected large numbers and led to stress responses and collective mourning. HTR's basic conditions include adversity that affected a large number of individuals, resulting in widespread adversity and collective mourning. The trauma was perpetuated by outsiders perceived to have nonbenign intent. HTR has influenced or shaped many of the difficulties experienced by today's AI, but with both qualitative and quantitative variations among tribe, communities, families, and individuals.

Although the impacts of historical trauma are very difficult to study in populations when this history extends over half a millennia and coincides with contemporary traumas, stresses, and adversities, it is suggested that both historical trauma and current adversities likely impact the development and biological, psychological, and social aspects of AI youth.

The context of the historical trauma varies according to circumstances and acculturation. Its manifestations will be judged by AI families according to AI values. **Box 1** illustrates some of these pan-Indian value tensions, presented here roughly in analogy to Erikson's developmental tensions, but without attempting to assign those tensions to any age ranges. The tensions described as "versus" are intended to show some areas in which traditional AI values vary from the majority/postcolonial cultures.

TREATMENT: PSYCHOPHARMACOLOGY

Research on medications for depression and suicidality among AI youth is very limited. In terms of availability of services, a 2003 study by Richardson and

> **Box 1**
> **Developing and balancing AI values in the postcolonial world**
>
> 1. Individuality versus membership
> 2. Selfishness versus generosity and gratitude
> 3. Microenculturation versus macroenculturation
> 4. Identity pride versus narcissistic pride
> 5. Resentment toward majority culture versus harmonious-enough living
> 6. Mindful of present versus mindful of past and future
> 7. Humility toward mystery/creation versus shame and poor self-concept

colleagues[15] found profound disparities of overall treatments and pharmacologic treatments among ethnic groups, with white children being the most likely to receive medication for depression and native or Hispanic youth least likely.

Limited data about pharmacologic treatment for depression in indigenous adults are reported with paroxetine, duloxetine, citalopram, venlafaxine, protriptyline, amitriptyline, and sertraline.[16-18] No similar data for AI youth are noted. Two studies from New Zealand, including adults and adolescents 15 years of age and older, found Maori and other islanders less likely than Caucasians to receive antidepressants.[19]

A 2016 study of 7.5 million people (all ages) with private health insurance found that about 1.2 million had received a psychiatric diagnosis, with 20.6% of AI and Alaska Natives, and 9.1% of native Hawaiians diagnosed. Despite their diagnoses, AIs were 20% less likely to have received pharmacologic treatments, all the more remarkable, given their superior adherence to the treatments that were prescribed.

Complementary and alternative medical treatments reported for depressed AI adults and children include ceremonies, spiritual treatments, herbals, and other interventions.[20] Herbals reportedly used for AI included valerian, ginseng, rhodiola, kava kava, palapalai, areca nut, lemon myrtle, passion flower, and lavender. Although the traditional healing practices of AI communities have not been subject to randomized, controlled trials, they are seen by many AIs as centrally important to health and healing. One study analyzed the combined and independent use of biomedical and AI traditional healing among AI adolescents and adults.

Complementary and alternative medical treatments may be offered with Indian-specific goals in mind, which may not correspond with those of the majority culture. The Indigenous healer Janice Longboat has stated that, "Healing the spirit ENABLES other healing" (personal verbal communication, 2003). Goals for these aspects of healing may be expressed to achieve some particular state of harmony, associated with wellness ("hozho" in Navajo, "dohi" in Cherokee).[21]

TREATMENTS: PSYCHOSOCIAL INTERVENTIONS

Variants on well-established psychotherapy, proven effective for the general population, such as cognitive-behavioral therapy (CBT), have been customized for Indian subcultures. A modified version of the CBT-based coping with depression for adolescents, was offered to a small pilot group of 8 rural AI youth and resulted in significantly lower depression scores at its end and 3 months later; anxiety scores were lower as well, but not to a statistically significant degree. Furthermore, the coping with depression for adolescents program was perceived as less stigmatizing.[22]

Depression and trauma are addressed by Honoring Children, Mending the Circle, a trauma-focused CBT program currently under study.[23] There is also a school-based CBT with promise, discussed in Settings for Treatment.

Settings for Treatment

Clinics and medical settings usually constitute the traditional setting for psychiatric treatment. Access to treatment among minority and underrepresented populations can be more problematic.

For certain minority and underrepresented children, school-based treatments are an effective way to provide mental health interventions, especially when families have barriers to other treatments (transportation, economics, and other variables). For AI children and youth, however, a unique barrier may exist for school-based treatment: this is the population with the largest proportion of children who are chronically absent from school, defined as missing 15 days a year or more; 22.5% are absent overall and 28% in high school.[24]

Although attendance may be less of an issue in Indian boarding school settings, there are other potential problems. Boarding schools provide therapy services during the school year, but these students do not receive care during the summer break. In 1 boarding school consulted by 1 of the authors, 4 children reportedly died by suicide during 1 summer break after returning to their reservations (Livingston, report of American Academy of Pediatrics Committee on Native American Child Health consultation, unpublished, 2011.)

YOUTH SUICIDE: INDIAN ISSUES

Unquestionably, the overall rate of death by suicides by AI youth is excessive and disproportionate to other populations. However, as child psychiatrist James Shore had advised long ago in 1975, tribal suicide rates may vary from 8 to 120 per 100,000. Epidemiologic data are scant. Clearly, some tribal groups fare better and some worse. It is certainly inappropriate to assume that homogeneity applies to prevention or treatment any more than it applies to prevalence.

One study compared suicidal ideation and suicide attempts in urban AI adolescents with those from a reservation.[25] One-fifth of the urban AI youth and one-third of those from the reservation reported suicidal ideation; suicide attempts were acknowledged by 14% and 18%, respectively. The groups did not share predictive correlates, and the authors suggested that different approaches might be advised to best understand these statistics.

Although depressive illness is not necessarily more prevalent in AI youth, suicide is, as previously noted. It is recommended nevertheless that the prevention of suicide should include the identification of any psychiatric illness and effective treatment for that illness. However, this measure does not suffice to decrease the incidence of suicide in AI populations owing to the multiple risk factors, etiology, and determinants.

A case-control study of Inuit suicide[26] identified the following as risk factors: experiencing child abuse, having relatives who died by suicide, substance abuse, impulsivity, and aggression. In another report, indigenous children in Chile were studied, with suicidal and nonsuicidal participants not differing on Children's Depression Inventory and anxiety scores, but significantly different on the variable of "involvement," with others and activities. Lower involvement was correlated with hopelessness and suicidal behavior, and higher involvement seemed to be protective.[27]

A large study of 11,666 AI youth in 8 Indian Health Service boarding schools found that 22% of girls and 12% of boys had attempted suicide, noting that 1 in 13 of those attempters eventually died by suicide.[28] This finding yielded an overall suicide rate of 31.7. Nonattempters had greater family and social connectedness, less suicide among family and friends, less history of abuse, and more exercise. Sexual abuse predicted male but not female suicide attempters. Female attempters were more likely to acknowledge bisexual fantasies. Although humiliation and shame were not specifically identified, clinical experience suggests a possible role for these experiences leading to humiliation and then to suicide attempts.

Berlin[29] compared several tribes, concluding that suicide rates were higher in those with the least adherence to traditional ways and AI religions. Novins and colleagues[30] studied 1353 high school students from 3 tribes, noting that no single suicide correlate was common to all 3 tribes, but suggested that culture can function as a protective factor. A measure of enculturation of youth was included in a survey titled, "Voices of Indian Teens."

A related issue that has been investigated is AI adoption by non-AI families. Johnson and Tomren[31] found that adopted-away AI children attempted suicide 6 times as often as other youth. A younger AI friend of the lead author said, "We are MADE for community." There are lots of reasons to hold this true for AIs. Clearly, there is a correlation between AI suicide with lack of enculturation, affiliation, participation, and tradition. Does this mean increasing those things will lower the suicide rate? The prospective studies certainly need to be done.

The possibility that HTR contributes specifically to depression and to suicide risk has been discussed, primarily from a theoretic perspective. Clinically, this should be assessed as a possible contributor, but it is difficult to know how precisely to use and interpret the information.

With reference to suicide prevention approaches in Hawai'i, Goebert and associates[7] have emphasized the importance of strengths-based approaches that enhance existing assets and relationships in families and communities; that unite communities around a common goal of suicide prevention through awareness and training; that involve youth in community-based efforts; and that reference cultural values and traditions. Following these approaches, which engender indigenization, communities can implement culturally relevant healing interventions that provide hope to youth who otherwise may have experienced marginalization and despair.

SUICIDE PREVENTION: ONE COMMUNITY'S APPROACH

The White Mountain Apache and the Center for American Indian Health at the Johns Hopkins Bloomberg School of Public Health has more than 30 years of collaboration in addressing health disparities. Infectious diseases were the greatest health disparity and focus of the initial collaboration. In the early 1990s, after a spike in youth suicide, the collaboration of the White Mountain Apache and Johns Hopkins began its focus on reducing youth suicide.

Initial efforts reviewed trends in suicide on the White Mountain Apache Reservation. Before the 1950s, suicidal behavior was rare. Spikes in suicidal behavior were initially in the 1980s, but were uncommon. The spike in suicide that occurred during the period of 1990 to 1993 signaled a dramatic turn of events. The average annual (age-adjusted) rate of suicide among White Mountain Apache tribal members was 44.7 per 100,000. There were a total of 45 suicide deaths and serious attempts over a 3-year period, including 7 deaths that occurred in a short 40-day period. In contrast with the pattern of suicide in the rest of the country, youth ages 13 to 28 years old were affected more commonly than older men, and hanging was much more common than gun-related suicide deaths.[4,32] In the early 2000s and in response to another spike in suicide among youth, tribal leadership took a unique step of mandating reporting of suicidal behavior to a suicide prevention task force in a manner similar to the reporting of infectious diseases. Under the plan, all tribal members were mandated to report suicidal behavior to the task force for the purpose of identifying those at risk but also to collect important data about patterns of suicide on the reservation and to develop tribal-specific prevention and intervention plans.[33] Results from the first 5 years of suicidal behavior surveillance (2001–2006) painted a sobering picture of suicidal behavior among the White Mountain Apache. The annualized rate of suicide was highest among youth 15 to 24 years of age at 128.5 per 100,000 which was 13 times the US all-races rate and 7 times the AI and Alaska Native rate over the same time period. Similar to rates in the rest of the country the male-to-female ratio was 5:1 for suicide, but in contrast with the rest of the United States where more females attempt suicide than males, suicide attempts occurred at a near equal rate for males and females. Hanging was the most common suicide method, and the third most common attempt method accounting for upward of 25% of suicide attempts. Similar to other studies of youth suicide, family and community members reported that family or intimate partner conflict was the most common precipitant to the young person suicide.[32] With continued surveillance of suicidal behavior, other patterns emerged. Mandated suicidal behavior reporting identified a developmental pattern of suicidal behavior that began early with suicidal ideation and that suicide attempts were most common in teens and young adults, who were most likely to die by suicide. In addition, youth who died or made a suicide attempt were frequently exposed to the recent suicidal behavior of peers or family members at high rates and that suicidal behavior often occurred in the context of alcohol use. Among those who were reported to the surveillance system were youth who were engaged in nonsuicidal self-injury (NSSI), a pattern of behavior not often described among AI populations. The NSSI rate of among was 600 in 100,000 overall, with children and young teens ages 10 to 14 years old disproportionately affected (3000 in 100,000). NSSI was more common among females (65%) and cutting was the preferred method (98%).[34] An additional finding from the surveillance system identified a pattern of alcohol binge use among youth that was described in terms similar to youth engaged in NSSI, which resulted in investigators suggested that binge drinking may be a form of NSSI for some AI youth.[35,36] (These factors may or may not be associated with depressive illness; further study is certainly needed.)

In keeping with the tribal mandate, a multilevel suicide prevention plan was implemented on the reservation. The universal prevention intervention consisted of raising awareness of suicide and particularly youth suicide in the community and the relevant risk and protective factors. For youth at risk for suicide, community elders launched a number of programs that attended to older children and younger adolescents using a strengths-based approach focusing on Apache traditions and cultural education. Applied suicide intervention skills training was implemented tribe-wide for those who were likely to come in contact with tribal members who were in distress or suicidal. Selected interventions for youth who attempted suicide included an emergency department-linked intervention for the youth and their family and case management services. A recent report documented a decrease in suicide rate from 40 per 100000 in 2001 to 2006 to 25 per 100,000 in 2007 to 2012 on the reservation during a time when rates in the United States were stable[37] or even potentially increasing.

A number of lessons can be learned from the White Mountain Apache suicide prevention program:

1. Tribal and other communities that experience disproportionately high rates of suicide can implement successful suicide prevention plans.

2. Surveillance community-wide in and of itself likely has a positive effect on suicidal behavior when combined with follow-up and case management.
3. Local data can lead to local solutions that may be more effective.
4. The engagement of tribal members in implementing the prevention program (task shifting of mental health prevention interventions) may be a model for other communities facing similar disproportionate levels of youth suicide.

CLINICAL RECOMMENDATIONS

The following are our clinical recommendations for child and adolescent psychiatrists providing care for AI children and adolescents pertaining to suicide and depression.

1. Screen and pursue identification of depressive and other affective disorders, psychosis, anxiety disorder, and substance abuse. When indicated, provide treatment interventions, medications, and psychotherapies. Provide evidence-based treatments to the extent possible, especially AI-specific interventions and adaptations.
2. Do not assume that adequate diagnostic assessment suffices for suicide risk assessment in indigenous youth; assess collaterals/supports, enculturation, and social isolation.
3. Treatment and prevention are better accomplished with the involvement of family, tribe, and AI/Indian community. This process requires consent procedures and may be time consuming and difficult, but is more resonant with AI values.
4. Assume that affiliation, participation, and enculturation have the potential to prevent Indian suicide and enhance mood quality and stability, especially for AI youth. Special attention should be given to lookout for loss or abandonment of existing affiliations and participation. Explore these factors to understand increased risk or early warning signs.
5. Identification and intervention for other possible suicide risk factors are essential, including those discussed in this article (birth weight, general health, inhalant abuse, nutrition, adoption, abuse, and other stressors).

Put the Gun Down, Cousin:

Because we don't have Indians to spare.

Because suicide and whiskey are gifts from the colonizers.

Because someone has cared, cares, will care.

Poem by Richard Livingston.

REFERENCES

1. Horden P, Hsn E, editors. The body in balance, humoral med in practice. New York: Berghahn Books; 2013.
2. Abbasi J. Why are American Indians dying young? JAMA 2018;319(2):109–11.
3. Beals J, Manson ST, Whitesell NR, et al. Prevalence of major depressive episode in two American Indian reservation populations. Am J Psychiatry 2005;162:1713–22.
4. Costello EJ, Farmer EM, Angold A, et al. Psychiatric disorders among American Indian and white youth in Appalachia. Am J Public Health 1997;87(5):827–32.

5. Guerrero AP, Hishinuma ES, Andrade NN, et al. Demographic and clinical characteristics of adolescents in Hawaii with obsessive-compulsive disorder. Arch Pediatr Adolesc Med 2003;157(7):665–70.

6. Andrade NN, Hishinuma ES, McDermott JF Jr, et al. The National Center on Indigenous Hawaiian Behavioral Health study of the prevalence of psychiatric disorders in native Hawaiian adolescents. J Am Acad Child Adolesc Psychiatry 2006;45(1):26–36.

7. Goebert D, Alvarez A, Andrade NN, et al. Hope, help, and healing: culturally embedded approaches to suicide prevention, intervention and postvention services with native Hawaiian youth. Psychol Serv 2018;15(3):332–9.

8. Yuen NY, Nahulu LB, Hishinuma ES, et al. Cultural identification and attempted suicide in Native Hawaiian adolescents. J Am Acad Child Adolesc Psychiatry 2000;39(3):360–7.

9. Else IR, Andrade NN, Nahulu LB. Suicide and suicidal-related behaviors among indigenous Pacific Islanders in the United States. Death Stud 2007;31(5): 479–501.

10. Guerrero AP, Fung D, Suaalii-Sauni T, et al. Care for the seafarers: a review of mental health in Austronesia. Asia Pac Psychiatry 2013;5(3):119–40.

11. Poznanski EO. The clinical phenomenology of childhood depression. Am J Orthopsychiatry 1982;52(2):308–13.

12. Costello EJ, Angold A, Burns BJ, et al. The greater smoky mountains study of youth. Arch Gen Psychiatry 1996;53(12):1129–36.

13. Hood KH, Lawrence JM, Anderson A, et al. Metabolic and inflammatory links to depression in youth with diabetes. Diabetes Care 2012;35(12):2443–6.

14. Whitbeck LB, Adams GW, Hoyt DR, et al. Conceptualizing and measuring historical trauma among American Indian people. Am J Community Psychol 2004; 33(3–4):119–30.

15. Richardson LP, DiGiuseppe D, Garrison M, et al. Depression in medicaid-covered youth, by race and ethnicity. Arch Pediatr Adolesc Med 2003;157:984–9.

16. Wardman D, Khan N. Antidepressant medication use among First Nations peoples in British Columbia. Am Indian Alsk Native Ment Health Res 2004;11:43–8.

17. Callazos F, Ramos M, Quereshi A, et al. Effectiveness of duloxetine in two different ethnic samples. J Clin Psychopharmacol 2013;33:254–6.

18. O'Malley SS, Robin WW, Leveson AL, et al. Naltrexone alone or with sertraline in Alaska natives. Alcohol Clin Exp Res 2008;32(7):127–83.

19. Exeter D, Robinson E, Wheeler A. Antidepressant dispensing trends in New Zealand. Aust N Z J Psychiatry 2009;43:1131–40.

20. Barnes PM, Bloom B, Nahin RL. Complementary and alternative medicine use in the US, vol. 12. Washington, DC: NHS report; 2007.

21. Leffler LJ. Under the rattlesnake: Cherokee health and resiliency. Tuscaloosa (AL): University of Alabama Press; 2009.

22. Lisug-Lunde L, Vogeltanz-Holm N, Collins J. A cognitive-behavioral treatment for depression in rural American Indian middle school students. Am Indian Alsk Native Ment Health Res 2013;20:16–34.

23. Bigfoot D, Schmidt SR. Honoring children, mending the circle: adaptation of trauma-focused cognitive behavioral therapy for American Indian and Alaska Native Children. J Clin Psychol 2010;66:847–56.

24. U.S. Department of Education. DOE pamphlet/brochure. 2016.

25. Freedenthal S, Stiffman AR. Suicidal behavior in American Indian adolescents. Suicide & life threatening behavior. New York: Guilford Press; 2004.

26. Chachamovich E, Kirmayer LJ, McCormick R, et al. Suicide among Inuit. Can J Psychiatry 2015;60:268–75.
27. Caqueo-Uziar A, Urzaa A, Demunta K. Mental health of indigenous children in Northern Chile. BMC Psychiatry 2014;14:11.
28. Borowsky IW, Resnick MD, Ireland M, et al. Suicide attempts among American Indian and Alaska Native youth: risk and protective factors. Arch Pediatr Adolesc Med 1999;153(6):573–80.
29. Berlin IN. Suicide among American Indian adolescents, an overview. Suicide Life Threat Behav 1987;17:218–32.
30. Novins DK, Beals J, Roberts RE, et al. Factors associated with suicide among American Indian adolescents: does culture matter? Suicide Life Threat Behav 1999;29:332–46.
31. Johnson T, Tomren H. Helplessness, hopelessness, and despair: identifying the precursors of Indian youth suicide. Am Indian Cult Res J 1999;23:287–301.
32. Mullany B, Barlow A, Goklish N, et al. Toward understanding suicide among youths: results from the White Mountain Apache tribally mandated suicide surveillance system, 2001-2006. Am J Public Health 2009;99(10):1840–8.
33. Cwik MF, Barlow A, Goklish N, et al. Community-based surveillance and case management for suicide prevention: an American Indian tribally initiated system. Am J Public Health 2014;104(Suppl 3):e18–23.
34. Cwik MF, Barlow A, Tingey L, et al. Nonsuicidal self-injury in an American Indian reservation community: results from the White Mountain Apache surveillance system, 2007-2008. J Am Acad Child Adolesc Psychiatry 2011;50(9):860–9.
35. Barlow A, Tingey L, Cwik M, et al. Understanding the relationship between substance use and self-injury in American Indian youth. Am J Drug Alcohol Abuse 2012;38(5):403–8.
36. Tingey L, Cwik M, Goklish N, et al. Exploring binge drinking and drug use among American Indians: data from adolescent focus groups. Am J Drug Alcohol Abuse 2012;38(5):409–15.
37. Cwik MF, Tingey L, Maschino A, et al. Decreases in suicide deaths and attempts linked to the white mountain Apache suicide surveillance and prevention system, 2001-2012. Am J Public Health 2016;106(12):2183–9.

Risk Versus Resiliency
Addressing Depression in Lesbian, Gay, Bisexual, and Transgender Youth

Brandon Johnson, MD[a],*, Scott Leibowitz, MD[b],
Alexis Chavez, MD[c], Sarah E. Herbert, MD, MSW[d,1]

KEYWORDS

- Lesbian • Gay • Bisexual • Transgender • Depression • Suicidality
- Gender dysphoria

KEY POINTS

- Lesbian, gay, bisexual, and transgender (LGBT) youth are at increased risk of depression due to stigma, discrimination, and victimization.
- Transgender youth often meet criteria for gender dysphoria, which may be associated with depression. This may additionally be alleviated by social and medical gender transition interventions (pubertal suppression and/or hormones).
- Targeting interventions to bolster supports in various environments (home, school, and community) is an important part of treating depression in LGBT youth in addition to other gold standard treatments.

INTRODUCTION

It has been widely established that youth who are minorities based on their sexual orientation and/or gender identity have a greater risk of negative mental health outcomes, including depression and suicidality.[1–6] Lesbian, gay, bisexual, and transgender (LGBT) youth have unique risk factors that predispose them to depression through the moderator of stigma. Experiences, such as family rejection, bullying, and lack of social acceptance, can contribute to negative health outcomes in this

Disclosure Statement: S. Leibowitz—Royalties from Springer. No further disclosures.
[a] Mount Sinai St. Luke's Hospital, Icahn School of Medicine at Mount Sinai, 411 West 114th Street, 2nd Floor, New York, NY 10025, USA; [b] THRIVE Gender Development Program, Nationwide Children's Hospital, The Ohio State University College of Medicine, 555 South 18th Street, Columbus, OH 43205, USA; [c] Department of Psychiatry, University of Colorado, Anschutz, 13001 East 17th Place, Building 500, 2E, Aurora, CO 80045, USA; [d] Department of Psychiatry and Behavioral Sciences, Morehouse School of Medicine, Atlanta, GA, USA
[1] Present address: 160 Clairemont Avenue, Suite 445, Decatur, GA 30030.
* Corresponding author.
E-mail address: brandondjohnson@gmail.com

Child Adolesc Psychiatric Clin N Am 28 (2019) 509–521
https://doi.org/10.1016/j.chc.2019.02.016
1056-4993/19/© 2019 Elsevier Inc. All rights reserved.

population. It can be difficult for clinicians to stay current with guidelines in a rapidly changing field, although the American Academy of Child and Adolescent Psychiatry Practice Parameter on Gay, Lesbian, or Bisexual Sexual Orientation, Gender Nonconformity, and Gender Discordance in Children and Adolescents can serve as a general guide.[7] This article discusses the current literature, describes the LGBT youth population, discusses the unique risk factors associated with this population, and identifies interventions to address both stigma and subsequent mental health outcomes.

TERMINOLOGY

Gender and sexuality are complex aspects of individuals' identities that include several components, including sex, gender identity, gender expression, and sexual orientation (**Fig. 1**). Although for many individuals, these identities align based on societal stereotypical grouping of categories (ie, male sex, male gender identity, masculine gender expression, and heterosexual orientation), for a significant subset of the population this is not the case. LGBT is an acronym that serves as an umbrella for several groups of individuals who have minority identities related to sexual orientation, gender expression, and/or gender identity. Although LGBT stands for lesbian, gay, bisexual, and transgender, there are many other identities that fall under the acronym.

Sex is a medical term determined by multiple factors, including internal anatomy (gonads), external anatomy (genitalia), genetics (chromosomes), hormones, and hormone receptors. Gender identity refers to a sense of self as male or female, having aspects of male and female genders, or neither. External genitalia typically are used at birth to assign a gender; this is known as the assigned sex at birth (ASAB). In Western culture, gender identity traditionally has been viewed as a binary system, including males and females. A more accurate depiction of gender identity reveals that gender lies on a spectrum, with many identities outside the binary. The term, *cisgender*, refers to when gender identity is aligned with ASAB. *Transgender* refers to incongruence

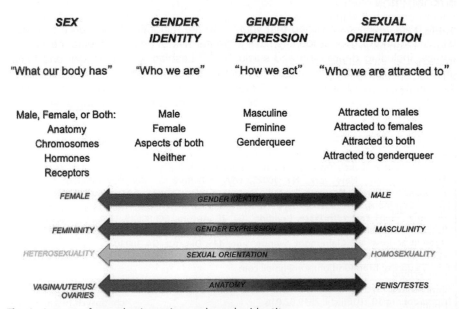

Fig. 1. Aspects of sexual orientation and gender identity.

between gender identity and ASAB. **Table 1** depicts more colloquial terms that describe relationships between gender identity and ASAB.

Differences in gender identity are not pathologic; however, some individuals who identify as transgender meet criteria for the *Diagnostic and Statistical Manual of Mental Disorders* (Fifth Edition) (*DSM-5*) diagnosis, gender dysphoria (GD). This diagnosis refers to the distress related to the incongruence between gender identity and ASAB. Diagnostic criteria include distress related to socially expected gender expression based on ASAB and related to the anatomic incongruence. The *DSM-5* describes both childhood and adolescent/adult subtypes of GD, with differing criteria.[8]

Gender expression refers to outward expression of gender through dress, speech, mannerisms, and behavior. Expression of gender is culture-specific, with socially constructed ideals of what is masculine or feminine within each culture. Just as with gender identity, gender expression falls along a spectrum from typically feminine to typically masculine expression. Although gender expression and gender identity are related phenomena for a given person (ie, gender expression often aligns with gender identity), they are not inextricably linked. Gender expression that is different from expected societal norms does not necessarily mean that an individual identifies as LGBT, although many on the LGBT spectrum have diverse gender expressions within their culture.

Children and adolescents with diverse expressions of gender, who do not currently identify as another gender, have been described by various terms in the literature, including *gender nonconforming*, *gender variant*, *gender expansive*, *gender diverse*, and so forth. For the sake of uniformity, this population is referred in this article to as *gender diverse*.

Sexual orientation refers to the gender (or sex) of the people to whom one is sexually attracted or aroused by. With heterosexuality (attractions and arousal patterns to a different gender) as the majority status, other sexual orientations fall under the LGBT spectrum. Queer is a historically derogatory term reclaimed by some LGBT individuals that is often used to represent those who identify as nonheterosexual and/or noncisgender but without a specific label denoting gender identity and/or sexuality. **Table 2** depicts more colloquial terms used to describe various sexual orientations. Sexual orientation and gender identity are distinct aspects of identity. For instance, transgender individuals can identify as any sexual orientation (in relation to their affirmed gender identity), making it important to recognize that some youth identify as both transgender and gay, lesbian, or bisexual.

Table 1	
Terms related to gender identity	
Term	**Gender Identity**
Cisgender	ASAB matches gender
Transgender	ASAB is the opposite of gender
Intersex	Any identity but with ambiguous sexual anatomy
Agender	Does not identify with gender
Bigender	Aspects of both male and female genders
Genderfluid	Different genders at different times
Genderqueer	Outside of gender norms—defies categorization of gender
Nonbinary	Neither male nor female but elsewhere on the spectrum

Table 2
Terms related to sexual orientation

Term	Individual's Gender	Gender Attracted to
Lesbian	Female	Female
Gay	Male	Male
Bisexual	Any	Male and female
Pansexual	Any	Any
Asexual	Any	None
Queer	Any	Nonheterosexual

METHODS

The authors highlight relevant literature and clinical guidelines related to LGBT youth and mental health outcomes, with a focus on depression and suicidal ideation as well as moderators of these outcomes in LGBT youth. The most widely known and relevant articles were used to compile data for this article. There is less research on transgender and gender diverse youth than on lesbian, gay, and bisexual (LGB) youth. In particular, the intersection of LGB and transgender or gender diverse identities has not been well studied. Where indicated, authors make a distinction between research that focuses specifically on LGB versus research on gender diverse identities.

EPIDEMIOLOGY

The number of people identifying as LGBT has been steadily increasing over the years.[9] Although many surveys have attempted to quantify the number of LGBT persons in the United States, differences in nomenclature and methodology have provided a range of estimates. These estimates of the adult LGB or LGBT population have ranged from 2.2% to 4%, or 5.2 million to 9.5 million adults.[10]

LGBT youth represent a significant percentage of young people, making the health disparities experienced by this population a serious and concerning problem. In the most recent Youth Risk Behavior Survey (YRBS) conducted by the Centers for Disease Control and Prevention,[1] 10.4% of high school students surveyed identified as LGB, which represents a larger percentage of teens than adults identifying as LGB.

UNIQUE RISK FACTORS FOR LESBIAN, GAY, BISEXUAL, AND TRANSGENDER YOUTH
Discrimination and Stigma

LGBT youth are at higher risk for depression, anxiety, suicide, and many other adverse mental and physical health outcomes.[1] When examining health disparities in minority populations, such as LGBT populations, it is important to consider the role that stress and stigma play to fully appreciate how these disparities are created, exacerbated, and perpetuated.

LGBT individuals can experience explicit legal discrimination (lack of same rights and protections as non-LGBT individuals) or noncodified discrimination through attitudes and behaviors used by the majority (bullying and exclusion) that restrict minority groups in the same manner.[11] Discrimination may prevent LGBT individuals from accessing important medical care either through refusal of care by the provider or through apprehension by the patient based on previous negative experiences.[12]

Chronic Stress and Internalizing Stigma

According to the minority stress model, discriminatory events lead to further expectation for future discriminatory events.[13] Persistent stigma creates a chronically elevated stress state in the individual, resulting in many negative mental and physical health conditions. When chronic stigma becomes internalized over time, this causes individuals to believe the discriminatory attitudes about them and leads to negative valuation of the self,[14] elevating the risk for depression. Internalized discriminatory attitudes can be directed toward one's own sexual orientation (internalized homophobia) or gender identity (internalized transphobia). Examples of internalized phobia are included in **Table 3**.

Family Rejection or Support

For all LGBT youth, a family's level of supportiveness is a major factor in a youth's self-esteem, health disparities, and overall well-being.[15] Unfortunately, gender diverse children are more likely to experience childhood physical, sexual, and psychological abuse by their parents.[16] Furthermore, LGBT youth from racial and ethnic minority groups experience parental rejection at a rate higher than racial majority groups.[17] Family rejection also may involve families sending a child to conversion therapy with the goal of changing the child's identity to cisgender and/or heterosexual. Efforts to change adolescents' identities through either parental efforts or conversion therapy have been associated with deleterious mental health and socioeconomic outcomes during young adulthood.[18]

Homelessness

In a 2012 study from the Williams Institute, 68% of LGBT homeless youth surveyed reported that family rejection was a major factor in their homelessness (by either running away or being forced out), making it by far the most commonly cited factor.[19] As many as 40% of transgender youth may experience homelessness at some point in their lives.[20] Lack of state funding, lack of local funding, and lack of federal funding were determined the top 3 barriers to preventing LGBT youth homelessness.[19]

Homelessness subsequently puts transgender youth at higher risk for many other negative outcomes. Homeless shelters or other types of emergency housing may deny transgender youth services outright due to religious beliefs or lack of comfort

Table 3
Examples of internalized phobia

Internalized Homophobia	Internalized Transphobia
"Men don't want to date other guys who are too 'faggy'."	"I'm not a 'real' man/woman."
"Women don't want to date other women who are too 'butch'."	"I don't want to transition if I can't pass because then I'll be a freak."
"I don't want my friends/family to meet my same-sex partner."	"I don't want to hang out with other transgender people if they don't pass."
"Gay relationships don't last as long as 'normal' relationships."	"If my friends or family don't use my name or pronouns it's okay as long as they don't kick me out of their lives."
"I refuse to hang out in LGBT spaces."	"Being transgender puts a burden on everyone around me and they are doing me a favor by accepting me."

in dealing with transgender populations.[20,21] When such emergency housing is available, they are more likely to experience victimization, including 50% or more of LGBT youth physically assaulted at larger shelters.[22]

School Environment

Targeting of LGBT youth can cause a hostile environment even in school. Data from the National School Climate Survey in 2011 found that large percentages of students felt unsafe due to their sexual orientation (63.5%) and gender expression (43.9%).[2] These unsafe feelings stemmed from high levels of verbal and electronic harassment and physical harassment or assault. The students who experienced higher levels of victimization due to their sexual orientation or gender expression had higher levels of depression than those with less victimization. Furthermore, the effects of LGBT-related school victimization persist and are strongly linked to negative young adult mental and physical health outcomes.[23]

Depression in Lesbian, Gay, Bisexual, and Transgender Youth

In summary, depression in LGBT youth is not a unique phenomenon that is unlike depression in any other youth. Whether there is a familial disposition, a break-up with a significant other, school pressure, or a loss of a family member, LGBT youth can suffer from depression for all of the same reasons as non-LGBT youth. Knowledge of the unique factors that may contribute to depression in LGBT youth is imperative, however, to understanding depression as a whole picture in this group.

DEPRESSION CHARACTERISTICS IN LESBIAN, GAY, AND BISEXUAL YOUTH

The mental health of LGB youth has been the subject of investigation for at least the past 30 years. Earlier research in the area of depression and suicidality in LGB individuals was done using convenience samples or selected population-based samples from 1 city or state. These older and less representative data found that LGB youth compared with non-LGB peers were more than 3 times as likely to have made a suicide attempt in the past 12 months.[3,4]

The 2017 YRBS showed some of the first data from a nationwide population-based sample of high school youth showing the prevalence of health-risk behaviors in LGB compared with non-LGB youth. The prevalence of most health-risk behaviors varied by the sexual identity and sex of a youth's sexual contacts.[1] Findings showed a striking difference on mental health measures between LGB and heterosexual youth. The YRBS asked about depression and suicidality to assess mental health risk with a question regarding feeling sad and/or hopeless with loss of pleasure for 2 weeks or more. This question was endorsed by 63% of LGB youth compared with 27.5% of heterosexual youth. Additionally, there were striking differences between the groups on measures related to suicidality (**Table 4**).

Whether there is a higher rate of actual suicide among LGB individuals is controversial because there are only a few psychological autopsy studies in the literature. Although there are not sufficient data to confirm a higher rate of completed suicide, there is evidence to suggest this could be the case.[24] More broadly, previous suicide attempts predict a greater likelihood of completed suicide, so it makes sense that LGB youth risk of completed suicide also is greater than that of their heterosexual counterparts.

Exploration of these nationwide data to understand the health risks faced by sexual minority youth still needs to take place. LGB youth also had higher rates of health risks

Table 4
Suicide-related outcomes reported by lesbian, gay, and bisexual youth in past 12 months on the Youth Risk Behavior Survey

Suicide-related Outcome	Rate Reported in Lesbian, Gay, and Bisexual Youth Versus Heterosexual Youth (%)
Seriously considered suicide	47.7 vs 13.3
Made a suicide plan	38 vs 10.4
Attempted suicide in the past 12 mo	23 vs 5.4
Suicide attempt requiring medical attention	7.5 vs 1.7

Data from Kann L, Olsen EO, McManus T, et al. Sexual identity, sex of sexual contacts, and health-related behaviors among students in grades 9-12—United States and selected sites, 2017. MMWR Surveill Summ 2018;67(No. SS-8):1–114.

related to driving, tobacco, alcohol, illegal drugs, exercise, and weight on the YRBS, but the differences were not as large as those related to depression, suicidality, and violence or victimization.[1] Understanding how these risk behaviors interact with the depression, suicidality, bullying, or violence experienced by sexual minority youth is important.

Protective Factors

There are many LGB youth who function well and are not depressed nor suicidal. Social relationships, self-concept, and coping style are known to be key factors in determining youth vulnerability to depressive symptoms.[25] So much of the focus on sexual minority youth has been on depression, suicide, victimization, and violence that clinicians do not always consider protective factors and resilience. For instance, family acceptance of LGB youth during adolescence has been shown to protect against depression, substance abuse, and suicidal ideation and behaviors.[15,26] Family connectedness seems to confer the most consistent protection against suicidal ideation and attempts among all youth regardless of sexual orientation. Stone and colleagues[27] found that although connectedness to adults outside the family was protective against suicidality for heterosexual youth, it was not protective for LGB youth. Furthermore, family connectedness was not more important for LGB youth, but it was the only type of adult connectedness associated with decreased suicide attempts in this population.

Additionally, sexual minority students living in states and cities with more protective school climates were found to have lower risk for suicidal thoughts, plans, and attempts. Protective school climates were defined as follows: having gay-straight alliances and safe spaces for LGBT youth, providing curricula on health matters relevant to LGBT youth, prohibiting harassment based on sexual orientation and gender identity, encouraging staff to attend trainings on creating supportive environments for LGBT youth, and facilitating access to off-site providers for health and other services targeted to LGBT youth. Sexual orientation disparities in suicidal thoughts were almost eliminated in states and cities that had the most protective school climates. Although the results were similar for suicidal plans and attempts, those measures did not reach statistical significance.[28]

Further evidence shows romantic involvement may be a protective factor for the psychological health of some sexual minority youth. One study of LGB youth found that romantic involvement was associated with lower psychological distress in lesbian and gay youth but with higher psychological distress in bisexual youth. The association between romantic involvement and psychological distress also differed by race/ethnicity, with romantic relationships more protective for black and Latino youth than white youth.[29]

Assessment and Treatment Interventions for Lesbian, Gay, and Bisexual Youth

There are important ways in which issues specific to sexual orientation can be addressed in depressed LGB youth. It is imperative to ask about the sexual identity of all patients; clinicians should not avoid this subject or assume they know the answer. If an adolescent identifies as LGB, then clinicians need to be aware of all the aforementioned risk factors and protective factors.

Treatment involves creating an individualized treatment plan to bolster protective factors and reduce risk factors. This should include targeting interventions to the various environments where the youth interacts. It is important to learn what resources are available for LGB youth within these environments so that a clinician can recommend appropriate supportive interventions (**Table 5** lists examples).

Interventions with parents can increase their knowledge and acceptance of their child and are vitally important for youth still living at home or still dependent on family. Youth who have received even some support from family regarding their sexual orientation have a more positive outcome in young adulthood.[26] Attachment-based family therapy has been preliminarily studied as an intervention for addressing the needs of suicidal LGB adolescents with promising data.[30] Respect for youths' need for confidentiality regarding their sexual orientation is important, because they may need time to explore and understand their sexual orientation prior to disclosure to family members. If youths have disclosed bullying or discrimination (electronic or in person), it may be important to help them know how to advocate for themselves or to involve parents in advocating for their child.

DEPRESSION IN CHILDREN AND ADOLESCENTS WITH GENDER DYSPHORIA

Although a majority of individuals with GD identify as transgender, not all transgender youth meet criteria for GD. Because there are evidence-based treatments specific to youth with GD related to gender transition, these youth are referred to as meeting criteria for GD rather than using the identity term, transgender. Depression in children and adolescents presenting with GD is important to identify, classify, and treat considering this population of youth is a high-risk and vulnerable group. The presence of depression in a youth who may, or definitely does, meet criteria for GD evokes several considerations: (1) the relationship between depression and GD in terms of

Table 5 Resources in different environments to support lesbian, gay, and bisexual youth	
Environment	**Resource**
Home/family	Family Acceptance Project Parents and Friends of Lesbians and Gays support groups
School	Gay-straight alliance Supportive faculty/administration Protective policies
Community	LGBT community centers LGBT support groups LGBT-friendly shelters
Online	Hotlines, text lines, chat lines like The Trevor Project

diagnostic clarity, (2) the clinician's ability to appreciate the relationship among various etiologic factors (gender identity related and otherwise) that is leading to depression for the particular individual, and (3) developmental differences between children and adolescents in terms of treatment.

Depression Characteristics in Gender-Dysphoric Youth

Youth with GD experience depression and co-occurring psychiatric disorders at disproportionate rates from cisgender peers. Spack and colleagues[5] described that in their sample of 97 referred adolescents, 44.3% had a prior history of psychiatric diagnoses, 37.1% were taking psychotropic medications, and 21.6% had a history of self-injurious behavior. Another study describing the baseline characteristics of 101 adolescents with GD seeking medical intervention found clinically relevant depression scores, as measured by the Beck Depression Inventory,[31] in 35% of the sample (24% in the mild–moderate range and 11% in the severe range).[6] Additionally concerning data showed that half of the 55 transgender adolescents recruited from a community center had reported suicidal ideations and 25% had reported at least 1 suicide attempt.[32]

Assessment and Treatment Principles That Apply to All Youth with Gender Dysphoria

The 2017 Endocrine Society guidelines recommend a comprehensive mental health evaluation using a biopsychosocial model prior to the use of gender-affirming irreversible interventions in minors.[33] Diagnostic clarity for GD can be complicated by depression in the following way: a youth may be depressed for another reason and sees gender transition as a pathway toward reducing depression. Alternatively, the depression may, at least in part, stem from GD and the internal and external factors associated with the diagnosis (ie, the lack of intrinsic comfort with anatomy, potential stigma, potential lack of family acceptance or hostile school climates, and so forth). Diagnostic clarity is important because, regardless of the presence of GD, there are gender-affirming medical treatments to consider with increasing degrees of irreversibility based on the World Professional Association for Transgender Health (WPATH) Standards of Care, 7th edition.[34] Withholding medical interventions that are at least partially irreversible (such as hormones) in hopes that other interventions (such as psychopharmacology) might improve a youth's depression is not a neutral act, particularly when the source of the depression is related to the lack of secondary sex characteristics of a youth's affirmed gender. Conversely, moving forward with irreversible gender-affirming interventions (hormones and surgery) with the intention of alleviating depression is not without risk. This is of particular concern when a youth's depression might impair a clinician's ability to accurately confirm the definitive presence of GD (eg, the youth is acutely suicidal). Importantly, the WPATH *Standards of Care for the Health of Transsexual, Transgender, and Gender Nonconforming People*, 7th edition, describes that psychological interventions (social gender transition) alone also may help alleviate GD as a first step.

Where the presence of GD is clear, clinicians should avoid premature closure via the assumption that depression is the direct singular result of a lack of social and/or medical gender transition. Assessing etiologic factors in a depressed youth with GD guides clinicians in prioritizing the timing and sequence of interventions, which include both those that are gender-affirming and treatment modalities used for all youth. It is prudent to understand the contributions of multiple etiologies, including the gender-sex incongruence itself, internalized transphobia, stigma, biological predisposition, and stressor-dependent and psychological or interpersonal factors.

Prepubertal Children with Gender Dysphoria

Assessment of prepubertal children to determine whether or not they meet *DSM-5* criteria for GD requires a child to have "a strong desire to be of the other gender or an insistence that one is the other gender (or some alternative gender different from one's assigned gender)."[8] Without meeting this criterion, children cannot be diagnosed with GD of childhood, no matter how many additional indicators are met. This has increased the specificity of the diagnosis to more accurately distinguish children who are truly dysphoric from those who are potentially only gender diverse in their expression but not identity.

There is no official consensus regarding whether or not social gender transition is the universal best course of action for prepubertal children with GD. The details surrounding the controversial nature of prepubertal social gender transition are best summarized elsewhere; however, clinicians must consider the etiology of depression when considering how to best proceed.[35] In some situations, social transition in this age group can lead children to feel as though they must keep their transition a secret, which over time may inadvertently lead to shame around their gender-sex incongruence. Conversely, children who have not transitioned may develop depressive symptoms as a result of not being able to live and be perceived as their authentic gender. Data on prepubertal children who have transitioned to their affirmed gender demonstrate comparable (low) rates of depression and anxiety compared with siblings and community cisgender control groups.[36] It is important, however, to interpret these data cautiously because there were no control groups of transgender-identified children with supportive parents who did not transition nor are the data longitudinal. Therefore, social gender transition in children remains complex. Collaboratively navigating the pros and cons of transitioning (including the pace at which a child transitions) with the families and children remains a commonly described individualized approach. This approach considers the lack of predictability for how a child will identify later in life[37] and addresses the importance of how a social transition will potentially alleviate depression symptoms in a particular child.[35]

Adolescents with Gender Dysphoria

Adolescence marks a time when youth may seek physical interventions as part of a gender transition process. This may present in the context of worsening GD as physical pubertal changes occur. Interventions are tailored to the emotional and cognitive capacity of the adolescent in terms of medical decision making. More irreversible measures are deferred until the adolescents can conceptualize more fully how a particular intervention will affect their physical bodies and emotional wel-lbeing. In the United States, adolescents rely on parental consent for hormonal treatment in most multidisciplinary treatment centers, which adds a layer of family dynamics inherent in the assessment and treatment of these youth.

Puberty suppression is indicated for younger adolescents who have begun to experience pubertal changes (at least Tanner stage 2) through the use of a GnRH agonist, which ultimately delays the production of sex hormones by the gonads.[33] This allows time for a GD adolescent to explore gender identity further without the pressure of the development of irreversible secondary sex characteristics that would likely worsen GD. The most recent hallmark prospective study suggesting positive mental health outcomes after medical interventions was done by de Vries and colleagues[38] in 2014. The Amsterdam team studied youth who received puberty suppression, then gender-affirming hormones, and subsequently gender-confirming surgery. Their cohort was found to have comparable psychological adjustment to cisgender controls groups in young adulthood.

The Endocrine Society recommends, as adolescents mature, the potential use of gender-affirming sex hormones for individuals continuing to meet criteria for GD in adolescents and adults.[33] Transgender female youth (assigned males at birth) receive estrogen to create feminizing effects whereas transgender male youth (assigned female at birth) receive testosterone to create masculinizing effects. The complexity of these interventions often is discussed in a mental health setting prior to initiation.

For depressed adolescents with GD, the timing of the initiation of any physical intervention often depends on an assessment of the acuity of the depression and the family's readiness to consent. Some adolescents seeking hormonal treatment have depression that is multifactorial in nature. As such, advising families that depression may not fully remit once hormonal interventions begin can help reduce future concerns in the event that depressive symptoms persist. Understanding that adolescents with GD become depressed for all the same reasons other adolescents do, in addition to the external and internal challenges of inherently being transgender, helps guide a provider to fully understand and treat the patient.

SUMMARY

LGBT youth have disproportionate health disparities, including higher rates of depression, than their non-LGBT peers. Available evidence repeatedly shows that these higher rates of depression occur in the context of stigma, discrimination, and victimization. Assessment of depression in LGBT youth must take into account these additional risk factors as they have an impact on a particular youth. Treatment includes addressing these factors in addition to using other gold standard treatments for depression. Emerging evidence shows that LGBT youth who are in more supportive environments have better mental health outcomes, making the role of the mental health provider as an advocate even more important in this population.

Further research is needed to better understand various aspects of working with depressed LGBT youth. This is perhaps most notable in the area of youth with GD, where complex medical decision making is currently based on limited outcome data. What seems most clear is that there is no 1-size-fits-all approach for working with LGBT youth. Forming collaborative relationships with both youth and their families allows clinicians to create an individualized treatment plan to address their unique needs.

REFERENCES

1. Kann L, Olsen EO, Mcmanus T, et al. Sexual identity, sex of sexual contacts, and health-related behaviors among students in grades 9-12—United States and selected sites, 2017. MMWR Surveill Summ 2018;67(No. SS-8):1–114.

2. Kosciw JG, Greytak EA, Bartkiewicz MJ, et al. The 2011 National School Climate Survey: the experiences of lesbian, gay, bisexual and transgender youth in our nation's schools. New York: GLSEN; 2012.

3. Garofalo R, Wolf RC, Wissow LS, et al. Sexual orientation and risk of suicide attempts among a representative sample of youth. Arch Pediatr Adolesc Med 1999;153:487–93.

4. Stone DM, Luo F, Ouyang L, et al. Sexual orientation and suicide ideation, plans, attempts, and medically serious attempts: evidence from local youth risk behavior surveys, 2001-2009. Am J Public Health 2014;104:262–71.

5. Spack NP, Edwards-Leeper L, Feldman HA, et al. Children and adolescents with gender identity disorder referred to a pediatric medical center. Pediatrics 2012; 129:418–25.

6. Olson J, Schrager SM, Belzer M, et al. Baseline physiologic and psychosocial characteristics of transgender youth seeking care for gender dysphoria. J Adolesc Health 2015;57:374–80.

7. Adelson SL. Practice parameter on gay, lesbian, or bisexual sexual orientation, gender nonconformity, and gender discordance in children and adolescents. J Am Acad Child Adolesc Psychiatry 2012;51:957–74.

8. American Psychiatric Association. Diagnostic and statistical manual of mental disorders. 5th edition. Arlington (VA): American Psychiatric Association; 2013.

9. Gates GJ. In U.S., more adults identifying as LGBT. In: Gallup, social and policy issues. 2017. Available at: https://news.gallup.com/poll/201731/lgbt-identification-rises.aspx. Accessed December 1, 2018.

10. Gates GJ. LGB/T Demographics: comparisons among population-based surveys. Williams Institute, UCLA School of Law; 2014.

11. Chavez A, Janssen A. Structural stigma in LGBTQ youth. JAACAP Connect, in press.

12. One Colorado Education Fund. Transparent: the state of transgender health in Colorado 2014. Available at: https://one-colorado.org/wp-content/uploads/2017/06/OC_Transparent_Download2mb.pdf. Accessed December 1, 2018.

13. Meyer IH, Link BG, Schwartz S, et al. Minority stress and mental health in gay men. J Health Soc Behav 1995;36:38–56.

14. Meyer IH. Prejudice, social stress, and mental health in lesbian, gay, and bisexual populations: conceptual issues and research evidence. Psychol Bull 2003; 129(5):674–97.

15. Ryan C, Russell ST, Huebner D, et al. Family acceptance in adolescence and the health of LGBT young adults. J Child Adolesc Psychiatr Nurs 2010;23(4):205–13.

16. Roberts AL, Rosario M, Corliss HL, et al. Childhood gender nonconformity: a risk indicator for childhood abuse and posttraumatic stress in youth. Pediatrics 2012; 129(3):410–7.

17. Richter BEJ, Lindahl KM, Malik NM. Examining ethnic differences in parental rejection of LGB youth sexual identity. J Fam Psychol 2017;31(2):244–9.

18. Ryan C, Toomey RB, Diaz RM, et al. Parent-initiated sexual orientation change efforts with LGBT adolescents: implications for young adult mental health and adjustment. J Homosex 2018;7:1–15.

19. Durso LE, Gates GJ. Serving our youth: Findings from a national survey of service providers working with lesbian, gay, bisexual, and transgender youth who are homeless or at risk of becoming homeless. Los Angeles (CA): The Williams Institute with True Colors Fund and The Palette Fund; 2012.

20. Ventimiglia N. LGBT selective victimization: unprotected youth on the streets. J Law Soc 2012;13(2):439–53.

21. Quintana NS, Rosenthal J, Krehley J. On the streets. Center for American Progress; 2010. Available at: https://www.americanprogress.org/wp-content/uploads/issues/2010/06/pdf/lgbtyouthhomelessness.pdf. Accessed on December 1, 2018.

22. Hunter E. What's good for the gays is good for the gander: making homeless youth housing safer for lesbian, gay, bisexual, and transgender youth. Fam Court Rev 2008;46(3):543–57.

23. Russell ST, Ryan C, Toomey RB, et al. Lesbian, gay, bisexual, and transgender adolescent school victimization: implications for young adult health and adjustment. J Sch Health 2011;81:223–30.

24. Plöderl M, Wagenmakers ER, Tremblay P, et al. Suicide risk and sexual orientation: a critical review. Arch Sex Behav 2013;42:715–27.

25. Martin-Storey A, Crosnoe R. Sexual minority status, peer harassment, and adolescent depression. J Adolesc 2012;35(4):1001–11.

26. Ryan C, Huebner D, Diaz RM, et al. Family rejection as a predictor of negative health outcomes in white and Latino lesbian, gay, and bisexual young adults. Pediatrics 2009;123(1):346–52.

27. Stone DM, Luo F, Lippy C, et al. The role of social connectedness and sexual orientation in the prevention of youth suicide ideation and attempts among sexually active adolescents. Suicide Life Threat Behav 2015;45(4):415–30.

28. Hatzenbuehler ML, Birkett M, Van Wagenen A, et al. Protective school climates and reduced risk for suicide ideation in sexual minority youths. Am J Public Health 2014;104(2):279–86.

29. Whitton SW, Dyar C, Newcomb ME, et al. Romantic involvement: a protective factor for psychological health in racially-diverse young sexual minorities. J Abnorm Psychol 2018;127(3):265–75.

30. Diamond GM, Diamond GS, Levy S, et al. Attachment-based family therapy for suicidal lesbian, gay, and bisexual adolescents: a treatment development study and open trial with preliminary findings. Psychotherapy 2012;49(1):62–71.

31. Beck AT, Steer RA, Brown GK. Manual for the Beck depression inventory-II. San Antonio (TX): Psychological Corporation; 1996.

32. Grossman AH, D'Augelli AR. Transgender youth and life-threatening behaviors. Suicide Life Threat Behav 2007;37:527–37.

33. Hembree WC, Cohen-Kettenis PT, Gooren L, et al. Endocrine treatment of gender-dysphoric/gender-incongruent persons: an Endocrine Society* clinical practice guideline. J Clin Endocrinol Metab 2017;102(11):3869–903.

34. Coleman E, Bockting W, Botzer M, et al. Standards of care for the health of transsexual, transgender, and gender-nonconforming people, version 7. Int J Transgend 2012;13(4):165–232.

35. Leibowitz S. Social gender transition and the psychological interventions. In: Janssen A, Leibowltz S, editors. Affirmative mental health care for transgender and gender diverse youth. Cham (Switzerland): Springer International; 2018. p. 31–48.

36. Olson KR, Durwood L, DeMeules M, et al. Mental health of transgender children who are supported in their identities. Pediatrics 2016;137(3):e20153223.

37. Steensma TD, McGuire JK, Kreukels BPC, et al. Factors associated with desistence and persistence of childhood gender dysphoria: a quantitative follow-up study. J Am Acad Child Adolesc Psychiatry 2013;52:582–90.

38. de Vries AL, McGuire JK, Steensma TD, et al. Young adult psychological outcome after puberty suppression and gender reassignment. Pediatrics 2014;134(4): 696–704.

Moving?

Make sure your subscription moves with you!

To notify us of your new address, find your **Clinics Account Number** (located on your mailing label above your name), and contact customer service at:

Email: journalscustomerservice-usa@elsevier.com

800-654-2452 (subscribers in the U.S. & Canada)
314-447-8871 (subscribers outside of the U.S. & Canada)

Fax number: 314-447-8029

Elsevier Health Sciences Division
Subscription Customer Service
3251 Riverport Lane
Maryland Heights, MO 63043

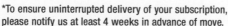
*To ensure uninterrupted delivery of your subscription, please notify us at least 4 weeks in advance of move.